THE DOCTOR'S WORLD

This is the story of the extraordinary life of Claver Morris and the society in which he lived. After his marriage at Chelsea in 1685, Claver Morris moved to Somerset where he established an outstanding reputation for his work as a physician. His diaries show us how he worked with apothecaries and surgeons, and travelled widely to treat all kind of patients, from the children of the poor to those of the landed gentry. The diaries also tell us about the joys and pains of Claver's personal and family life, and of his various intrigues.

Claver Morris was a man of many talents: immensely enterprising, knowledgeable, sociable and loving. His house was always filled with music, guests and entertainments. Yet he was often faced with disputes and troubles partly of his own making – as when he courted a bishop's daughter, or stole some land to build his Queen Anne house.

The Doctor's World provides a unique portrait of a physician living and working through the political and religious turmoils that beset the nation at the turn of the eighteenth century. Tales of medical treatments, clandestine marriages and self-serving priests are entwined with famous acts of treason and rebellion, and the pleasures and tragedies of daily life.

This meticulously researched book will appeal to all readers of social, political, medical and family history.

Paul Hyland is an award-winning teacher and Emeritus Professor of History. He is a specialist in Eighteenth Century Studies and editor of *The Enlightenment: a Sourcebook and Reader*, published by Routledge.

THE DOCTOR'S WORLD

The Life and Times of Claver Morris, 1659–1727

Paul Hyland

Routledge
Taylor & Francis Group
LONDON AND NEW YORK

Front cover image: Detail from Wells Cathedral, by Thomas Shepherd (1792–1864): © Newport Museum and Art Gallery/Bridgeman Images NWP153584.

First published 2023
by Routledge
4 Park Square, Milton Park, Abingdon, Oxon OX14 4RN

and by Routledge
605 Third Avenue, New York, NY 10158

Routledge is an imprint of the Taylor & Francis Group, an informa business

British Library Cataloguing-in-Publication Data
A catalogue record for this book is available from the British Library

Library of Congress Cataloging-in-Publication Data
Names: Hyland, Paul, 1953- author.
Title: The doctor's world : the life and times of Claver Morris, 1659–1727 / Paul Hyland.
Identifiers: LCCN 2022025851 (print) | LCCN 2022025852 (ebook) | ISBN 9781032367644 (hardback) | ISBN 9781032367651 (paperback) | ISBN 9781003333654 (ebook)
Subjects: LCSH: Morris, Claver, 1659-1727. | Physicians--England--Somerset--Biography. | Medicine--England--History--18th century. | Somerset (England)--Biography.
Classification: LCC R489.M67 H95 2023 (print) | LCC R489.M67 (ebook) | DDC 610.69/5 [B]--dc23/eng/20220706
LC record available at https://lccn.loc.gov/2022025851
LC ebook record available at https://lccn.loc.gov/2022025852

ISBN: 978-1-032-36764-4 (hbk)
ISBN: 978-1-032-36765-1 (pbk)
ISBN: 978-1-003-33365-4 (ebk)

DOI: 10.4324/9781003333654

Typeset in Bembo
by SPi Technologies India Pvt Ltd (Straive)

CONTENTS

LIST OF ILLUSTRATIONS

ACKNOWLEDGEMENTS

It was long ago, on a trip to Virginia, that I came across Laurel Thatcher Ulrich's *A Midwife's Tale: the life of Martha Ballard based on her diary, 1785–1812* (New York, 1990). I was hooked. Ulrich showed how, through 'the very dailiness, the exhaustive, repetitious dailiness' of Martha's humble record of her work in Maine, the life of a whole community could be evoked. I had been reading *The Diary of a West Country Physician AD 1684–1726,* edited by Edmund Hobhouse (1934) and was wondering how much of the original dairy, 'for the most part a bald record of events', Hobhouse had reproduced. After examining the manuscripts it was clear that about 20 per cent of the original diary had been published, plus a tiny fraction of a much larger body of accounts.

Like Martha's 'plain, matter-of-fact' daily notes, Claver's 'bald record of events' were private and full of what most historians who had looked at Martha's diary saw as 'trivia'. But Claver's writings revealed his distinctive character and voice, and showed that he, like Martha, believed that 'living was to be measured in doing. Nothing was trivial.' Faced with well over half a million words in the manuscript diaries and accounts, and a cast of thousands, thanks to Ulrich I thought it might be possible to tell the doctor's tale.

I am especially grateful to the late Paul Hobhouse and to his wife, Jeannie Hobhouse, for enabling me to work on the Claver Morris manuscripts, and for encouragement and patience during the long gestation of this book. Niall Hobhouse tracked down a book of Claver's accounts that had been missing for over seventy years and provided tremendous support through the final stages of research. Staff at Drawing Matter, Shatwell Studios in Somerset, where the manuscripts are held, have also been exceptionally helpful, and I am particularly grateful to Niall Hobhouse for permission to reproduce extracts and images from the manuscripts, and to Craig Stevens for much of the photographic work herein.

Special thanks are due to Dr Harry Johnstone, Emeritus Fellow of St Anne's College, Oxford, for sharing the findings of his research into Claver's musical activities, and to Dr Roger Rolls, for sharing his knowledge as both a medical doctor and historian. Over the years, I have benefitted greatly from the support of many university colleagues, most notably Dr Roberta Anderson, Professor Alan Marshall, Rachael McDonald and Nicky Wilson. I am also grateful to the late Dr Dennis Gibbs MRCP, at Oxford, for providing me with information about Claver's books, and to Lesley Seal, librarian at Bath, for spotting that it was probably Claver's reputation for using herbal remedies that led to him being given an album of over two hundred botanical drawings based upon the *Codex Bellunensis.*

I have also been helped by citizens of Wells, where I grew up. As well as school-friends, I should like to thank Pat Robinson, a former mayor who shared her knowledge of the city; William Smith, a former archivist of Wells who drew my attention to sources that I might otherwise have overlooked; and David Walker, curator of the Wells and Mendip Museum, who kindly took photographs for me of the Symes map of the city. I am grateful for the help of staff at the Cathedral School, the Chapter Office, the Public Library, and the Wells and Mendip Museum. Further afield, I should like to thank staff at Bath Record Office, the British Library, Dorset History Centre, the National Archives, North Devon Record Office, the Public Record Office, and Somerset Heritage Centre.

When I first put pen to paper, Philip Rowe and Michael Claydon of Bath, and Sian Rogers of Altrincham, were kind enough to read some early drafts, and I am grateful for their advice. When the work was completed, or so I thought, Dr Barbara White read everything meticulously. For the many improvements she graciously advised, I am deeply grateful. As the book proceeded to production, staff at Routledge were always very helpful and professional. In particular, I should like to thank Michael Greenwood and Louis Nicholson-Pallett. I should also like to thank Yassar Arafat at SPi Global and especially Nick Brock for his excellent work and advice as copyeditor.

Finally, without my wife, Pauleen, who has shared all the joys and pains of bringing Claver's world to life, there would be no book at all. What appears here (at least in all the best bits) is as much hers as it is mine. *X*

Paul Hyland, Bath.

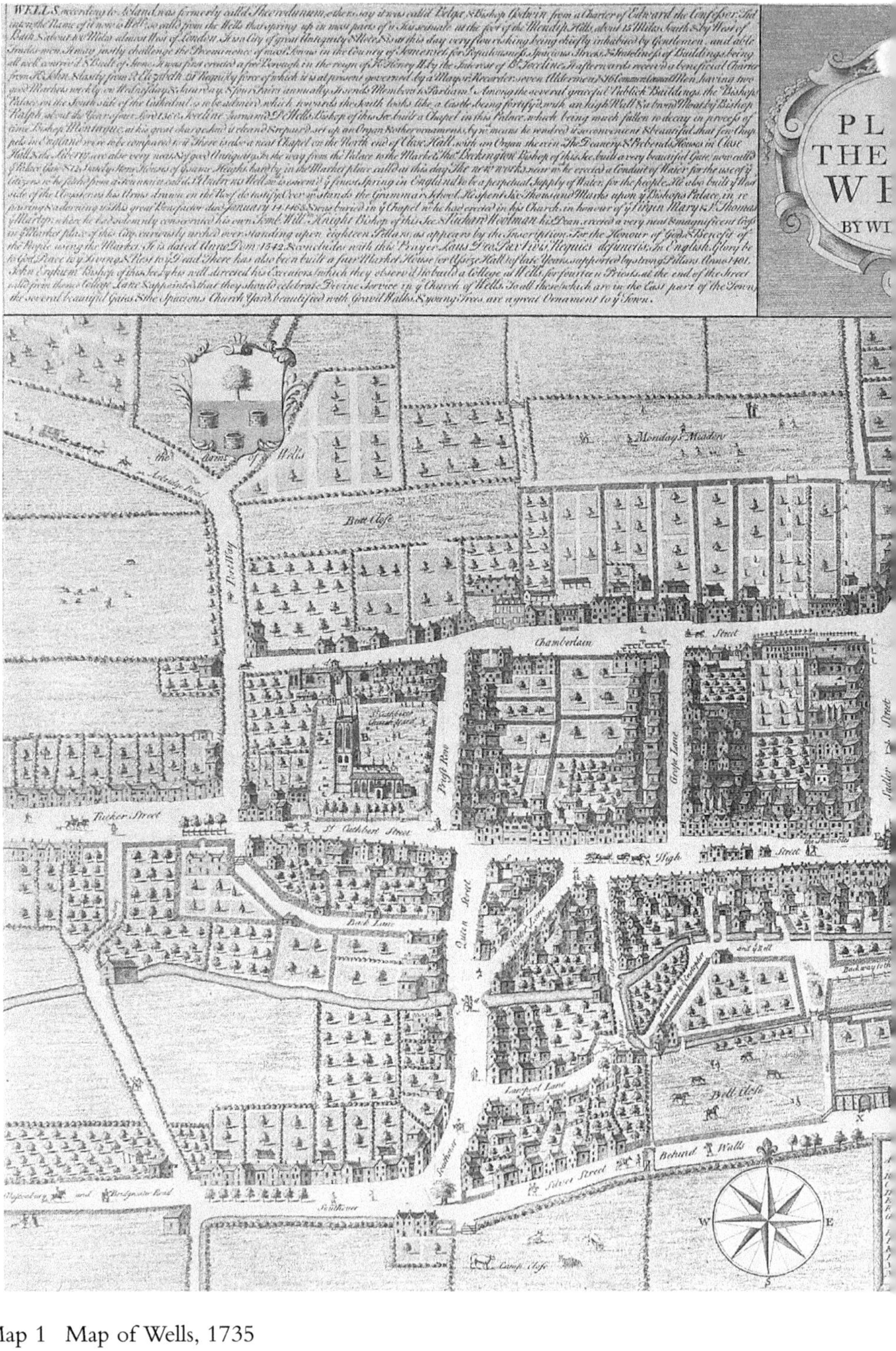

Map 1 Map of Wells, 1735

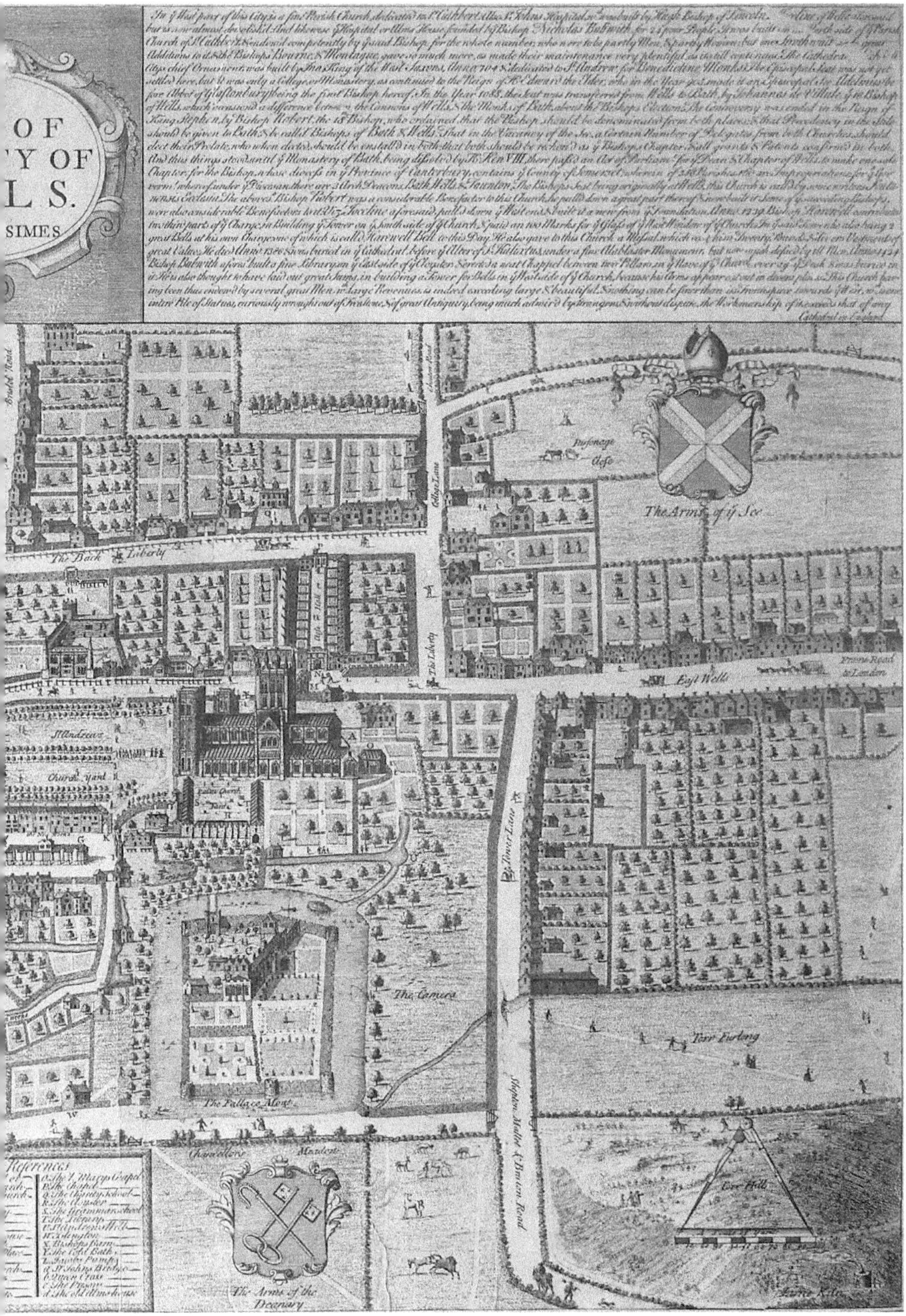

OF
TY OF
L S.
SIMES
The Back Liberty
The Liberty
College Lane
Parsonage Close
The Arms of ye See
East Wells
Frome Road to London
St Andrews Church yard
Tower Lane
The Camery
The Pallace Moat
Torr Furlong
Torr Hill
Shepton Mallet & Bruton Road
The Arms of the Deanary
References

FAMILIES & FIGURES

ANNE (QUEEN): daughter of James II, reigned 1702–1714.

ARCHER: Edmund, married to Elizabeth, was archdeacon of Taunton, and later of Wells.

AYLESBURY: William, a clergyman, married to Frances.

BAMPFYLDE: a gentry family from Devon. John was married to Margaret, the daughter and heir of Francis Warre of Hestercombe, near Taunton. Sir Coplestone Bampfylde was John's brother.

BARON: a large Wells family including: the brothers, Matthew (a mercer) and Charles (an apothecary), both mayors; and William and Martha of New Street, and their daughters Hester, Anne, Martha and Katherine.

BATHURST (RALPH): dean of Bath and Wells.

BEAL (HANNAH): one of Claver's maids.

BERKELEY: a gentry family with several branches. At the Pylle branch, near Shepton Mallet, colonel Edward Berkeley was married to Elizabeth (née Ryves). Their children included: Maurice, MP for Wells, who did not marry; Elizabeth, who did not marry; and William, who married Anne, the daughter of Sir Edward Seymour. At the Maiden Bradley branch, near Bruton, Sir Maurice Berkeley, 3rd viscount Fitzhardinge, had two daughters by his wife Anne (née Lee): Eleanor, who married Hugh Montgomery, 2nd earl Mount Alexander; and Jane, who married James Gendrault.

BRAGGE: a gentry family from Devon. William I (m. Mary Drewe) had four daughters (Mary, Anne, Elizabeth and Margaret) and a son and heir, William II (m. Edith Larder). William II and Edith had several children, including their son and heir, William III, who did not marry.

BRAILSFORD (MATTHEW): dean of Bath and Wells, who did not marry.

BRICKENDEN (THOMAS): a residential canon of Wells. His son, Edmund, was also a vicar.

BRIDGES (HARRY): the son of Sir Thomas (squire of Keynsham), and the father of James.

BRYDGES: Marshall was a residential canon and chancellor of the bishop's court, married to Frances (née Creighton). His brother, William, was a barrister.

BULL: a large gentry family from Shapwick near Street. Henry, a barrister, married Elizabeth, by whom he had three children: Henry, Elizabeth, and Eleanor. Eleanor married George Dodington, and her son, Henry, inherited the Shapwick estate.

BURLAND (JOHN): gentleman and heir to the manor of Steyning in north Somerset.

CHAMPION (GEORGE): Claver's senior man-servant.

CHARLES II: returned from exile at the Restoration in 1660, he ruled until 1685.

CHEYNEY (THOMAS): residential canon and bishop Ken's chaplain.

CHICHESTER: Sir Arthur Chichester (3rd bart.) married Elizabeth Drewe. Their eldest son, Sir John (4th bart.) married Anne, the daughter of John Leigh of Newport.

CLARK (WILL): Claver's man-servant.

CLAVER: a farming family from Dorset. Hannah was Claver Morris's mother. James, an apothecary in Salisbury, was Claver's cousin.

COMES (RICHARD): a gentleman attorney of Wells, married to Sarah, by whom he had several sons.

COWARD: William, a wealthy lawyer and MP for Wells, was the father of William (also an MP for Wells) and Bridget, who married George Hamilton.

COXE: John, of Leigh in Wiltshire, married Margaret (née Hippisley) of Ston Easton manor. They had several children, including Ann, Susannah, and their son and heir John Hippisley-Coxe.

CREECH (THOMAS): vicar of Butleigh and the chapelry of Baltonsborough, near Glastonbury.

CREIGHTON: Robert, married to Frideswide (née Piers), was the precentor of Wells cathedral. Their children included Robert (a schoolmaster), Katherine (m. Henry Layng), Margaret (m. John Pope) and Frances (m. Marshall Brydges).

CUPPER (RICHARD): a Wells apothecary and shopkeeper. His son, Richard, was also an apothecary.

CURTIS (JOHN): Claver's man-servant.

DAVIE: Frances, daughter of Sir William, was married to Sir George Chudleigh of Devon, by whom she had several children.

DAWE: Edmund I, lord of the manor at Ditcheat, was married to Anne (née Salmon), by whom he had several children including: Edmund II (m. Martha Hill), Anne (m. George Farewell), Elizabeth (m. Robert Jeanes), Charles (the father of Nancy and Elizabeth), and Thomas. Edmund II had several children, including his heir, Hill Dawe.

DREWE: a gentry family from south Devon. Edward was a canon of Exeter cathedral and archdeacon of Cornwall.

EDWARDS: Thomas, an attorney and MP for Bristol and Wells, was married to Mary who inherited a fortune from her uncle, Edward Colston.

EVANS: a Catholic family in Wells. John and Anne Evans of the Liberty had a daughter and heir, Mary.

FAREWELL: George, rector of South Cadbury, was married to Anne Dawe by whom he had two sons, George and Thomas. He also had a brother, Nathaniel, married to Susan Coker, and a sister Ann, who was married to the choral vicar Farewell Perry.

FOX (BARUCH): a wealthy mercer from Sherborne.

GENDRAULT: James, a Huguenot refugee, married Jane, a daughter of Maurice Berkeley, 3rd Viscount Fitzhardinge. Their children were Charles, Jane, and Ann.

GEORGE I: the first Hanoverian king, ruled 1714–1727.

GODDARD (EDWARD): a Dorset gentleman, married to Claver's sister, Hannah, by whom he had a son, William.

GOULD: Sir Henry, of Sharpham Park near Glastonbury, was a Justice of the King's Bench, married to Lady Sarah (née Davidge). Their son, Davidge, was a barrister, and their daughter, Sarah, was married to Colonel Edmund Fielding, by whom she had seven children, including Henry and Sarah Fielding.

GREENE: family and relations of Grace Green, living in London, Middlesex and Wiltshire.

GWYN (FRANCIS): was married to his cousin, Margaret Prideaux, from whom he inherited Forde Abbey in Dorset.

HAMILTON: George, a son of the 6th earl of Abercorn, was married to Bridget Coward of Wells, by whom he had eleven children.

HARDRES (THORESBY): citizen of London and guardian of Grace and Elizabeth Greene.

HARRINGTON: a large gentry family of talented musicians. John Harrington, lord of the manor at Kelston, had many brothers and sisters, including Henry, William, Robert, Edward, and Helena, who married Lawrence Huddleston, the rector of Kelston.

HEALY: William, married to Mary, was a doctor of Law and clerk to the dean and chapter. Their children included Mary (m. Thomas Cook, rector of Thorncombe), Phyllis (m. Francis Warre, rector of Cheddon Fitzpaine), and Richard, the vicar of St Cuthbert's, who was married to Mary.

HELYAR: an old gentry family from south Somerset. William I married Rachael Wyndham. Their son, William II, married Joanna Hole by whom he had seven children. Their son, William III, married Mary Goddard.

HILL: Samuel, married to Grace, was rector of Kilmington and archdeacon of Wells. Their children included two sons: William, a choral vicar and vicar of Dulverton; and Sam, who also became rector of Kilmington.

HIPPISLEY: Preston married Susannah (née Yorke), and their daughter Margaret (m. John Coxe) was their heir.

HOOPER (GEORGE): bishop of Bath and Wells. His daughter, Abigail, married John Prowse.

HORNER: Thomas, of Mells near Frome, was married to the heiress Susanna Strangways. Their daughter, Elizabeth, became their heir.

HUGHES (WILLIAM): chancellor of the bishop's court, married to Cecilia, and father of several children.

IRISH: a gentry family from the Liberty, Wells. John (a son of Matthew), a mercer in the Market Place, was married to Elizabeth. They had two daughters, Grizelda and Elizabeth.

JAMES II: the Catholic brother of Charles II, reigned 1685–1689. Married to Mary of Modena, he was the father of 'The Pretender', James Francis Edward Stuart (born 1688).

JEANES: Robert, of West Pennard near Glastonbury, was married to Elizabeth Dawe.

KEEN: Christopher, a merchant from a gentry family, was married to Jane (née Berkeley), the widow of James Gendrault, and later to Rose Aldworth. Sarah Keen (daughter of Francis) was married to William Westley.

KEN (THOMAS): Bishop of Bath and Wells.

KIDDER (RICHARD): Bishop of Bath and Wells, and father of Susanna and Anne.

LAYNG: Henry, subdean of the cathedral and later archdeacon of Wells, was married to Katherine, a daughter of Robert Creighton.

LEIGH: John, of Newport on the Isle of Wight, was married to Anne Bragge. Their daughter, Anne, married Sir John Chichester.

LONG: George, son of the republican Sir Lislebone Young of Downside, was married to Mary, daughter of Marmaduke Jennings. Their children included William, Elizabeth and Deborah. William's children included William, Elizabeth, Frances and Anne.

LOUIS XIV: King of France, 1643–1715.

LUCAS (CHRISTOPHER): a surgeon in Wells.

MALET: William, a Wells attorney, was married to Margaret Bailey, by whom he had a daughter, Ann.

MARTIN: a gentry family of East Pennard, near Glastonbury. Gerard was married to Mary, but they had no children.

MATTOCKS (GEORGE): a barrister of the Liberty in Wells, married to Martha, with a daughter, Mary.

MILLS (HENRY): the headmaster of Wells Grammar School.

MITCHELL (MOLLEY): one of Claver's longest-serving maids.

MOGG: a gentry family from Farrington Gurney. John and Dorothy had several children, including Richard and Dorothy, who married Thomas Churchey of Wincanton.

MUTTLEBURY: a Catholic family of Wookey manor, near Wells. Thomas and Mary had many children.

NEWCOURT: John and Mary of Ivythorn manor near Street, had a son and daughter.

NEWMAN: Francis Holles Newman of North Cadbury, had nine children with his wife, Eleanor Mompesson. Of these, his heir Francis (Frank) married Dorothy Gifford but had no children. Nor did another son, Henry, rector of South Cadbury. But a further son, Charles, married Hannah Sandys and had five children.

NOOTH: James was a clerk and a choral vicar. Jane, his wife, was a nurse and midwife.

PENN (WILLIAM): Quaker, writer and founder of Pennsylvania.

PHELIPS: Somerset landed gentry. Edward inherited Montacute House from his uncle who was married to Lady Edith. He married his uncle's daughters, first Ann (by whom he had two daughters, Anne and Bridget), and then Elizabeth (by whom he had a son and heir, Edward).

PIERS: a large family descended from William I, bishop of Bath and Wells (d. 1670). His son, William II, archdeacon of Taunton (d. 1682), married Mary Coward. Their first son, William III, was married to Katherine, daughter of William Coward. Their second son, Captain Thomas, married Mary and had one surviving son, Thomas. Their daughter Frideswide married Robert Creighton, the precentor. William III and Katherine had a son, William IV, who became MP for Wells and had several children.

PITT: William, of Kensington and Cricket Malherbie in Somerset, was married to Jane. Their only son, Samuel, was married to Mary Speke.

POPE (JOHN): vicar of St Cuthbert's, Wells, was married to Margaret, a daughter of Robert Creighton.

POULETT: Francis (second son of John Poulett, 1st baron of Hinton St George) was married to Catherine, the sister of the precentor Robert Creighton.

PROWSE: John, from a gentry family near Axbridge, was married to Margaret Bragge, and later to Abigail Hooper, the bishop's daughter.

REBOTIER (ELIAS): a Huguenot refugee who was Bishop Hooper's chaplain and the rector of Chelwood.

ROGERS: Mary was a midwife, and her husband, George, a choral vicar.

SACHEVERELL (HENRY): High Church preacher and chaplain of St Saviour's, Southwalk.

SALMON: William was a wealthy draper who, like his father and grandfather, was a mayor of Wells. His brother, John, was an apothecary.

SANDYS (EDWYN): archdeacon of Wells and rector of Yeovilton. He had six children by his wife, Elena.

SELLECK (JOHN): archdeacon of Bath. He had a sister, Joan, and several children, including John and Nathaniel.

SEYMOUR: an aristocratic family with several branches. Anne, the only daughter of Sir Edward Seymour, married William Berkeley of Pylle, the younger brother of Maurice. Lady Katherine, a daughter of Charles Seymour, 6th duke of Somerset of Petworth House, Sussex, married Sir William Wyndham.

SHIRLEY (NICHOLAS): a Dorset gentleman, married to Claver's sister, Ruth.

STARR: Richard was one of Claver's tenants, and Anne was his sister.

STEARE (ROBERT): a mayor of Bridgwater.

STRODE: a large gentry family with branches at Downside, Shepton Mallet and Pilton. Edward (Ned) of Downside had many children, including Edward, John, Elizabeth and Mercy (m. Francis Wyndham).

TAYLOR: a large family in Wells, including John, an apothecary, and the children of Robert and Frances Taylor: Robert, a grocer; Charles, a builder; Joseph, a grocer; Benjamin, an innkeeper; and Frances.

TREVELYAN: Sir John, of Nettlecombe Court, was married to Susanna, by whom he had several children.

WESTLEY: William, from a gentry family, was clerk to the dean and chapter. His first wife was Sarah (née Keen), and his second wife was Frideswide, widow of Edmund Brickenden.

WHITE (ANNE): the nanny for Grace and Elizabeth Greene.

WILDING (BENJAMIN): headmaster of Sherborne school.

WILLIAM AND MARY: ruled as joint sovereigns from 1689 until Mary's death in 1694, after which William ruled alone until 1702.

WILTSHIRE (GEORGE): a choral vicar.

WYNDHAM: a large landed gentry family with several branches. Thomas, of Witham Friary near Frome, was MP for Wells. His nephew, Sir Edward, of Orchard Wyndham near Exmoor, was the father of Sir William Wyndham who married Lady Katherine Seymour, a daughter of the 6th duke of Somerset.

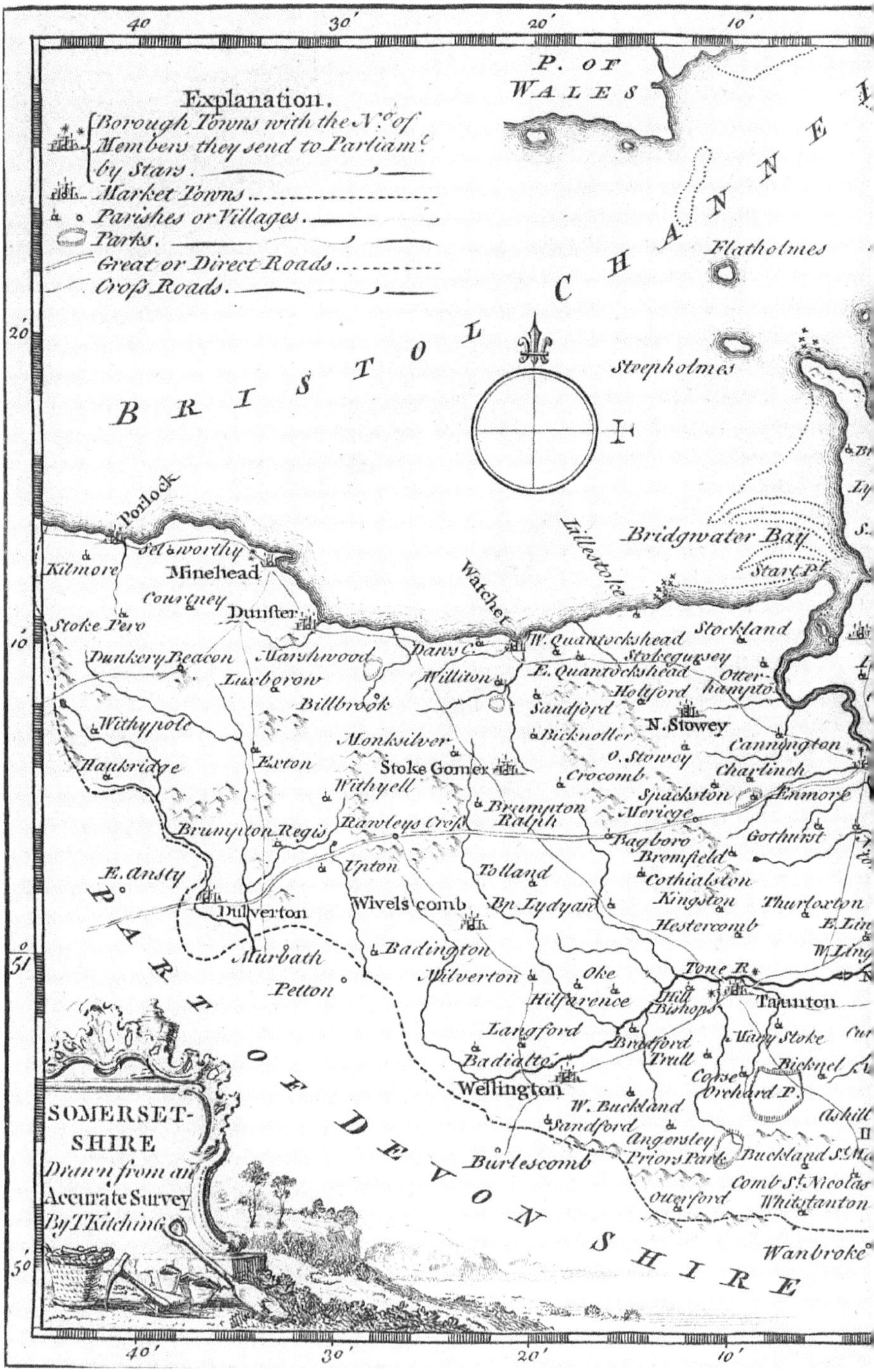

Map 2 Map of Somerset, *c.*1749

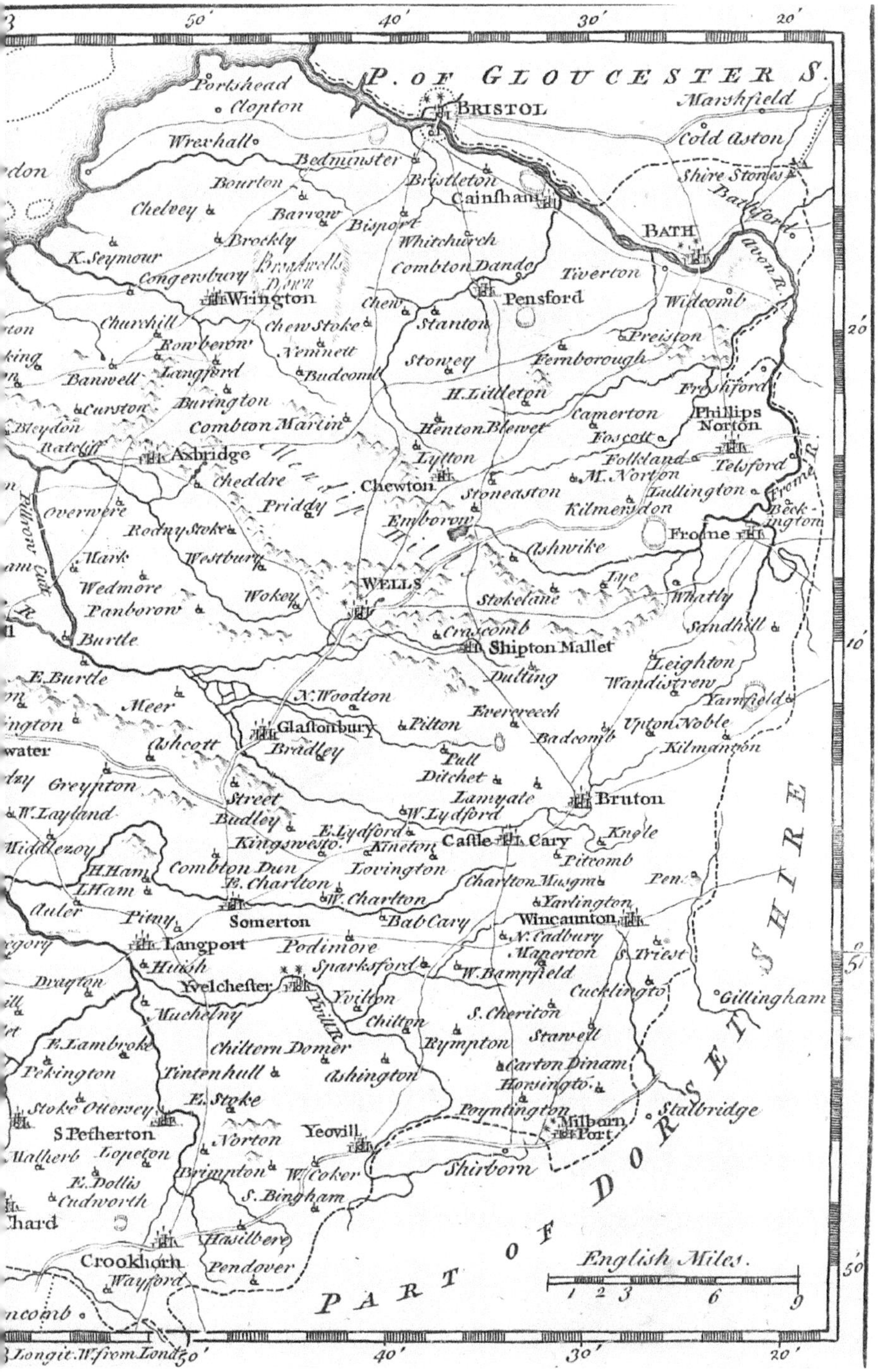

50'
40'
30'
20'
P. OF GLOUCESTER S.
Portshead
Clopton
BRISTOL
Marshfield
Wrexhall
Bedminster
Cold Aston
Bourton
Bristleton
Cainsham
Shire Stones
Bathford
Chelvey
Barrow
Bisport
Brockly
Whitchurch
BATH
Avon R.
K. Seymour
Broadwells Down
Combton Dando
Tiverton
Congersbury
Wrington
Pensford
Widcomb
Churchill
Chew
Chew Stoke
Stanton
Preiston
Rowberow
Nemnett
Stowey
Fernborough
Banwell
Langford
Budcomb
Freshford
Curston
Burrington
H. Littleton
Camerton
Phillips Norton
Bleydon
Combton Martin
Henton Blewet
Foscott
Ratcliff
Axbridge
Lytton
Folkland
Telsford
Cheddre
Chewton
M. Norton
Frome R.
Overwere
Priddy
Stoneaston
Lullington
Rodny Stoke
Emborow
Kilmersdon
Beckington
Mark
Westbury
Ashwike
Frome
Wedmore
Wokey
WELLS
Stokelane
Iye
Whatly
Panborow
Sandhill
Burtle
Crascomb
Shipton Mallet
Leighton
E. Burtle
Dulting
Wandistrew
N. Woodton
Yarnfield
Meer
Evercreech
Glastonbury
Pilton
Upton Noble
Ashcott
Bradley
Badcomb
Kilmangton
water
Pull
Greynton
Ditchet
Street
Lamyate
Bruton
W. Laylund
W. Lydford
Budley
E. Lydford
Knole
Middlezoy
Kingswesto.
Kineton
Castle Cary
H. Ham
Combton Dun
Lovington
Pitcomb
L. Ham
B. Charlton
W. Charlton
Charlton Musgra
Pen
Auler
Yarlington
Pitny
Somerton
Bab Cary
Wincaunton
Langport
Podimore
N. Cadbury
Maperton
S. Triest
Huish
Sparksford
W. Bampfield
Drayton
Yvelchester
Yvilton
Cucklingto
Gillingham
Ivill R.
Muchelny
Chilton
S. Cheriton
E. Lambroke
Chiltern Domer
Rympton
Stawell
Pekington
Tintenhull
Ashington
Carton Dinam
Horsingto.
E. Stoke
Stoke Otterey
Poyntington
Milborn Port
Stalbridge
S. Petherton
Norton
Yeovill
Malherb
Lopeton
W. Coker
Shirborn
E. Dollis
Brimpton
Cudworth
S. Bingham
Chard
Hasilbere
Crookhorn
Pendover
English Miles.
Wayford
1 2 3 6 9
PART OF DORSET SHIRE
ncomb
Longit. W. from Lond. 50'
20'
10'
0
51
50

PART ONE

1659–1697

1

GRACE

It was a three-mile ride from the heart of London through Westminster and across the fields to Chelsea. On other days, the reports of highwaymen lurking on the commons might have led some travellers to prefer the safer but longer up-river journey to the village. But, on Tuesday 13th October 1685, the progress of the coaches carrying the wedding party of Claver Morris and Grace Greene from their homes and lodgings in the city was not interrupted.

Before arrival at the old brick church there was much to see along the autumnal riverbank: the fine houses of courtiers and merchants, the 'physic garden' of the Worshipful Society of Apothecaries now boasting two new cedar trees, and the foundations of the new Royal Hospital. These were all signs of Chelsea's appeal to people well beyond the small farmers, artisans and servants who made up the body of the population. Inside the church the appeal was even more apparent: there was a cornucopia of monuments to former residents, from the chapel and tomb of Sir Thomas More to the marble sarcophagus of Lady Jane Cheyne, a recently-departed benefactress.[1]

Looking around, Claver Morris and his guests would have known that 'Chelsy near London', as he put it, was by any measure a long way from his father's parish, deep in Dorset. But at the age of twenty-six, as an Oxford-educated Bachelor of Medicine and *Extra Licentiate* of the Royal College of Physicians, hard-working and ambitious, he had everything before him. So did Grace Greene, who was just twenty-two. As the daughter of John Greene, a woollen draper and member of the Clothworkers' Company of London, Grace had grown up in the city. She was still a baby when the Great Plague had taken an official toll of 68,596 souls in London during the autumn of 1665. A year later, the Great Fire, blamed on 'barbarous Papists', had destroyed 13,200 houses, St Paul's Cathedral and most of the city's churches. This included the two houses that her father owned off Fleet Street,

DOI: 10.4324/9781003333654-2

in the parish of St Dunstan in the West. During the re-building, Grace's mother, Mary, had rented a house in Chelsea, and it was here in the hamlet of Knightsbridge that she died on 18th May 1674. She had died so quickly it was necessary for those present – her mother Elizabeth Tyrell, her maid Anne White, and Bernard Skelton, a local clerk – to compose a 'Memorandum' on her dying wishes.[2] They expected this would stand in place of a signed last will and testament, and it did.

Aside from small bequests to servants and relations, Mary Greene left everything to be divided equally between her young daughters, Elizabeth and Grace. As with most orphans, their prospects depended as much upon the character of their relatives as upon the size and nature of the inheritance. Among their relations, Mrs Tyrell was granted an annuity of £10 and released from a debt of £50. She would take at least a passing interest in her granddaughters' development over the next few years. So would aunts and uncles from the Willoughbys and the Greenes; old gentry families from little villages near Salisbury. Aunt Willoughby and Captain Greene would be fully reimbursed for the costs of accommodating and feeding the girls during occasional visits they would make in the years ahead. So, the daily joys and troubles of bringing up the girls fell largely on the shoulders of their mother's maid, Anne White. Starting with two bibles and two silver spoons, she would oversee the purchase of all the silk and cotton gowns, petticoats, aprons, stockings, scarves and hoods, as well as the coats, gloves, shoes and all the other 'necessary things' needed 'for ye children' over the next ten years. She would accompany the girls on visits to their relations in Wiltshire, and nurse them through their illnesses. By 1685, after ten years of looking after them, Anne ('Nan') White would have known the girls as though they were her own.

Alongside her expenses, Nan White received wages of £10 a year, plus an initial gift of £10 from Mary Greene's estate. This was sufficient to secure her loyalty and even to allow her to make some savings. So, by the time of Grace's wedding Nan could afford to lend an out-of-pocket Claver Morris £20 – something that she would surely not have done had she thought him an unsuitable match for Grace. A few months later, when Grace and Claver were still both short of cash, she did the same again, this time lending them each ten shillings and £5. Claver was not rich, but more important to Nan was the fact that standing at the altar was a healthy young man from the West Country: a man of middling stature and good family; a firm believer in the Church of England; well mannered, well-educated and well dressed; highly sociable, generous, inventive and inexhaustible; maybe a little vain and certainly strong-minded, but almost certainly in love with Grace.

For all Nan White's industry, legal responsibility for the girls and the management of their inheritance was entrusted to executors: Mr Joseph Hall, a mercer, and Mr Thoresby Hardres, a linen draper and fishmonger, both citizens of London. As Joseph Hall did not trouble himself with any kind of work for the estate, it was vital that Thoresby Hardres should be trustworthy and capable of presenting fair accounts of money spent for occasional scrutiny by the Court of Aldermen in London. His first task was to orchestrate the funeral arrangements. These were extensive, including the hire and purchase of coaches, hearse and coffin to carry Mary Greene and all the mourners from Knightsbridge to the Guildhall for overnight 'watching', and then for a half-mile procession to St Botolph's in Aldersgate. In all, the making of mourning clothes and gloves for Elizabeth and Grace, the payments to the parish, plus a £1 sermon and other costs amounted to over £114. £50 of this was spent on mourning clothes and £20 on mourning-rings, including a special one for Nan White. These costs could be met quite comfortably from the cash that Hardres gathered in the 'ready money' of coins and gold left in Mary's home, the sale of her household goods, her silver-plate and lace, and the collection of small debts. But this was just the beginning of his work.

At a time when orphans' legacies were often squandered or stolen, there could be no doubt that Mary's trust in putting her daughters' future in the hands of Thoresby Hardres needed to be well placed. The principal assets were two houses off Fleet Street in Crane Court: one on the east side leased to a merchant Mr Samuel Lawrence for £50 a year, and a slightly smaller one, 'the lesser house' where the Greenes had lived, on the west side, now let to the earl of Suffolk for £40. Another resident, Dr Nicholas Barbon (son of the radical Puritan, Praise-God Barebone), a physician-turned-property-developer after the Great Fire and a builder of new houses in Crane Court, owed £60. Thereafter, two other £200 loans made to the young linen-draper John Dennett – who Hardres would call his 'loving friend', and with whom Elizabeth and Grace would occasionally stay – were the only other major assets of Mary Greene's estate.

After accounting for the costs of house repairs, legal fees and taxes, there would be an income of about £100 each year; a respectable sum for a family from the 'middle orders' of society. Hardres soon set about securing this, signing longer leases on the houses and recovering the loans to Barbon and Dennett so that £400 could be invested at a better rate in the Chamber of London, run by the city corporation. In all these steps he was sure-footed.[3] But having no wife or children of his own to call upon for advice, he might well have felt less confident about the paternal responsibilities that Mary Greene had placed upon him, possibly very unexpectedly.[4]

As soon as he had retained Nan White to care for the girls and moved them to a home in Hackney, the most pressing question that Hardres faced was what to do about their education. Based upon centuries of religious teaching and patriarchal thinking that women were less capable of reasoning than men, and best suited to supporting life in the domestic sphere, the proper education or 'embellishments' of a girl were usually considered as being very different from those needed for a boy, particularly if the boy were to be sent to university. But a good education was no less important for girls of a middling or higher rank if they were to attract the kind of husbands of which their families might approve.

Within two months of their mother's death, Hardres had enrolled Elizabeth and Grace in Robert Woodcock's new boarding-school for girls, paying £2 in entrance fees and another two for 'dancing, writing, cooking and singing'. Seeing the girls regularly, occasionally with treats – 'two muffins', 'a bottle of scent for Grace', 'wine and a lobster' – Hardres could chart their progress and justify the expense of about £22 per year on each girl's board and lodging. As they grew older, so their need for more pocket money grew, and by the spring of 1685 Hardres was giving each of them a very generous £5 every month. Robert Woodcock, their schoolmaster, was also doing well. Having married another teacher, Deborah Littleton, daughter of the rector of Chelsea, in 1683, he had moved his school to a large house in Chelsea village.[5] But in the summer of 1685, all was not so well.

There was nothing unusual about the annual cycle of births and deaths across the 132 parishes of London and Westminster in 1685. Every year there were more burials than baptisms. This was due to the piles of human and animal excrement that were deposited in the streets; the choking smoke from the coal fires of homes and industries; the overcrowded houses, burial pits and graveyards; and the leaking of cesspits which contaminated the sources of fresh water. Such living conditions spawned a host of stomach problems: worms, diarrhoea and dysentery. Diseases such as typhoid, meningitis and asthma were also prevalent, as was rickets due to the lack of sunlight in most streets.

Periodically, there were outbreaks of diseases such as plague and smallpox. And there was a regular loss of mothers and babies' lives in childbirth, and of almost everyone from common infections of the teeth and gums. In the published *Bills of Mortality* for 1685, listing a total of 23,222 burials for the year, most were attributed to common causes: 'Ague [malaria] and Fever' (3,832); 'Consumption and Tissick [tuberculosis]' (3,502); 'Convulsion' (3,420); 'Flux [diarrhoea] and Small Pox' (2,496); 'Griping in the Guts' (2,203); 'Aged and Bedridden' (1,163); and 'Teeth' (1,138).[6] There were no deaths due to plague, and of the major causes of death, only 'Teeth' sufferers were likely to have called upon a barber-surgeon, for an extraction if they could afford one.

In the summer of 1685, before his wedding, Claver paid an apothecary £5 for medicines for Grace's sister, Elizabeth, and Grace called for visits from the surgeon Henry Tonge.[7] But, whatever medical treatment Elizabeth received, she did not survive. To pay for the funeral in July, Grace borrowed £100 from Tonge, a sum that Hardres guaranteed. At the age of twenty-two, Grace would now inherit the whole of her mother's legacy, and as a single woman she could enjoy the financial independence of owning her own property, taking an occupation or running her own business if she wished. But as soon as she married, all of this would change. The whole of her inheritance would be transferred to her husband. It was a high price to pay for the greater social standing that a married woman normally possessed, especially as Claver had so little money of his own. But Grace did not demur. Following the fashion among the wealthy, on 19th September, Grace and Claver were granted permission to marry without the announcement of their marriage banns, either in the city or at Chelsea.[8]

In choosing Chelsea for her wedding, Grace was returning to the place where her family had settled after the Great Fire; the place where she grew up with her sister and where they prayed together in the church. In recent years she had also been taught in Chelsea by Deborah, the rector's daughter and her husband, Robert Woodcock. The rector, Dr Adam Littleton, had himself moved to Chelsea to set up as a schoolmaster, supplementing his income as a prebend of Westminster and Chaplain-in-Ordinary to the king. In 1669 he had delivered the sermon at the funeral of Lady Cheyne, and in the following year he was made a doctor of Divinity on account of his 'extraordinary merit' and 'ready facility in preaching'. Yet it was as a scholar and linguist of rare learning that he was most widely known. His works included *Solomon's Gate, or, An Entrance into the Church* (1662); a catechism on the Lord's Prayer and Ten Commandments; a large dictionary *Linguae Latinae* (1678); and three volumes of *Sixty One Sermons Preached Mostly upon Public Occasions* (1680) dedicated to his parishioners at Chelsea.[9]

From these and other texts there could be no doubt about the nature of Littleton's opinions. But even if Grace and Claver had never read any of his works or heard him preach, they would certainly have known of his views by reputation. In almost every respect his views were unsurprising: Littleton was a devout believer in the Church of England and a fierce defender of its liturgy in the face of what he believed were the foolish errors and dreadful assaults of Protestant nonconformity and Popery. On one subject, however, his views were shocking.

Put simply, Littleton believed that 'the woman has equal rights with man'. He never tired of explaining that God had intended 'the Equality of Woman's Merits and Rights with Men'. For Littleton, women were just as intellectually capable as men, even though men had fashioned a society in which 'Vertue and good Education were undervalued, and Wealth is become the Lovely Thing, and all the Shafts of Men's Desires are Tipt with Gold and Silver'. Such extraordinary views went even further than those expressed a few years later by the Anglican campaigner for women, Mary Astell. And being a young resident of the parish, she would have heard them preached by Littleton.[10] They would have been at the heart of his message in his marriage sermon too, and whether or not Grace and other members of the congregation were paying much attention, when it came to sermons, Claver was always listening.

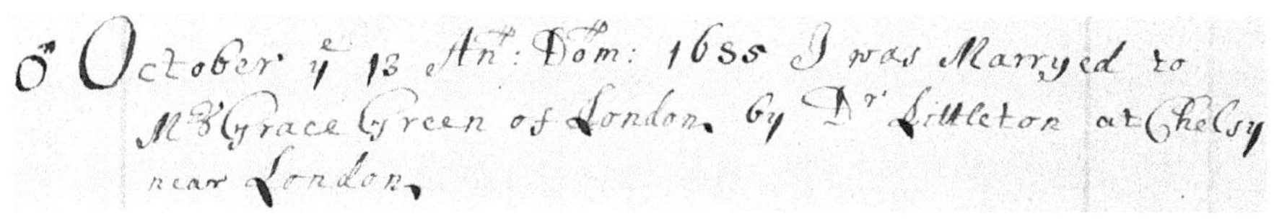
♂ October ye 13 Ano: Dom: 1685 I was Marryed to Mrs Grace Green of London by Dr Littleton at Chelsy near London.

FIGURE 1 Marriage to Grace Greene, 1685
This is Claver's first entry in the book of accounts he received from Thoresby Hardres

2

CLAVER

When Claver Morris was born at Bishop's Caundle in Dorset on 1st May 1659, the celebrations at his baptism would have proceeded with solemnity and caution. As one of only two sacraments (alongside Holy Communion) to survive from the Reformation, the fundamental importance of baptism as the foundation for a Christian life was not in question.[1] But as almost every aspect of how it should be conducted was contested, and the ancient festival of May Day had been banned by parliament, with maypoles reckoned 'a Heathenish vanity generally abused to superstition and wickedness', any sign of feasting, singing or dancing on this day would be sure to attract attention.[2] So too would the unusual decision not to give the baby a good Christian name. There was no mystery here, for everybody in Bishop's Caundle knew that Hannah Claver was the baby's mother, and that Claver families had been living and working in Lydlinch and neighbouring parishes for generations.[3] And where two old families came together through marriage, it was not uncommon for a son to be christened with his mother's maiden name. Even so, William Morris's decision to honour his wife's maiden name – one that was still associated with illicit paternity in the records of the parish[4] – was bound to set tongues wagging.

There had been no rector at Bishop's Caundle since 1646 when, at the height of the Civil Wars, the incumbent Henry Watkins had been ejected from his living. Like many other clergy, he had been ejected for his opposition to the revolution that was underway.[5] Dorset had not suffered any major battles, but the royalist garrisons, sieges and marches that had swept across the county since 1642 were quite sufficient to have fed the deep religious and political divisions that had taken root. Inevitably, amidst all the fighting and incessant looting, by 1645 there was also exhaustion, not least among the common people of Dorset living in the Vale of Blackmore, south of Salisbury. Here, the three villages of Claver's youth – Bishop's Caundle, Lydlinch and Manston – lay in the gently undulating landscape of the Vale.[6]

DOI: 10.4324/9781003333654-3

At the height of the war in Dorset, on 25th May 1645 several thousand 'miserable inhabitants' armed with clubs and swords had gathered to formulate their 'Desires and Resolutions' in a humble petition to the king. Lamenting that 'the true worship of Almighty God and our Religion are almost forgotten', and believing that 'Destruction, Famine and utter Desolation will inevitably fall upon us, our wives and children', the Clubmen begged the king and parliament for 'a happy Peace, and accommodation of present differences without further effusion of Christian blood'.[7] Charles I agreed, for although the Clubmen, led by local clergymen and Thomas Young, an eloquent attorney from Manston, wore white ribands as a mark of their neutrality, they were clearly more on the side of tradition than revolution. Oliver Cromwell was less patient with their complaints and ordered his dragoons to attack 'the poor silly creatures' on the chalky grasslands of Hambledon Hill, overlooking Blackmore Vale. After the killing of a dozen and the surrender and pardoning of several hundred, the Clubmen did not set forth again.[8] Yet not everyone was intimidated or defeated. Parliament still had its supporters among the Dorset villagers; men such as John Veale of Bishop's Caundle who lent £140 to the new regime, including 'one fatt oxe at the price of eight pounds' for 'the service of the State'.[9]

Claver would have heard these local stories of resistance and defiance in his childhood, especially from his father for whom the Civil Wars had been a defining experience. Having left Oxford University to serve as a standard-bearer for a royalist troop of cavalry, when the Civil Wars were over, William Morris had entered the church as a curate (an assistant priest) in 1651. He was not the first to serve in place of the ejected rector at Bishop's Caundle. Two other curates had preceded him, the latter with a stipend of just £18 from a parsonage worth £70 a year.[10] But, however small the salary, considering William's royalist sympathies and service, he was fortunate to be appointed to any clerical position. His marriage to Hannah, the daughter of William Claver, a prosperous farmer from Lydlinch, may well have helped, and later in 1651, at the age of nineteen she gave birth to their first daughter, Ruth. Another daughter, named Hannah, was born in 1655; a son William in 1657; and finally Claver in 1659.[11]

As William had been curate of Bishop's Caundle for eight years before the birth of Claver, he would have known every one of his two hundred parishioners and most of their secrets and beliefs. He would also have known what they thought about the beheading of the king in 1649, Cromwell and the puritanical Republic: the abolition of the bishops and the House of Lords, the rise of militarism and the foreign wars, the levels of taxation, and all the ways in which the local community had learned to cope with a world turned upside-down. Like most of his parishioners and the country as a whole, William would have quietly prayed for a restoration of the monarchy. And on 1st May 1660, exactly a year after Claver's birth, the House of Commons voted to invite Charles II to return. Two years later, William was ordained a priest and was on the move to St Nicholas's church in Manston.

In many respects, Manston, with its seventeen tax-paying households, was just like Bishop's Caundle; a little larger in population, with hamlets and small farmers dedicated to working the meadows, open fields and manorial estates of Blackmore Vale.[12] As in the much larger parish of Lydlinch, wool, corn and dairy produce were vital to the local economy and way of life. But the most valuable exports were the cattle that had been fattened on the 'verie good Pastures' of the Vale before being driven over Salisbury Plain to feed the beefy appetite of London.[13]

In the farming community a price was put upon the heads and eggs of the animals and birds that might compete with people for the precious food resource. So, the slaughter of 'vermin' – from sparrows, crows and herons, to foxes, otters and badgers – was often paid for by churchwardens as required by Tudor laws. The common belief that hedgehogs secretly drank milk from the udders of recumbent cows throughout the night meant that the cull of hedgehogs, at tuppence apiece, was probably severe. And at Manston, where the river Stour was 'full of good Fish', there was an additional activity from which Claver and his siblings could help earn their keep. From their parents' point of view, however, it was the prospect of a rectory with five good hearths (the third-largest house in the parish) that drew them from Bishop's Caundle to the tiny church of St Nicholas at Manston.[14]

Riding the high tide of conservatism that rolled in with the Restoration, the Cavalier Parliament was determined to restore bishops and the Church of England, and to root out what it saw as the radical Protestantism that it held responsible for the nation's sins and sufferings during the Republic and Civil Wars. Under the Act of Uniformity in 1662 – which required all clergy and schoolmasters to accept the Thirty-nine Articles of Anglican faith and everything in the Book of Common Prayer – there was a new round of ejections as about 1,000 clergy (a sixth of the total) and teachers lost their livings. These clergy and their congregations, mostly Presbyterians, were now often called 'Non-conformists' or 'Dissenters' from the Church of England, though many still hoped that they would be able to rejoin the Church if further Protestant reforms could be achieved. At Manston, Claver's father had no difficulty in declaring his allegiance to the crown and acceptance of the Act of Uniformity when he was ordained a priest in 1662. As at Bishop's Caundle, the rector of Manston, John Ryves, had been ejected from his living in 1646, leaving his wife to petition for payment of the standard compensation (one fifth of the rector's income) to support herself and her thirteen children.[15] But, in 1662, John Ryves still held a legal entitlement.

Under the terms of the agreement, William Morris could only enjoy the full fruits of the parsonage, reckoned to be worth £80 a year, if he first paid £60 a year to Ryves. Considering that William had to undertake all of Ryves's duties, and even to provide 'sufficient mansmeate [beef] and horsemeate' for the rector should he ever visit, this was not a generous deal.[16] But, knowing that Ryves was nearly seventy, William was looking to the future, and two weeks after Ryves's death, in September 1665 William, now forty-two, became the rector. Without any great family or inheritance to support them, William and Hannah, who was ten years younger than her husband, must have worked hard to make the most of the barns, stables, orchards, gardens and dove-houses of their rectory to create a good home for their four children, then aged between thirteen and six. By 1672 they could afford to buy a five-hundred-year lease on over twenty acres of land at Abbas Combe, twelve miles away, for £144.[17] This would raise their income to a figure well above that of most families in the region. They also acquired a long lease on a parcel of land at Felton in north Somerset, where their daughter Ruth also managed to acquire five acres. For this, in 1678, she confidently signed a lease (with Claver as her witness) for a yeoman to pay her ten shillings rent, and thereafter a shilling every year.[18]

Though prosperous by common standards, even with the help of friends and relations there was no money for any expensive schooling of the children, so William and Hannah must have taken this upon themselves. In March 1673 their eldest son William was enrolled at St Edmund's Hall, Oxford, aged fifteen. But he would not complete his studies: in December 1675 he died and was buried at Manston on Christmas Day, with the whole parish in attendance.[19] In the following spring, Claver entered New Inn Hall at Oxford, aged sixteen, graduating with his Bachelor of Arts in 1679 and a Master of Arts in 1682.[20] Such opportunities were not open to his sisters, but their education was not neglected. Both would make 'good matches', each with a substantial marriage portion of £500. Ruth would marry Nicholas Shirley of Bagber, and Hannah, Edward Goddard of Marnhull; men from old gentry families living in the villages nearby. Ruth had 'a very weak constitution' and she died in 1683, just two years after her marriage. But Hannah would live long enough to have two children by Edward Goddard, a boy and a girl whom she christened William and Ruth after her lost siblings.[21]

By the time Claver became a Bachelor of Medicine shortly after his 26th birthday, he had been a student at Oxford for nine years. Even in his most recent terms as a student of 'Physic' (Medicine), his studies would have been highly academic, focusing on Latin and Greek, mathematics, natural philosophy (physics), chemistry and botany. Above all, he was expected to attend lectures twice a week by the Regius Professor of Physic on the works of Galen and Hippocrates, and to listen to formal disputations on the nature of illnesses and their treatments according to the ancient texts. This required a deep appreciation of how the four elements of all matter (and their primary qualities) – Earth (cold and dry), Fire (dry and hot), Air (hot and wet), and Water (wet and cold) – corresponded with the four fluids or 'humours' of the human body and its mental state: Black Bile (melancholic), Yellow Bile (choleric), Blood (sanguine), and Phlegm (phlegmatic). For it was generally believed that all illnesses arose from an imbalance of these humours which could be most readily diagnosed from a physician's examination of the smell, sediment, swim, colour, crown, and sometimes the taste, of a patient's urine.

Alongside this examination a physician would probably conduct a case study of the patient's medical history; their diet, bowel movements and 'regimen'. He might also cast a horoscope to see how the position of the moon and planets might have influenced the patient's health – as in Saturn's association with melancholia and gout. Any physical examinations (such as to determine whether the patients were cold, hot, moist or dry) also proceeded along these lines, which usually led to bloodletting and to the prescription of a great range of vomits, purges and enemas, regarded as fundamental to the treatment of most conditions.[22]

Since the Restoration, among some physicians there had been less emphasis on the role of astrology in medicine – though the efficacy of the relationship was still strong in the minds of many practitioners and was commonly upheld in almanacs.[23] In particular, some physicians were less interested in the position of the moon and stars during bloodletting, but had a growing interest in botanical gardens and in human anatomy, based upon the observation of dissections performed on the corpses of executed criminals. There had also been a growing challenge to traditional thinking, through the followers of Paracelsus, the sixteenth-century Swiss mystic and physician. Paracelsus had denounced most of Galen's theories, claiming that there were just three principles – sulphur, mercury and salt (all combustible, volatile and residual when heated) – in God's Creation and the Book of Genesis, and that different kinds of salt in the body were responsible for different kinds of disease. According to Paracelsus, therefore, diseases were not due to imbalances of the humours.

Paracelsus also believed that particular organs of the body were related to particular planets and metals, and that chemistry (with the aid of fire) was key to understanding nature. His followers (iatrochemists) were often physicians at universities in Europe and, like Claver, were keen to conduct experiments to produce chemical treatments alongside, or in place of, the traditional Galenic herbal and organic recipes. But, for all these developments and a few fundamental discoveries, such as those revealed in William Harvey's treatise on the circulation of the blood in 1628, at Oxford and Cambridge the advance of medicine as a modern science had been slow by comparison with the leading universities overseas.[24]

In England, a university-educated physician, a gentleman and a man of learning, was expected to be able to reason, knowledgeably and eloquently, about the nature of all illnesses. He would provide patients with prescriptions and advice (including advice about their lifestyle or 'regimen') for the use of specific medicines and cures, normally leaving the manual labour of making and mixing medicines and drugs, or cutting flesh and bone, to apothecaries and surgeons. The physician was expected to be a man who worked primarily with his head, rather than with his hands. In this traditional hierarchy of physicians, apothecaries and surgeons, the relationships between these key practitioners – as well as all manner of nurses, midwives, tooth-drawers, bonesetters, diviners, eye-surgeons, wise-women, herbalists and healers – could be co-operative, though it was often confused and fraught.[25] And it was greatly aggravated by the growth of quacks (often unqualified practitioners and itinerant conmen) pedalling popular remedies, 'panpharmacons' and other medicines, and performing operations up and down the country.

The apothecary was generally reckoned to be a tradesman, responsible for procuring ingredients and preparing and selling medicines, either according to the physician's prescriptions or according to a customer's request. Customers could find hundreds of ready-made pills and potions, as well as luxuries such as coffee, tea, chocolate and other exotic items believed to have health benefits, on the shelves of the apothecary's shop. Having split from the Grocers' guild, apothecaries had obtained a charter to form their own Worshipful Society in 1617 with the exclusive right to dispense medicines within seven miles of London. But this did not endear them to the Royal College of Physicians which objected to apothecaries dispensing medicines without a physician's prescription. Naturally, the apothecaries countered that physicians should not be allowed to make and dispense their own medicines – as Claver would often do. Even so, most physicians and apothecaries were keen to protect the integrity of their work and incomes from the damage done by common people diagnosing their own illnesses and making their own medicines; which, of course, they had done since the dawn of time. But the growing popularity and availability of medical texts translated from Latin into English, threatened to undermine the medical men's monopoly of knowledge.[26]

While an apothecary was a tradesman in the public mind, a surgeon – with his great array of strange and special instruments for bloodletting, treating wounds and fractures, and undertaking internal operations, amputations and extractions – was a kind of craftsman. He was a practitioner of one of the two crafts still regulated in London by one authority, the Company of Barber-Surgeons, despite a request from the surgeons in 1684 for a formal separation. At Salisbury in 1676, putting similar crafts together, the city's silk weavers (cutters and stitchers) were also incorporated within the Company of Barber-Surgeons. Here, the widows of all three craftsmen were fully entitled to continue 'the art or mysterye' of their husbands' business. But only the widows of barbers and surgeons were permitted to increase their skills and knowledge by 'mak[ing] an anottomy' of the body of a condemned person after execution.[27]

The superior status of physicians was most clearly demonstrated by the fact that neither apothecaries or surgeons were required or expected to have had a university education, though apothecaries were supposed to have a little Latin so that they could read a physician's instructions. But apothecaries and surgeons were expected to have served several years of apprenticeships before admission to their associations. They were also expected to be able to provide testimonials, which were sometimes needed to obtain a bishop's license before they began their practice; though in the diocese of Bath and Wells a license could normally be obtained with no more effort than putting a signature to an oath subscribing to the Thirty-nine Articles of the Church of England.

As it was generally accepted that no health could be preserved or illness cured without God's help, a bishop's license was meant to confirm the applicant's religious worthiness as much as their medical competence. Midwives and nurses (who were not required to have had any formal education, and had no trade association to promote their interests) were also encouraged to apply for licenses. When granted, these served as evidence of their holder's good character and ability; and, in emergencies, a midwife might even be permitted to conduct a baptism. But there were plenty of practitioners who went unlicensed. Some, such as the self-certifying physician Robert Shoot of Yeovil in Somerset, were then prosecuted in the bishop's court. Having been told that he could not practice surgery without a license, it was reported that he told the court 'he cared not a fart and a turd for the bishopp nor his licence'.[28]

In 1685, with his license from the Royal College of Physicians and his Bachelor's degree in Medicine, Claver Morris was fully qualified to work as a physician. His cousin, James Claver, son of William and Margery Claver of Bishop's Caundle, was four years older and well-established as an apothecary in Salisbury.[29] It was while staying with James that Claver probably first met Elizabeth and Grace when they were visiting their relations at Knoyle and Donhead Lodge, on the road between Salisbury and Manston. Staying with James also meant that Claver could spend time learning about the business of a medical practice directly from his cousin, before undertaking the difficult task of setting up his own. He could also gain practical experience of the hundreds of complex and often dangerous processes involved in making medicines, and even experiment with some concoctions of his own. And at Salisbury he was just thirty miles from his family home.

For all these advantages, Claver was still in no position to set up the kind of practice that would attract the patronage of wealthy clients. Even in a large and prosperous city such as Salisbury with a population of seven thousand, there was too much competition. And in the seething metropolis of London with its half a million citizens, a number growing at a terrifying rate each year, the challenges were even greater. Without a wealthy patron or family tradition in medicine, Claver needed money as well as time to build a practice. But after so many years of study, he had no capital or income other than the gifts of £5, £10 or £15 that his mother and father gave to him throughout the year. To make a living, he needed to be married to someone who had money of their own.

After their wedding in October 1685, Grace and Claver remained in London, staying for the winter in the smaller of the two houses that Grace had inherited at Crane Court, with a view to moving to a new home in the spring. In addition to the £100 that Grace had borrowed from the surgeon Mr Tonge to pay for her sister's funeral, Claver had borrowed a further £50 from him, and on 3rd November he met Thoresby Hardres to review the guardian's accounts. In the eleven years since Grace and Elizabeth were orphaned, Hardres had received exactly £1,804 and five shillings income from properties and investments, and had spent £1,836 and ten shillings on the children, leaving a final balance of £32 and five shillings owing. More importantly, the principal assets of the estate – the deeds and leases of the two houses in Crane Court, and two bonds worth £500 – were still intact.

Now, with the help of loan of £45 from his parents, and the wedding gift of £20 per year from their land at Felton, Claver had the means to repay debts. At the end of the month he rode to Salisbury to pay back £55 that he owed there, including £12 to his cousin. But it would be another year before he was in the clear. Little gifts from his parents totalling £80 were still forthcoming, but to stay afloat he needed to borrow another £90 from friends of his family at Manston, plus £55 from his married sister, Hannah. So it was with understandable relief at the end of a three-week trip in November 1686 that he could say, 'when I came out of London I did not owe either Mr Hardres or Mr Tong, or Any other Man or Woman there one Farthing'.[30] But he really only had Grace to thank for that.

3

THE CATHEDRAL CITY

It was probably during their first winter together, in London, that Grace and Claver decided that the cathedral city of Wells was the right place for them to settle. The city, founded at a natural spring and site of ancient pilgrimage, was no longer the largest town in Somerset, as it had been in the Middle Ages. But it was still a very busy place, specialising in the making of men's woollen stockings, and especially important as the seat of the diocese of Bath and Wells which covered the whole county. Nestling on the southern skirts of the Mendip Hills, Wells lay between the hill-farming, sheep-grazing villages to the north (where the caves and gorges of the Mendips had been mined for lead, calamine, zinc, iron and coal since Roman times) and the open rich pasturage of the marshy moors of Avalon immediately to the south. Here, the butter, cheese, leather and other produce of the dairy farms was often mixed with the rearing of hens, ducks, geese and pigs. And, one way or another, most families also worked on the harvesting of barley for malt; of reeds and rushes for thatching and baskets; and of teasel flower-heads, dried for use as combs to cleanse and tease the nap of wool.

There was a long coastline twenty-five miles north-west of Wells that could be reached by travelling along the foothills of the Mendips through Cheddar and Axbridge, and there was an important port at Bridgwater further south along the coast. Closer to Wells, towards Wiltshire in the east, lay all the manufacturing towns and villages that were the hub of the West Country's great woollen industries. Historically and economically, Wells was therefore a natural centre for the region, and it was renowned for the 'good company' of wealthy citizens and local gentry who chose to live there.[1] It was also just forty miles, a long day's ride in good weather, from Claver's old family home at Manston.

When Grace and Claver arrived at Wells to set up home and a physician's practice, it was the spring of 1686. At first, they stayed with their friend Richard

DOI: 10.4324/9781003333654-4

Cupper, a forty-six-year-old apothecary and shopkeeper who had lost his first wife ten years before, and who endured the misfortune of being famous for his red hair – commonly seen as a sure sign of secret wickedness.[2] Cupper lived with his sixteen-year-old son and second wife in what was still known as Bishop Bekynton's 'New Works'; a 200-year-old terrace of twelve stone-built houses on the north side of the marketplace, backing onto the cathedral green.[3] The south side of the marketplace was largely occupied by the Red Lion inn and by an equally old, gabled and bay-fronted coaching inn known as the Crown. On its west side, the marketplace was open to Sadler Street and the High Street which provided the only access through which a horse and cart could pass through the town.

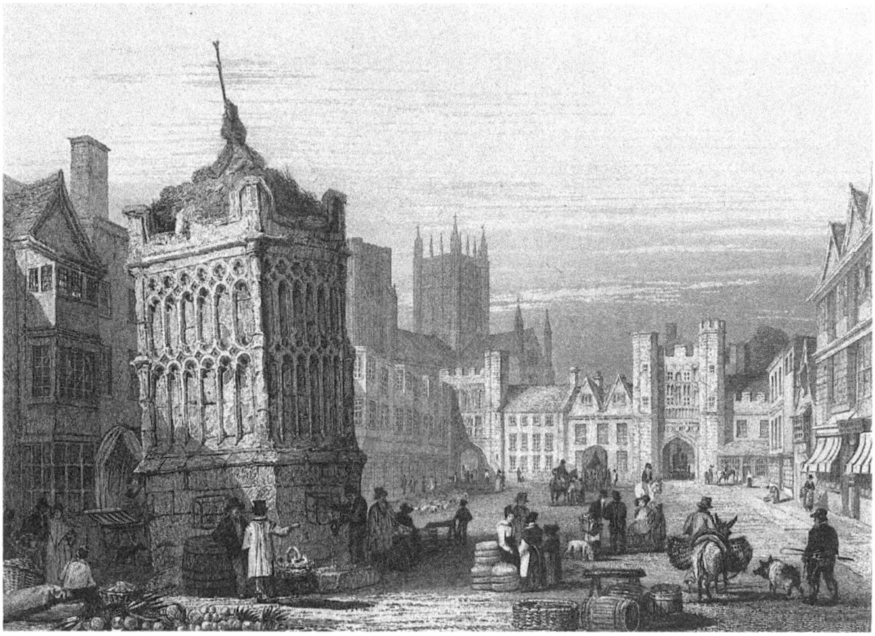

FIGURE 2 The Market Place, Wells
On the north side, behind the great Conduit, is the row of shops and houses known as Bekynton's 'New Works'. On the far side, Penniless Porch leads to the cathedral green, and the Palace Gate leads to the bishop's residence. Part of the Crown Inn can be seen on the south side. In Claver's day, a High Cross and Assize Hall, stood in the middle of the marketplace

Directly outside Cupper's house and shop, close to the High Cross, stood another of Bekynton's creations; the great stone Conduit building. The Conduit was designed to provide a ready source of drinking water for the people and a much-needed means of keeping the city clean by releasing water into the gutters running down the High Street. Towards the bottom of the High Street a left turn after the Christopher inn would lead into the poorest quarter, Southover, and then to Glastonbury, six miles across the moors. But, straight ahead, at the end of the High Street, the Conduit water continued its journey down the spine of the town, along St Cuthbert Street and Tucker Street until it reached the city's western limits. Here stood the largest church in Somerset, St Cuthbert's, serving not only the city's guilds, its mayor and council and surrounding hamlets, but also – being the city's only parish church – the great majority of its three thousand inhabitants.

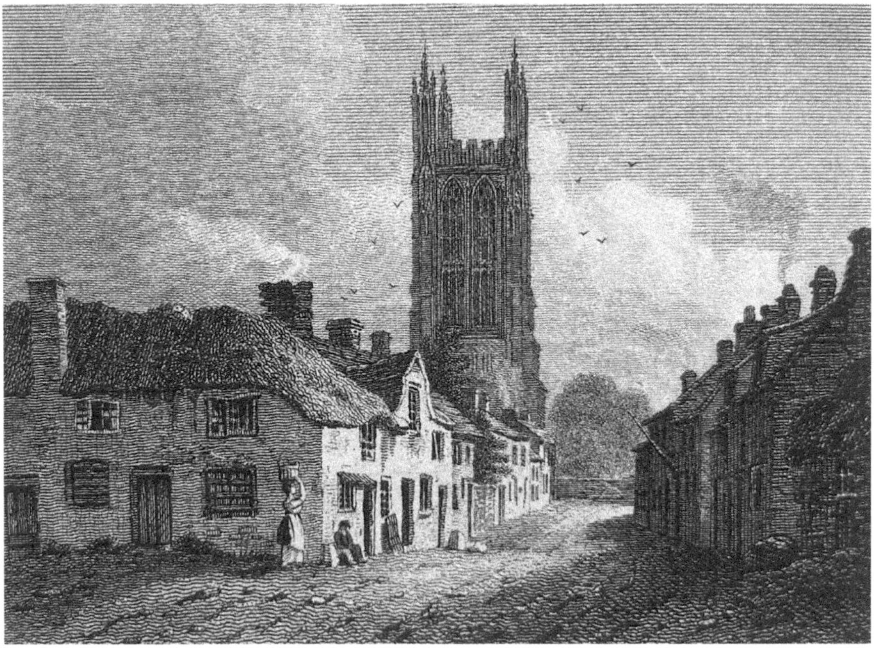

FIGURE 3 St Cuthbert Street and Church, Wells
Looking up St Cuthbert Street from the west end of the city

Many of the oldest and most prosperous working families had built good houses among the inns, tenements and shops that were squeezed into this western body of the city. And next to St Cuthbert's, in Chamberlain Street and Priest Row, several homes had also been built for some of the city's poorest residents. In the fifteenth century, Bishop Bubwith had built an almshouse with a guildhall and a chapel for twenty-four poor men and women. Bishop Still had added a hostel for six more, and from the legacy of a mayor in the seventeenth century, a third almshouse had been built for ten elderly women, providing each with a parlour, bedroom and small garden. But these almshouses, like the town pump 'Jacob's Well', the city's slaughter-houses and its prison in the cellars of the City Arms, were all at the bottom or west-end of town, and this was not at all where Grace and Claver had set their sights. They even looked beyond the marketplace where, in the 'New Works' on the north side, several genteel families, such as the Keens and the Westleys, lived next to successful woollen drapers, lawyers and pharmacists like Richard Cupper. There were clergymen living here too, and on the south side, near the Crown, the eccentric archdeacon Edwyn Sandys had just finished building himself a grand new home.[4]

In this rich social mix, those shopkeepers who could afford to live at the centre of the city's commerce were clearly able to derive a profit from their location. For them, the sounds and smells of the place, plus the blood and dirt of the pigs and other animals brought in for slaughter on market days, were just a necessary part of business. And there were other benefits. News and public information was disseminated from the tower room of the High Cross at the entrance to the market, where the bishop's bailiff read out notices and proclamations and received petitions. There was also a Market Hall, the old Exchequer building, which stood in the middle of the Place. The Hall, a long wooden structure built on twenty stone pillars, had recently been restored to provide more shelter for stallholders on the open-sided ground floor, and two chambers on the first floor for meetings of the mayor and corporation. The ground spaces were designed to be enclosed with boards to meet the needs of justices and court officials during the courts of assizes and quarter sessions – though the judges continued to complain about the cold and damp.

The assize was always welcome. It brought a train of visitors to the city who 'filled it like a faire'; spending money in the markets, shops and inns. When a national survey was conducted in 1686 to determine the number of guest beds and stables that were available in each town and county (in case they were needed by the army), it was reckoned that the eighty inns and alehouses of Wells had 402 guest beds and 599 spare stables. This was much more than any other town in the West Country, except Bristol.[5] Wells was therefore a very popular destination for visitors and lodgers even when the assize was not in session. And it was certainly profitable at times when the assize was held. For the general entertainment of five judges for a few days during the 'Bloody Assizes' of September 1685, the mayor and corporation paid Richard Cupper over £19 on behalf of local labourers and traders.[6]

Not everyone was welcome. There were always rogues and vagrants who needed to be punished or moved on, and for such offenders the corporation usually kept its gallows, pillory and ducking-stool in good repair. Before Grace and Claver had arrived, five 'lewd women' were ordered to be whipped for an hour on market day for having had 'bastard children borne of their respective bodies'.[7] It was not without good reason that an alley off the High Street was named 'Grope Lane'. But there were plenty of other problems too.

Maintaining standards in what was generally regarded as a clean and tidy city was not easy. The water and shambles wardens were sworn to look after the lead pipes and fittings of the Conduit and to ensure that only wholesome flesh and fish were brought in for sale. Yet they struggled with these simple tasks. At the quarter sessions they reported that 'the ancient channel or watercourse running down the High Streete' was frequently diverted for private use by 'great bayles of soyle and dung', and that some people simply swept their dirt straight into the streets 'to the great nuisance and annoyance of inhabitants'. For this, offenders would be fined a shilling.[8] Years later, in response to similar complaints, it was ordered that 'noe

Butcher or other person kill any beast or catle in the publick streets ... or empty any Belly in ye same, or at ye conduit or att any other place unless it bee att the Common Slaughter houses belonging to ye Citty'. The penalty set for this offence was six shillings and eight pence, but the problems did not go away.[9]

It was probably only at times of extraordinary unrest that the everyday annoyances of living in or near the marketplace may have outweighed the benefits in the minds of residents. For those who enjoyed the excitement of being at the centre of the city's fairs and festivals, its elections and seasonal celebrations, there was no better place to live. What everyone could agree upon, however, was that on passing through either of the two grand gateways built by Bishop Bekynton on the east side of the marketplace you would be entering a quite different world.

The first and most imposing entrance, built with a house on either side, was a three-storey tower called the Palace Gate, or more commonly the 'Bishop's Eye'. Here, behind two great timber doors there was a green and tree-lined paths circling the moat and crenellated walls of the bishop's private residence. To the right, the paths led to the open fields and deer park that were part of his estate. Straight ahead, by the tall wall of the cathedral cloisters, the paths led around a horsepond to the drawbridge and portcullis of another gatehouse; this one guarding the twelve acres of land within the palace walls.

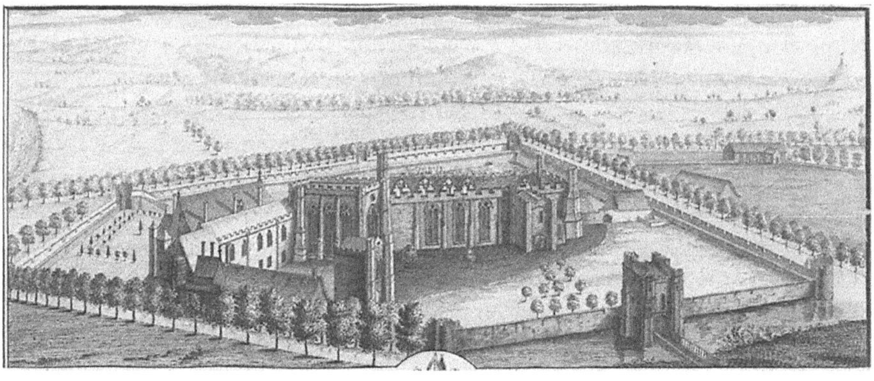

FIGURE 4 The Bishop's Palace, c.1733
Looking south from the cathedral, the engraving shows the bishop's chapel and residence, the tree-lined moat and drawbridge, and Glastonbury Tor on the horizon (top right)

There was simply no entry over the moat and into this domain without an invitation; and unless Claver established a reputation as a good physician and citizen it was unlikely that he would ever receive one. Begun in the thirteenth century by Bishop Jocelyn – who, by legend, had slain a milkmaid-eating dragon – the palace had been extended to include a new wing by Bekynton, more gardens, a grandly decorated chapel, and a great hall built to entertain medieval kings. A little beyond the moat's gatehouse, a path led to the ever-bubbling springs of St Andrew's Well, an ancient site for the pilgrimages that marked the origins of the city. This was also the place from which fresh water was fed into the palace moat, into the streams that drove the bishop's mills, and into the pipes that ran under the 'New Works' and into the market Conduit.[10]

The second arched gateway, Penniless Porch, at the north-east corner of the marketplace, was a more modest opening; a place where, for as long as anyone could remember, the city's beggars had always been permitted to solicit alms. But it was no less important as a border post, marking, since 1207, the boundary between the authority of the city and the Liberty of St Andrew. In the city, the corporation guarded its territory so tenaciously that when William Sherston (Claver's patient) was elected mayor, his election led to a dispute. The problem was that his house straddled the boundary between the city and the Liberty. This meant that if he was reckoned to reside inside the Liberty, he was not entitled to serve as mayor. And even if he made a door from his house to step directly into town, this would not be an acceptable solution. For he could not exercise any authority as mayor from inside his own house, if the house itself were deemed to lay outside the city's jurisdiction.[11]

Inside the Liberty, an area of over fifty acres including the cathedral and its precincts, the residents were free from the laws and taxes levied by the city and the bishop. Instead, they were governed by rules of conduct set out in canon law under the jurisdiction of the clergy of the diocese of Bath and Wells.[12] This meant that even some statutory offences, such as failure to attend church services or to take Holy Communion, were tried by the dean and chapter (the cathedral's governing body). Sentencing was often more lenient too, as Elizabeth Loxton of the Liberty found in October 1685 when, having been 'brought to bed about a month since of a base male-child begotten on her body by one Thomas Moore, who is since fled', she was not put in the stocks, washed in the bishop's moat or whipped half-naked through the streets, but just required to do a prayerful penance.[13] Being an 'extra-parochial township', the Liberty was also outside the parish of St Cuthbert, and for most residents this was vital. In effect, it meant that the cathedral was their parish church, not just for baptisms, burials and weddings, and for worship, but as the centre of the local community.

After centuries of building, most places in the wide streets of Liberty were owned and leased as part of the large portfolio of properties belonging either to the dean and chapter or to the bishop's see. Most were usually granted at low fixed rents to senior clergy for their lifetime or for forty years. Some properties were owned privately, and some of the nominally 'residential' clergy chose to live elsewhere (and could make good money from the subletting of their houses to other tenants). So, the privileges afforded by living in the Liberty were not confined to those clergy who had great patrons or who had been appointed to high positions. Many of the larger houses were occupied by the families of wealthy citizens or local gentry and their servants. Yet the total number of residents was never great enough to prevent everyone from knowing everyone else in person. With a little effort and much gossip, it was possible to learn plenty of things about everyone else's business, for this was not a community in which anyone could expect to remain anonymous.

In April 1686, the news that a newly-married couple – a smart and highly sociable young physician and his wife from London – were about to take up residence would not have gone unnoticed.

It was a five-minute walk from Richard Cupper's shop through Penniless Porch towards the house in which Grace and Claver planned to live. The Porch led directly onto a wide expansive green from where, between the rows of trees, the great west face and flanking towers of the cathedral could be viewed. Unlike its sister church, Bath Abbey, which had been run by Benedictine monks, the cathedral had survived the Protestant Reformation virtually unscathed. The immense Catholic tableau of over 360 life-size statues – including the 9 orders of angels, 85 scenes of nude figures rising from the dead, and the Madonna and Child above the central door – was still intact.[14] After four hundred years, most of the blue, gold and scarlet paints that had coloured the original tableau had worn away, as had most of the facial features of the statues. Much of the damage done to the windows and statues during the Civil Wars when troops had plundered the cathedral was also now beyond repair. But, for all this damage to the fabric, much more remained unscathed. Gazing at the west front in 1686, the cathedral still looked like a gigantic decorated casket within which, alongside its own treasures, most of the surrounding city and its people might be placed with room to spare.

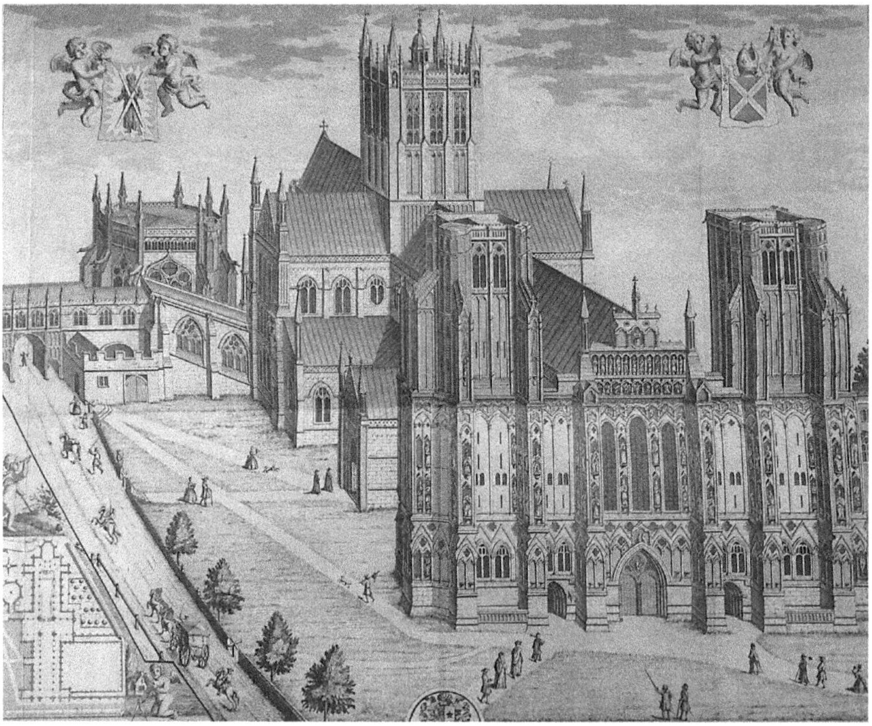

FIGURE 5 The West Front of the Cathedral, c.1730
The top of the octagonal Chapter House can be seen behind the Chain Gate across St Andrew Street

At the far corner of the green, next to Brown's Gate marking another border point between the city and the Liberty, the old Mitre tavern was a popular place for Claver and his friends to meet. From here on a clear day at sunset they could watch the sandy-coloured limestones on the face of the cathedral turn to shades of pink. From the Mitre, walking along St Andrew Street next to the green, a house and courtyard had been built for the dean and his staff. Further along there were grand houses built for the chancellor and archdeacon. After the street passed under the arches of the Chain Gate (an ornately-enclosed footbridge linking the cathedral with the little terraced houses in the gated community of the Vicars' Close) there was a medieval Tower House which was the home of another senior dignitary, the precentor.

At the end of the street, beyond the cathedral precincts, lay the tenements of East Wells; a small district renowned for its poverty and alehouses, where miners of the Mendips lived and drank. From here, there were two roads from the city. The first, heading east, followed the twisting valley of the river Sheppey to the cloth-working towns of Shepton Mallet and Frome, six and sixteen miles away. The second road led twenty miles to Bath where a traveller could pick up the stagecoach to London, 110 miles away.

It was not necessary to pass through East Wells to reach the house in which Grace and Claver planned to set up home. From the Tower House where the recently widowed precentor Dr Robert Creighton resided with his five young children, the high wall around his garden continued into the East Liberty, a gently rising street with half a dozen fine houses leading to Grace and Claver's at the top. Here, on the edge of Wells, the towers and bells of the cathedral could be seen and heard above the long chimneys of the Vicars' Close, and past another line of fine properties along the Back Liberty, Claver and Grace would hope, one day, to be able to afford to drive their own coach and horses into town.

4

THE PHYSICIAN

In the Middle Ages, when it was customary for wealthy Christians to build chapels and leave legacies to pay for the chanting of masses for their souls, Grace and Claver's large house had been a college with lodging for fifteen chantry priests. Since 1547, when chantries were abolished as Popish indulgences, the house had become a private residence, changing hands several times before being purchased for £106 by William Evans, master of the Cathedral Grammar School, in 1609.[1] William's son had inherited the house in 1632 and was still living there when he died in 1683. But his son and heir, John, preferred to live at Burcott manor in a hamlet on the edge of Wells. This meant that the old chantry house was unoccupied until Anne his wife decided to let it to Grace and Claver from Lady Day, 25th March 1686. The Evans family did not need the money for they were well known as an old gentry family with land and estates in and around the city and far beyond.[2] Yet they were also renowned for something else: Catholicism.

Although they were recusants (registered non-attenders at Church of England services) the Evans family had tried to keep a low profile for many years; steering clear of politics as far as possible, paying fines for non-attendance, and accepting their exclusion from holding any public office. But in 1641, when the House of Commons demanded that all adult males over the age of eighteen should sign the Protestation Oath promising to maintain and defend 'the true reformed Protestant religion expressed in the doctrine of the Church of England, against all Popery and popish innovation', John's father had refused. He was not alone: there were seventeen other Catholic men in Wells who did not sign, and three of these lived in the Liberty. They all stood out – especially the wealthiest, the Evans family – against the 869 adult males of Wells who signed.[3] Throughout the Civil Wars, the Republic and the Restoration, the Evans family continued their tradition of steering clear of politics and they offered no support for royalist armies or conspiracies. But when great waves of fear and anger washed across the country soon after the accession

DOI: 10.4324/9781003333654-5

of the Catholic James II in 1685, it seemed most unlikely that there could be any happy outcome, for anyone. Like other Catholics, to protect their lives and properties the Evans family might well need friends.

For Grace and Claver the annual rent of £13 for the old chantry house, plus an annual two-shillings 'chimney money' tax for each of its seven hearths, was very reasonable. But before they could move in, renovations and cleaning were needed throughout the kitchen, parlours, brewhouse, necessary house, stables and walled garden. Their new home also needed refurbishing. Throughout April, shopping trips were made to the best drapers, ironmongers, cabinet-makers and glassblowers of Bristol and Wells, where Grace and Claver purchased everything from silver spoons and pewter platters to leather chairs and lanterns. In this spending spree, hundreds of yards of plain white calico, purple-printed dimity, linens and woollens were chosen, as well as 200 pounds (over 90 kilograms) of the softest feathers, just to furnish the three main bedrooms.

There were also personal items that required transport from Manston, Salisbury and London – as well as a small monkey, a fashionable amusement. Grace alone had half a tonne of things, including her bed and a box bought for the carriage of a picture of her grandmother. Her friend Nan White, who had cared for Grace after the death of her mother, had travelled with her to Wells, though not with so much baggage, as her trunks only weighed 100 pounds. By the end of April, when they had moved in, all that was needed were the deliveries of wine for the 'strangers' and 'visitants' that were expected for the house-warming parties. They were not disappointed. After four deliveries of wine, a few weeks later Claver topped up the cellar with over eighty pints of claret.

After so many years of training, it was important for Claver to establish his reputation in Wells as soon as possible. At the village of Wedmore, nine miles away, there was a surgeon, John Westover, who often prescribed medicines and treated local families. On his farm he had also built a special barn or 'madhouse' for the confinement of 'inpatients' suffering from mental illnesses, and he was making a modest living.[4] But this was no competition for Claver's ambitions as a qualified physician. Confident of success, on 5th May 1686, the first anniversary of his Bachelor's degree in medicine, he began recording what he hoped would be a growing list of people who would be willing to pay 'For my Advice & Prescriptions in Physick'. His first entry was for 'John Walsh of Holcomb', who had brought his son for treatment. The 'Childe which had Ascarides come from him about 6 foot long' was suffering from a relatively common condition considering the prevalence of intestinal worms among young children. Claver's fee of two shillings and sixpence reflected the relative ease of treatment, and probably the fact that most physicians recognised that medical interventions for children often needed to be gentle.[5]

Claver treated four more patients in May, and received a ten-shilling fee paid by John Evans, his landlord, on behalf of Anne, his wife. But at this rate, he was not going to make a living as a physician. In June, his closest neighbour, Catherine, wife of the eighty-year-old Honourable Francis Poulett, called on him, but this was only to administer to her maidservant for ten-shillings.[6] On 16th June, captain Piers

[Peirs], a twenty-year-old grandson of a former bishop of Bath and Wells, became the first person to pay a whole guinea for medical advice. The captain would pay another guinea five days later, even though he was on his deathbed and leaving behind a heavily pregnant wife.[7]

Claver's fees (when he charged) were not excessive – ranging from two shillings and sixpence for poorer patients to a guinea per consultation for the wealthy and the gentry, plus any travel expenses – but there was no rush for his services. He was rarely called upon to make long journeys, though in July he rode with Grace for six hours to prescribe for her cousin, Mrs Edith Davies at West Knoyle in Wiltshire, taking a gift of four silver salt-cellars. With so little demand for his services, he had time to make his own medicines, rather than rely on the 'chemicall preparations' he previously ordered from his cousin James Claver. In May he purchased:

- ***oyl of amber***, made from fossilised tree-sap, used 'to cure the suffocation of the uterus', and 'excellent against fits of the mother, epilepsy, convulsion, palsy, lameness, numbness, wounds of the nerves etc'[8];
- ***saccharum essence***, made from the juice of cane sugar, believed to be 'good in all diseases of the lungs', for cleansing cuts and easing pain;
- ***resin of jalap***, made from the tubers of the Mexican plant and frequently used to make boluses to treat gout or dropsy (swellings of the head or limbs); and
- ***resin of scammony***, made from the tuberous roots of the Syrian plant, used to make strong purgatives, and especially to kill worms in children.

These were all standard herbal ingredients for the production of traditional medicines according to William Salmon's 880-page translation of the Royal College of Physicians' famous *Pharmacopoeia Londinensis. Or the New London Dispensatory* (1682). But Claver showed no interest in the equally familiar use of animal ingredients such as

- ***goat's urine***, dropped into the ears to cure deafness;
- ***dried bone of stag's heart***, taken to prevent miscarriages;
- ***dried mole's heart***, taken to treat ruptures, 'most effectual in May';
- ***oyl of winged ants***, for drinking to excite lust;
- ***dried fox lungs***, drunk to treat coughs and colds;
- ***ashes of a black cat's head***, blown into the eyes to cure eye diseases; and
- ***legs of the male tortoise***, which 'being cut off alive a little before the change of the moon, and bound to the part affected, the right to the right, the left to the left' leg, would be a cure for gout.[9]

Favouring herbal and chemical treatments above those based on the use of animal ingredients was indicative of Claver's commitment to the rise of science over superstition. But this may have cost him a few patients, and throughout the summer he was still only making a handful of prescriptions. In July, when Grace and her maid Hannah Best were taken ill, he called on Cupper for the 'physick' (medicine), and they soon recovered. A week later he paid ten shillings for more ingredients to make his own:

- ***ens veneris***, 'essence of Venus'; a mixture of copper and ammonium chloride, regarded as 'a noble and worthy anodyne', 'easing all manner of pain and strengthening the parts dedicated to generation';[10]
- ***hepatica oyl,*** made from the liver-shaped leaves of the plant, mostly used to treat liver diseases, to provoke urine and as a cure for yellow jaundice, rickets and gonorrhoea;
- ***vitri antimony,*** a toxic infusion of the glass of antimony, a silvery-white metalloid used to promote sweating, vomiting and purging, 'best made on Sundays when the moon is in Pisces or other watery signs'.[11] It was also widely used as 'an antidote to Plague' and as 'a cure for the green-sickness in virgins' (a disease, associated with weakness and a pale complexion, that was widely believed to afflict unmarried young women, due to a lack of iron or sexual intercourse); and
- ***aqua fortis,*** 'strong water', nitric acid prepared by distilling potassium nitrate with sulphuric acid, and used to dissolve silver and other metals.

These were powerful chemicals of a kind that Claver often preferred to 'languid medicines' and, in keeping with his convictions, he purchased a double-strength distillation of nitric acid. He could use this to dissolve the brass filings that he purchased, making a treatment to cleanse sores and ulcers. He also purchased clove-water from Cupper; believed to protect against the plague, and 'to cure new wounds and old ulcers, emend the corruption of bones, and ally tooth-ach'.[12] And he bought essence of jasmine, 'an excellent perfume' which, taken internally, would 'warm and comfort the womb, and cure the schirrous [tumour] therof'.[13]

For all these purchases and days spent making medicines, he still needed more people who were prepared to put their lives and those of their loved ones in the hands of a relatively unknown and inexperienced twenty-seven-year-old physician. To build a reputation would take time and it would depend upon word of mouth about his social standing, family connections and personal and religious conduct; and trust in his professional knowledge and abilities, especially his discretion. By the time he rode to London after his wedding anniversary in October 1686, however, he was still only prescribing for three or four people every month.

The main purpose of the trip was to settle the outstanding matters of Grace's inheritance, and this was duly done, leaving Claver delighted that he had paid his debts, except to his family and friends. Between the business meetings, there was time to pay for lessons on the violin, and to do some shopping. He needed a scabbard for his sword, a new setting for his diamond ring, and a frame for a picture of Lady Jane Fisher — the young woman who had played a heroic part in the escape of Charles II after his defeat at the Battle of Worcester in 1651. He also liked to keep abreast of fashions, so he ordered a woollen coat with Persian silk linings and frosted gold buttons; deep-blue breeches; pairs of worsted and copper-coloured silk stockings; a campaign wig with curly sidepieces; a beaver-fur hat and a walking cane. He also bought presents: doe-skin gloves and a lace petticoat and gold-net cap for Grace; a settee and gloves for this mother; an apple-roaster for his sister Hannah; and (perhaps mindful of his unfortunate red hair) a twenty-five-shilling periwig for Richard Cupper.

During his stay in London, Claver also took the opportunity to add to his learning, buying the latest books by physicians who, like himself, were keen on the therapeutic use of chemical ingredients. These Latin texts were:

- ***Opera Pharmaceutica Chymica*** (Leipzig, 1686), by the young German iatrochemist Michael Ettmulleri, who pioneered the idea of injectable medicines, though there was still no alternative to injecting veins by use of goose feathers;
- ***Encyclopaedia Medicinae Theoretico-Practicae*** (Amsterdam, 1686), by Johannes Dolaus, a German physician who was warning that sick infants should not be purged, except by the natural qualities of breast milk;
- ***Tractatus de Febribus Intermitentibus*** (Hague, 1684), by John Jones, a lawyer and physician who had just been appointed Chancellor of Llandaff Cathedral, most famous for his work on fevers; and
- ***Arcana*** (Utrecht, 1680), by Lazare Riviere, a former Professor of Medicine at Montpellier University whose *Practice of Physick*, translated by Nicholas Culpeper in 1655, had already appeared in over twenty English-language editions.

Alongside these hefty tomes in the trunk of goods that Claver packed for home was a newly-bound edition of John Playford's *Courtly Masquing Ayres: Containing Alamanes, Ayres, Corants, Morisco's, Jiggs etc of Two Parts* (1662). This was a collection of popular dance-tunes for viols and violins. It was much smaller, cheaper and more popular than any of the other books, but in Claver's hands it would fill him with delight.

5

THE MONMOUTH REBELLION

On his return to Wells in November 1686, Grace and Claver began to prepare for winter. Recent winters had been severe, especially during the Great Frost of 1683–1684 when, with 'small pox very prevalent and mortal', the Thames had frozen for three months. The icy weather had supported fairs and sports 'like a carnival on the water', but it took a heavy toll on birds, animals and people that froze to death.[1] Somerset fared no better. On the hills above Wells, 'people did die so fast, that it was the greatest part of their work to bury the dead; it being a day's work for two men' to make a grave. The drifts were so deep that 'some of the snows remained at Mendip till Midsummer'.[2] Fortunately, the Morris household was quite small; just Grace's companion Nan White, her housemaid Hannah Best, and Claver's apprentice-boy who was, in effect, another servant, plus themselves. But all needed to be fed, clothed, cared for and kept warm, the costs of which fell entirely upon Grace and Claver, and the work very largely upon Hannah and the boy.

Since Hannah and the apprentice depended upon the generosity of their employers for almost everything – from the quality of their diet to the clothes they wore and the hours they worked – they were paid a pittance; twelve shillings and sixpence every three months for Hannah, and a little less for the apprentice-boy. But Grace and Claver were not mean in their treatment of their servants. Both enjoyed spending money and not only on themselves, and they were probably regarded as far too generous in having items such a £3 pair of new shoes made for a mere apprentice-boy. Ninety-two large sacks of coal (at ninepence each) would keep everybody warm throughout the winter, and fifty-two bushels of barley malt (at three shillings and sixpence for the best) would be sufficient to brew at least

DOI: 10.4324/9781003333654-6

fifteen gallons of small beer for safe drinking every week. Their only other regular expenses were food for the household at about eleven shillings a week; hay for the horses; and an occasional hogshead (51 gallons) of Somerset cider for £1, plus gallons of brandy, claret, sherry and white wine that were delivered almost every month – some of which was reserved for medicines.

One of the most popular 'cure all' medicines, 'a most Excellent Preservative of Man-kind', was 'Daffy's Elixir', created in the 1640s by a Leicestershire vicar, Thomas Daffy. After his death in 1680, his son had made money by turning the cordial into a household name. He claimed to have sole knowledge of the secret formula, but it was not difficult to reproduce the sweet and warming taste of the original, or its laxative effect.[3] So Claver was following the fashion for this medicine when, in December 1686, he started making his own version, consisting of two gallons of brandy and a few pinches of dried senna, coriander, liquorice, aniseed, elecampane, ginger roots and raisins. He did not call it an elixir, but simply and more honestly his 'Cathartick Liquor', and he made a similar tonic with even greater quantities of white wine. But still he had few patients. In the six weeks leading up to Christmas there were just four: Madam Sellick, sister of the archdeacon of Bath, for her young niece; Mrs Packer for her friend Mrs Morgan, the wife of a wealthy woollen draper; and Mrs Sarah Westley, at first for herself and then for her husband, William.

The Westleys lived in the 'New Works' of the marketplace, one house away from Penniless Porch. So it was a five-minute walk for Claver, down the East Liberty and around the cathedral, to attend to them. William, a fifty-one-year-old big-hearted man, was from old gentry stock, his father Thomas having left Essex in the 1630s to join his friend (Bishop Piers) as vicar of St Cuthbert's. Both men had been removed from office during the Civil Wars and had been reinstated after the Restoration. Sarah Westley was also from the gentry: her father, Francis Keen, had been keeper of the bishop's second palace at Banwell on the Mendips, and her mother, Jane, was still living in the house next door. In the 1670s Sarah had borne William five children, four girls and a boy, but none had lived for long. The twin girls had been buried together in one coffin and, most recently, the last surviving child, the son, had been buried at the age of four. Whatever pains Sarah and William were now enduring, by the time Claver left them on Christmas Eve 1686, they were on the mend. They had paid him six guineas for his advice and prescriptions, but they had also found a doctor they could trust, and in the process a good friend.[4]

Like Richard Cupper a few doors away, the Westleys had been children during the great turmoils of the Civil Wars, but living in the marketplace in 1685 they had been eye-witnesses to events that would haunt Wells and the West Country for generations. The story, which lost nothing in the telling, was well-known to the nation. Despite growing fears of Catholicism, throughout the 1670s and '80s parliaments and plots had failed to prevent the accession of the proud Catholic James II to the throne on the death of his brother Charles in February 1685. Even so, Charles II's eldest illegitimate son, James Scott, the duke of Monmouth, the 'darling of his father and the ladies', was unwilling to accept the rule of a new Catholic king. After sailing from Holland and landing at Lyme Regis, he raised an army of Protestant nonconformists and workers from the cloth-manufacturing towns of Somerset and Devon. In June, at Taunton, he proclaimed himself the rightful king and protector of the people.[5]

At Wells on 18th June 1685, as a sign of loyalty to the crown, the city's corporation and the dean and chapter both granted money to support the royal forces being marshalled by the lord lieutenant of the county. The chapter recorded this was 'in order that the cathedral church may be seen in some way to take its part so far as it can in these difficulties'.[6] Yet a small detachment of Monmouth's army arrived a few days later with scythe blades fixed to eight-foot poles, their 'cruel and murthering weapons'. Their aim was to gain more recruits, possibly from among the miners of East Wells.[7] There were now inflated reports of 10,000 'Clubmen' on the moors, ready to join up. But when the whole rebel army arrived in Wells on 1st July, though still sizeable, it only numbered about 5,000 men.

According to the government's official newspaper, the *London Gazette*, at Wells the rebels 'robbed and defaced the Cathedral Church, Drinking their Villainous Healths at the Altar', and 'plundered the Town, ravished the Women and committed all manner of Outrages'. It was also later noted that some of the rebels, assisted by a local woman, 'searched the poor people's coffers' at the city's almshouse. Less dramatically but more reliably, the rebels seized the wagons left by the king's dragoons, tore lead from the roof of the cathedral in order to make musket balls, and stole a ceremonial silver verge or wand. From the dean and chapter's meeting in the afternoon – or, rather, the meeting of chancellor Holt and the notary Nicholas Neblett, as all other members of the chapter were either laying low or out of town – it was recorded that the 'rebel fanatics' had also 'almost utterly destroyed the organ, and turned the sacred building into a stable for horses'. Frideswide Creighton, wife of the precentor who was out of town, was unlikely to have been frightened, but she was sufficiently intimidated to pay a rebel officer £20 in order to prevent the canons' houses along the cathedral green from being pillaged.[8] On 2nd July the rebel leaders left, heading west across the moors to Bridgwater, and taking two days to reach their destination due to the incessant rain.

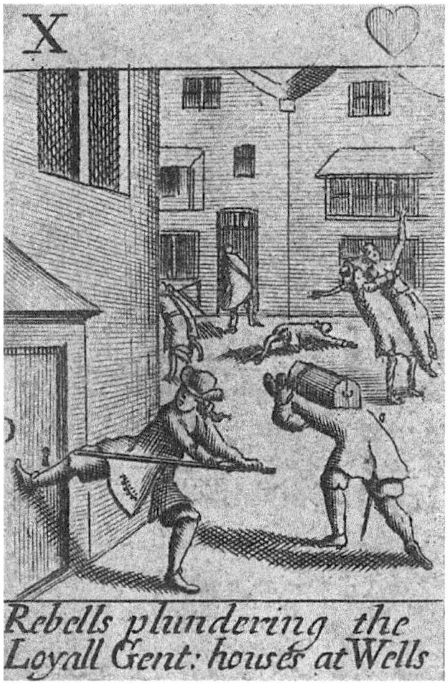

FIGURE 6 Rebels in Wells, 1685
A pack of playing cards depicting scenes from the rebellion was published in London a few months after Monmouth's execution

On the night of 5th July they attacked the royal army at Westonzoyland, and by the morning they had been defeated. In the battle, a former bishop of Wells, Peter Mews, 'the bombardier bishop' as he was known, played a vital role in harnessing his coach-horses to the royal cannon so that they could be drawn up to fire into the rebel ranks. Dozens of those captured now faced summary execution, and 'man-catchers' were paid five shillings for every fugitive they caught. Monmouth himself was caught in Dorset, and on 15th July, after five strokes of the axe in London he was clumsily beheaded. On their way home from Sedgemoor on 6th July the Wiltshire militia stopped at Glastonbury to hang six captives before marching on to Wells. There, as hundreds of prisoners, many of them under twenty-one, were held in St Cuthbert's and the bells of the church were rung in celebration, a thanksgiving service led by Peter Mews, now bishop of Winchester, was held in the cathedral, and all its bells were also rung. After the service, another five prisoners were hanged.[9]

Whatever relief or distress the citizens of Wells and the West Country felt after the defeat of the rebellion, they must have expected that in the months ahead their spirits would begin to lift. But there was much more to come. A royal regiment under the command of Colonel Edward Berkeley was now stationed at the bishop's barn to deter any disturbances as the city prepared for the arrival of the young Lord Chief Justice Baron Jeffreys and four other senior judges of the Western Assize. By the time they arrived at Wells, their final stop, on 23rd September (three weeks before Grace and Claver's wedding), everyone knew what to expect. A month earlier, at the opening of the assize at Winchester, Dame Alice Lisle, an eighty-year-old widow and loyal subject, had been tried for innocently providing a Dissenting minister (a fugitive) with a night's lodging at her home. Convicted of treason, she was sentenced to be burnt at the stake; but following an appeal to the king, her sentence was commuted to beheading.[10] As the Western Circuit moved on to Salisbury, Dorchester, Exeter, Taunton and Bristol, condemning hundreds of rebels to hanging or transportation, a stream of dreadful stories about Judge Jeffreys and 'the Bloody Assize' were seared into local memories.

At Wells and other towns, the numbers awaiting trial were so large the prisoners were encouraged to plead guilty to speed up the proceedings. In his opening address Judge Jeffreys always stressed that the king would pardon those who pleaded guilty; and to prove his point at Dorchester, when a batch of thirty prisoners claimed to be not guilty, twenty-nine of them were immediately condemned. Under the guise of helping the accused, the town clerk of Wells, David Trym, legal officer to the mayor and corporation, had 'wheedled them to confess' at Ilminster gaol, before handing his examinations to the judges. And at Wells, when Colonel William Mangell had the audacity to plead 'Not Guilty', he was hanged straight away as an example to the rest.[11]

Sitting in the discomfort of the recently-but-poorly refurbished Market Hall and suffering severely from the pain of his kidney stones, Judge Jeffreys could be relied upon to dispatch the business of the day with his customary contempt for evidence and the law. While the accused were brought to trial in batches from their temporary accommodation in the cathedral cloisters, Jeffreys also had plenty of time to rest. He might try some of the 200 gallons of ale and sixty bottles of the very strong and bitter 'October' beer (cellared for at least a year) provided for the judges' refreshment, and then send reports on his work to the king and royal court – which looked on with approval.

On a single day in Wells, 23rd September 1685, 518 prisoners were accused of levying war against the king, nine of aiding and assisting the rebel cause, and six of uttering seditious words. Of these, ninety-nine were sentenced to death in towns across the county, including seven in the marketplace itself: Thomas and William Durston, yeomen from Axbridge; William Meade, a local glover; Abraham Bond from Chard; Robert Doleman, a husbandman from Langport; John Shephard, a husbandman from Compton Dando near Bath; and the outspoken Colonel Mangell. The twenty-one-year-old Jacob Tripp from Axbridge, and John Bird of Beckington near Frome were not due to be hanged at Wells. But when they both caught 'a very malignant infectious feaver' (typhus), 'hand-bolted' together in the city gaol, it was feared that Tripp, 'being unconscious', would not survive a journey back to Axbridge. He was hanged in the marketplace instead.[12]

Of all the prisoners tried at Wells, only twenty could afford a pardon, usually costing about £60; though it may be that some prisoners who could afford a pardon chose not to ask for one. Men like George Bisse of Martock, a gentleman and lay leader of the local Presbyterians, who had been arrested (wrongly, so he thought) for assisting the rebel cause. His lawyer advised him to plead guilty and pay £250, but he was still convicted of high treason. Saved by the persistent efforts of his wife, he was eventually pardoned for £400 and released in March 1686.[13] Other prisoners were kept in custody and fined or whipped for their seditious words. But the majority, 383, were sentenced to transportation. This meant ten years' servitude in 'some of his Majesties southern plantations, viz. Jamaica, Barbados, or any of the Leeward Islands', and 200 of those tried at Wells were shipped to the colonies for the benefit of the Governor of Jamaica. At a starting price of £10 or £15 per head, it was a highly profitable business, so the queen herself, Mary of Modena, was given a hundred convicts, though she wanted more.[14]

Perhaps believing that the time had come to show a little clemency, on 10th March 1686, James II issued a General Pardon, noting that 'many of those who joyned themselves in that Rebellion being poor Labourers and Handicraftsmen' they had been seduced by 'Ill-disposed Persons of greater Note and Quality'. He then added a list of 135 men and 43 women, most still in hiding, who were 'excepted'. One of these was Thomas Oram, a woolcomber from Wells. His kinsman, John, another woolcomber, had already been transported; but both were pardoned in July 1686. Other local men were not. John Carter and Richard Chinn were both tried at Wells, but sent to Bath and Shepton Mallet to be hanged.[15]

By the time that Grace and Claver arrived in Wells in the spring of 1686, most of the material damage of the rebellion had been repaired: £500 was being spent on repairing the cathedral's roof and the silver verge had been replaced with a new one made by the local goldsmith John Penny. Although she had died in December 1685, leaving behind a husband and five children, the precentor's wife Frideswide Creighton had been reimbursed for her well-spent £20 to protect the canons' houses along the cathedral green from pillage.[16] Yet Grace and Claver could not have travelled far without being confronted by the carnage. Well over 300 people had been hanged, disembowelled, beheaded and quartered. Under the sheriffs' instructions, the body parts had then to be boiled in brine and dipped in tar in order to preserve them, before being set on poles or spikes to be exhibited at the towns and landmarks of the region.[17] At Weymouth on the Dorset coast 6 heads and 12 quarters were to be displayed at the grand pier, the windmill, the bridge and the town hall, and another 6 heads and 34 quarters were to be presented to parishes nearby.[18] Even in little Bishop's Caundle, where Claver had been born, the parish paid the expenses for the 'fetching from Sherborne and hanging up the Quarter of the Traitor'.[19]

6

MOTHER & CHILD

Wells – like Bath, Bristol, Exeter and Salisbury – had not been a hotbed of recruitment, though many of the surrounding towns and villages had been more sympathetic to Monmouth's call. But as Claver rode out on his young horse to visit patients, whichever road he took there were hundreds of families, including royalist ones, who were now in mourning or nursing wounded soldiers. If he headed east, within an hour or two he would be among the cloth-working towns and Presbyterian communities of the Frome, Bruton and Shepton Mallet region. If he rode south and west to Glastonbury and across the moors of Avalon, he would come to Taunton and all the towns of South Somerset, Devon and Dorset from which Monmouth had drawn so much support. Whatever ailments or misfortunes the people were suffering, Claver was willing to prescribe. It was his nature and his duty, and in his financial interests too. So he treated members of rebel families such as the Bisses and the Chinns, and even the Strodes of Downside who had harboured Monmouth after his defeat. On the royalist side, he would visit several notoriously 'loyal' figures such as the 'wheedling' lawyer David Trym, whose sickness required a long course of treatment that cost £4.

Yet, at Easter 1687, when Claver sat at his desk to take annual stock of his financial accounts, he could see that he needed to raise his income. The house-keeping, under Grace's jurisdiction, was economical enough; just over £28 plus coal and malt for almost a year since they arrived in Wells. But on top of this there was rent, taxes, clothes, wine, wages and all manner of other expenses in lists that ran over so many pages Claver could not bring himself to add them up. Even allowing for the exceptional costs of furnishing the old chantry house and the income received from the Crane Court rents and from his family's gifts, the balance between the 'Money Laid Out' and the 'Money Received' was sobering. In the past year, Claver had earned just over £38 for all his 'Advice & Prescriptions'.

DOI: 10.4324/9781003333654-7

Both as a firm believer in the Church of England and as a physician, it was important for Claver to practice his religion by regular attendance at church services. In church, he could pray not only for himself, his family and friends, but also for his patients. Whatever medicines and treatments he devised, he knew that there could be no hope of healing anyone's mind or body without God's blessing. It was widely believed that some pains and diseases had been sent by God as punishments or warnings, or as tests of faith and forbearance. But, in the natural world of His Creation, God had also provided the materials from which – through the intercession of a good and worthy person – cures and consolations could be found. In prayer, Claver's Christian faith and medical duty came together in a way that was entirely meaningful and very practical – exactly as he would wish. Rising early to attend matins in a magnificent cathedral at 6 a.m. on several days each week would be no hardship, even though he was often late to bed. After the service he would meet his friends, sometimes over breakfast. He was also often called to work on Sundays. In all of this he would be seen observing the kind of conduct that was expected of a dutiful new doctor; one who truly cared about his patients.

This was important because, in 1687, most of Claver's regular patients were still closely connected to cathedral business. His friend William Westley was chapter clerk – responsible for keeping the records (in English or Latin) of the meetings of the cathedral's governing body – so he was perfectly placed to keep Claver abreast of all clerical affairs and to recommend the doctor's services. William's wife Sarah was also a friend and an exceptionally valuable patient, paying over eighteen guineas for medical treatments throughout the year. Living next to the Pouletts, Claver's neighbours in the Liberty, the Selleck family were also important patients. As archdeacon of Bath, the seventy-seven-year-old Dr John Selleck was responsible for the welfare of a fifth of the 383 parishes in the diocese of Bath and Wells. He had been ejected from his Somerset rectory during the Civil Wars after showing great loyalty to the crown in the reign of Charles I. For this he had been rewarded with the archdeaconry in 1661 and, in the following year, an important diplomatic mission to free (with a ransom of £10,000) 162 English sailors captured by pirates at Algiers. Having a legalistic and cantankerous disposition, he was not the easiest of patients. Even so, the fact that he, his sister, Joan, and his sons all called upon Claver for prescriptions and advice could only enhance the young doctor's reputation.[1]

Other patients included Edwyn Sandys, the forty-three-year-old archdeacon of Wells who, like Dr Selleck, was one of the principal dignitaries of the cathedral. As rector of Yeovilton and other benefices, he had been made an archdeacon in 1683 with responsibility for over half the parishes of the diocese. Strong-minded, eccentric and disputatious, not least over the new house that was being built for him in the marketplace, it was said that he hated children and that he 'never would baptise an infant, nor see one of his own several children till they were eight or nine years of age'. He did not call on Claver personally for advice, but his wife did; both for herself and for her son.[2] So did Mary Healy, wife of the thirty-two year-old Dr Richard Healy who was the cathedral librarian, communar and master of the fabric as well as William Westley's hard-working assistant as deputy chapter-clerk. Mary had called for Claver when her five-month-old son was sick in November 1687. Claver could not save the baby, but Mary remained his patient, and he became a 'dear friend' of her husband.[3]

In the summer of 1687, there was joyful news when Grace discovered that she was expecting her first child. Aside from the replacement of her maid with a new one (earning ten shillings more each year), there was no great change to the pattern of life at the old chantry house. In response to letters and messages received, on some days Claver would visit patients. On most days, however, his time was spent at worship, seeing patients at home, reading or writing letters and prescriptions in his study, preparing medicines in his laboratory, brewing beer in the parlour, playing the violin, or meeting friends and patients – most of whom lived within a few minutes' walking distance of his home.

Some cases entailed several visits to related families, such as the descendants of a former bishop of Bath and Wells, William Piers. One branch of the family living in New Street required treatments, as did the family of Katherine Piers, who lived in the Archdeacon's House on the cathedral green. Katherine had given birth to a son in May 1685, but a year later, she, her husband and their infant were all seriously ill. The sickness running though the Piers families in Wells had taken a toll on several of the former bishop's grandchildren and a great-grandchild in the previous year. But this time Claver could say that, under his advice, everyone recovered.[4]

At Christmas, Claver bought himself a 'mute violin', adding to his growing collection of musical instruments. With no children of their own, his closest neighbours, the Honourable Francis Poulett and his wife Catherine, had become Grace and Claver's friends, but when the eighty-year-old Francis became ill in January, Claver could not save him.[5] However, Catherine was not left entirely on her own as she was the sister of Robert Creighton, the precentor who had lost his wife the year before. So, Catherine now had five young motherless children (a nephew and four nieces) to keep an eye on. Living at the Tower House, close to the cathedral, meant they were within easy reach for both Catherine and Claver to care for them.

The social standing and influence of Creighton meant that keeping the children healthy was a great responsibility and opportunity. The children's grandfather had been a famously fiery Scottish preacher and chaplain to Charles II during his exile in France, taking his twelve-year-old son, Robert, with him for several years. After the Restoration, he was appointed professor of Greek at Cambridge, then dean of Bath and Wells, and briefly the bishop before his death in 1672.[6] Two years later, Robert, his son, was appointed the precentor. Like his father, Robert had also been a professor of Greek at Cambridge. He also harboured a strong antipathy towards Protestant nonconformity to the Church of England which he expressed at every opportunity and in publications such as *The Vanity of the Dissenters' Plea for their Separation from the Church of England: a sermon preached before the King at Windsor, Sept 10th 1682.*

As precentor, Robert Creighton was in charge of the music and liturgy of the cathedral. He was responsible for the choir, the choirmaster, the organist and the training of the choral vicars. But, due to the age or absence of several of the other major dignitaries of the cathedral, Creighton's power and influence was far greater than his nominal status might suggest.[7] Still only fifty in 1688, he was also exceptionally able and ambitious – especially for his children.[8] This was not someone that a young newcomer such as Claver could afford to cross. So it was fortunate that they had things in common, including a classical education and faith in the Church of England. Most of all, however, they shared a love of music.

By the 1680s the precentor had already composed several of his nine church services, and fourteen anthems that could be sung in the cathedral. Nor were his interests confined to sacred music, for he also composed lute pieces, vocal items and dozens of trios and sonatas that could be performed on any secular occasion.[9] Nothing could have been sweeter to Claver's ear. He did not need to live in Wells to practice his religion or to work as a physician: he could do both in other places, as long as there was somewhere to worship and sufficient people who were willing to pay for his advice. But to hear and sing good music every day, or several times each day, and to be able to talk and practice with a coterie of other music lovers made living in a cathedral city something special and essential. With five Creighton children to educate and entertain, Claver would relish playing and singing with them to their father's tunes or to the jigs and courantes of the *Courtly Masquing Ayres* – songs and dances that could be enjoyed by people of all classes. Grace too, like any well-educated lady, would know how to sing and dance for entertainment. However, she needed to take more care now that she was with child.

On Tuesday 20th March 1688 at the old chantry house, Grace gave birth to a baby girl. Both mother and child were healthy, so there was no need to rush to a christening in the cathedral, and within a few days they were both strong enough to make the forty-mile trip to Manston. There, at the rectory, Claver's parents, William and Hannah, were waiting. On Wednesday 28th March, standing before his congregation at St Nicholas's church the Reverend William Morris proudly baptised his granddaughter, Mary; named in honour of Grace's mother, Mary Greene.

Claver did not stint on the celebrations, but he was sober enough to return to Wells and resume his practice in mid-April. A few weeks later, he bought a cradle and hired a coach to fetch Grace and Mary home in comfort. While Grace was nursing Mary, Claver resumed his business treating regular patients and a few new ones, including 'a strang woman' who paid five shillings for his help. He also found time to tally up his annual accounts. Since March, he had employed two maids for Grace, and the house-keeping bills had risen to £35 a year. But by far the biggest change was in his annual income from 'Advice & Prescriptions', which had almost doubled to nearly £73. This was a sign of his growing reputation and it augured well. But in July, when Mary was only four months old, she suffered from a sickness that – despite anything Grace, Claver, Nan White and others could do, or say in prayers – would leave her helpless. On 27th July she died. The following day she was taken back to Manston where she was wrapped in a lace shift and shroud and placed in a coffin for burial. The great bells were tolled in Manston and in Wells, and gloves, sweets and wine were handed out in both places. Before her burial, Grace and Claver took a keepsake, a lock of Mary's hair.

While they mourned the loss of their baby, the attention of the nation was focused once again upon how to cope with the obdurate old Catholic king. In April 1688, James II had re-issued his Declaration of Indulgence: suspending all penal laws enforcing conformity to the Church of England; permitting freedom of worship for Catholics and Dissenters; and ending the requirement for men to be communicants of the Church of England in order to hold public offices. As his Catholic second wife, Mary of Modena, had given birth to five children during their fourteen years of marriage (though none had lived), it was believed that, when James died, the throne would pass peacefully to James's Protestant half-sister, Mary, who was married to the young champion of Protestantism in Europe, Prince William of Orange. But after a visit to Bath, the Catholic Queen, whose pregnancy was not widely known, unexpectedly gave birth to a healthy son. When James Francis Stuart was born on 10th June at St James's Palace, the prospect of a Catholic heir plunged the kingdom's nations into crisis.

Rumours were spread that the baby was not the Queen's and that he had been smuggled into the bedchamber in a warming pan. The stories were not true, but William of Orange would not miss his chance. Riding on a wave of anti-Catholicism, on 5th November – auspiciously marking the centenary of the 'Protestant wind' when God had blown the Catholic Armada onto the rocks, and the day on which the country had been saved by the discovery of the Gunpowder Plot – William landed at Torbay in Devon. He had 14,000 troops ready to march with him through the West Country and into London. After a few skirmishes, James II's much larger army deserted, and by Christmas he had fled to France, leaving William and Mary to reach a settlement with parliament. In all this 'Glorious Revolution' as it would soon be styled, there could be no doubt that the fate of the whole kingdom was at stake. But this was not what was at the front of Claver's mind.

At the end of December 1688, suffering from a violent disease, Grace had become dangerously ill. To Claver, she seemed 'transfixed by the same weapon' that had seized her baby daughter. He hired a nurse, Mary Conduit, for five weeks in the hope that she could help, but Grace died on Monday 14th January 1689. Her friend and neighbour, Catherine Poulett, who had lost her own husband the year before, and the Longs of Downside, who were also friends, provided coaches to carry Grace's body to Manston. As with her baby's funeral, on 18th January the bells of Wells cathedral and St Nicholas's church were rung, and mourning-rings, gloves, wine and spices were handed out. In keeping with tradition, a little dole money was given to the poor in Wells and twelve dozen cakes were baked to be given to the Manston needy. During the service, dressed and wrapped in lace, Grace was laid to rest in a grave under the communion table. Torches were needed to carry out this work, as it was such a dark and freezing day.

A few weeks later, when Claver had returned to Wells, he opened his ledger to record the bare facts of the occasion. His quill was heavy with black ink as he tried to write neatly and in much larger letters than he was used to, adding a few flourishes to decorate the script: 'For the Interment of one of ye Best and Kindest of Wife's Who Dyed January ye 14, & was Buryed Jan. 18 1688/9'. After the word 'Dyed' he drew a small crescent to mark the fact that this was a Monday, and the moon was entering its first quarter.[10]

7

VISITS TO NEW PATIENTS

After the 'long frost and deepe snow' of another winter when the Thames froze over, Claver set out for London on Monday 4th March 1689. The days were longer now and the ancient roads, so deeply rutted by the traffic of carriages and carts, were less likely to be icy for the horses. Lodging at the coaching inns along the Great Road over the chalk-lands of the Wiltshire downs and the heavy soils of the Thames valley, even with fair weather Claver would not expect to reach the capital much before Thursday evening. He made the journey on his trusted ten-year-old bay gelding, 'very strong grown' with 'a Starr on his Forehead'. His apprentice-boy rode the four-year-old, a 'Sandy Grey' with one white sock and a black-braided mane. As soon as they reached London, Claver bought himself a periwig, a new pair of boots, a new riding sword, a silk handkerchief and, most importantly, another mourning suit.[1]

It had been three and a half years since Grace and Claver had lived together briefly at her family home in Crane Court, and it was almost three years to the day since they had left London to set up home in Wells. Since then, the 'lesser house' on the west side of the Court had not been well maintained, and the aim of Claver's visit was to oversee its renovation. He rented rooms and stabling nearby, just outside the old city walls. This was just a few minutes' walk over the open sewer of the river Fleet and the building of the new cathedral of St Paul's. The whole district was notorious for the hustle and bustle of its trade in every line of business. This included the harbouring of stolen goods and fugitives. Most recently, the notorious highwayman William Davies, who had preyed on travellers over Salisbury Plain for forty years, had been arrested for the murder of a local butcher.[2] Here, among all the taverns and coffee houses and publishers and printers' stalls squeezed into the streets around St Paul's, Claver would be among the first to hear the latest news. Among the current stories was one about Judge Jeffreys that would have attracted

DOI: 10.4324/9781003333654-8

his attention. Having been arrested and kept in the Tower of London since his failed attempt to flee to France, the 'Widdows and Fatherless Children' of Dorset, Somerset and Devon were now petitioning parliament that 'the vilest of Men, may be brought down to the Counties aforesaid' to face justice at the hands of 'the good *Women* of the *West*'.[3]

The loyal newspapers were reporting that towns and cities across the country were 'ringing bells, lighting bonfires and showing all other imaginable Expressions of Joy' in celebration of parliament's proclamation that William III and Mary II would soon be crowned 'joint sovereigns'. In truth, parliament had little choice as William made it clear that he would not be a Regent or Prince Consort: 'He could not submit to be tied to the apron strings even of the best of wives'.[4] Everyone knew that war with France was coming. This was an inevitable outcome of Louis XIV's ambitions and his refusal to see William of Orange as anything better than the leader of the Protestant heretics of Europe. In fact, war had already started.

On 12th March, James II, Louis XIV's cousin, had landed at Kinsale with 6,000 French troops determined to regain his kingdoms, and there were reports from Bristol that 'in all the Western Ports great Multitudes of distressed *English* Protestants from *Ireland'* were arriving in a 'most deplorable' condition. They told stories of how 'at *Dublin* the Protestants were all disarmed, and their Horses taken from them, and many of them plundered and cruelly treated by the Soldiers, who had likewise seized on both the Cathedrals and the Colledge'.[5] A few days later, when a boat arrived at Liverpool from Drogheda with no passengers, the reports were even more disturbing: the Catholic soldiers were not permitting any Protestant 'Man, Woman or Child to come away'.[6]

After catching up on the news, Claver would have read the short advertisements, several of which would certainly have caught his eye. One was for a workshop in Bishopsgate where the instrument-maker Richard Mears was selling 'All Sorts of fretted Instruments, especially Lutes and Viols, fitted with exact and perfect Stops'.[7] Another was for a new pamphlet, *Obedience Due to the Present King, Notwithstanding our Oaths to the Former.* This reviewed the tortuous debates in parliament and the country over whether James II (despite his declarations to the contrary) could be said to have 'abdicated' his divine right to the throne, thus leaving a 'vacancy' that could be filled. After searching desperately for any legal, historical or religious excuse that could be deployed to justify the taking a new oath of allegiance to William and Mary, the author concluded limply 'we have no liberty left us, either to *dispute* the King's [William's] *Title*, or deny him our *Duty*. Give unto *Caesar* the things that are *Caesars*'.[8] But this was an argument that suited James II and his Jacobite supporters just as well.

Almost every day there were personal stories too; usually about horses, dogs, valuables and jewellery that had been lost. Less often, there were reports of robberies by highwaymen on Putney Heath, or by footpads holding up the Oxford coach. Occasionally, there were calls for the capture of servants who had run off with stolen goods; like the French footman who, 'having a pale Face, lank black hair, and a long Nose with a Wart upon it', might be caught with fifty guineas taken from the fabulously wealthy Duchess of Mazarin, 'an extraordinary beauty and wit' and former mistress of Charles II.[9] But there were far more advertisements for the recovery of servants who had run away for reasons that were not disclosed. For a few, the chances of making an escape were good, especially if they could get away from London.[10] But for others, such as Ned, 'a Negro man of a Tawny Complexion, with Mosse Hair, middle stature' and 'a Down Cast Look', as 'he walks with his chin in his Bosom, having a piece of one of his Ears cut off, with a Brass Collar about his Neck', the chances of a new life were, at best, remote.[11] In every case, a guinea was the reward for the discovery and return of a lost dog, horse or slave.

For Claver, there was little consolation in the personal loss he was enduring. He bought himself a copy of the magnificent new folio edition of the King James Bible, a new binding of the Book of Common Prayer, a flute and a bassoon. He bought three guineas' worth of drugs for his patients, and he went to talk with Thoresby Hardres, the guardian who had known and cared for Grace for most of her life. He had no other friends or relatives to call upon in London, and no presents to buy and carry home. So, once the roof of the lesser house had been re-tiled, its windows, doors and walls repaired and new closets, dressers and shelves fitted for the sum of £25, there was no reason to extend his stay. In early April, before the celebration of the coronation of William and Mary at Westminster Abbey on the 11th, and the death of Judge Jeffreys from kidney failure a week later, he paid for his accommodation; three guineas for four weeks' stabling and lodging, and ten shillings for his apprentice-boy. He gave another five shillings to the servants at the inn and set out on the journey home to Wells.

Although the old chantry house was much quieter now, after a month's absence there were plenty of regular patients for Claver to see and a growing list of new ones who were calling for a visit. As his reputation grew, many of his new patients were now from wealthy families across the West Country. They would write to him on their own behalf or for a loved one, explaining their condition and asking him to visit as soon as possible, for he was most unlikely to diagnose, advise and prescribe until he had conducted at least one examination. Thereafter, his apprentice-boy could deliver letters, messages and medicines, and collect any payments due. But normally there was no alternative to Claver riding out, often for the best part of a day, including Sundays, in order to see his patients. He would then stay in their house or at an inn nearby and rest his horse before returning home the following day, often calling on friends and other patients as he returned.

In fair weather and in any season, he would expect to make two or three such journeys every week, often covering well over a hundred miles. So his horses needed to be fresh and sturdy, and regularly re-shod by the farrier John Joyce in order to tackle the 'long miles' of badly decayed stone roads, rough farm-tracks, marshy lanes and slippery river crossings for which the whole county was renowned. When the horses were tired or sick, John Joyce would also try to cure them, leaving Claver to hire a horse for a shilling every day.

Travelling with cases carefully packed with glass flasks for the analysis of urine, cloths and bandages, and a selection of surgical instruments and medicines according to what he knew or might anticipate about a patient's condition, Claver also needed to be fit and well himself in order to cope with the physical demands that travel, often in haste, would make. At times, he also needed to be brave. For although physicians were often mocked by satirists for their greed and indolence, and their indifference towards their patients' suffering,[12] they only had one notable defence against infection – the physician's cane. Having filled its perforated silver head with aromatic herbs and powders, Claver would hold this to his nose to mask any foul smells, 'bad air' or miasma, arising from his patients. And as miasma was believed to be the vehicle for the transmission of contagious diseases, so it was hoped that this simple practise would afford protection.

By May 1689, at the age of thirty, Claver had already made one of the longest journeys of his career when, in the previous autumn, he had visited the former Cavalier, Sir William Walrond at Bradfield House, a large manor in Uffculme, ten miles from Tiverton in Devon. There was nothing that Claver could do to save Sir William, a single man of forty-nine, and he was buried in the spring. Like everyone else across the West and much further afield, Claver would have known that the Walrond name had become associated with great shame in most people's minds. This was due to the heartless actions of Sir William's heir and penniless brother, Colonel Henry Walrond JP, who lived twenty miles away in the village of Isle Brewers, near Taunton. Here, in 1680, after a protracted pregnancy a poor woman of good character and the mother of five children had given birth to conjoined twins. Though joined at the chest, the girls had 'two female faces' and 'beautiful, fair and pleasant aspects'. They would 'suck together', being 'equally desirous of Nourishment', and they were 'equally sensible of their Grief and Pain'. But what was most astonishing to everyone was not the fact that they were born, for *lusus naturae* or 'freaks of nature' were well known. Much harder to understand was why they had not died soon after birth; rather, they seemed to thrive.[13]

At first, the family and villagers 'knew not what to think', but the girls were soon taken up into people's arms. They were baptised Priscilla and Aquila (after the early Christian missionaries) and became so popular that hundreds of people came every day from far away to see them and leave gifts. Clay plates were made as souvenirs, and a report of their birth was submitted to the Royal Society for publication. Their fame was further spread by the printing of sensational accounts of the 'Monstrous' and 'Prodigious' births, in which it was also noted that at that time a cow nearby had died while giving birth to conjoined calves.

For the vicar who had christened Priscilla and Aquila, they were a terrible portent of Monmouth's unnatural rebellion. But for Henry Walrond and his accomplice, Sir Edward Phelips of Montacute House, they were simply an opportunity to make money. Henry and Edward were already well known in Somerset for the pleasure they took in persecuting Quakers, but nobody expected them to steal the twins for exhibition. When the girls died soon after, large Lambeth Delft plates were made at Bristol depicting the kidnappers and their crime, in the hope that this would accelerate arrests. The pair were indeed caught and prosecuted for abduction but, being gentlemen, they managed to escape conviction.[14]

The Church was generally satisfied that each of the twins possessed a soul, but it was their survival over several years that most fascinated and confounded public and medical opinion. For Claver, this was more than a story about the need for faith when faced with the mysteries of Nature, which was God's creation. It was also a call to work hard; to put the powers of reasoning and discovery that God had bestowed on mankind to good use in 'doing well'. There was great suffering in the world for sure, to which, even if there were no cure, a physician should be able to provide relief or consolation. But for Claver, life was never intended to be 'a vale of tears'.

He had no time for the whole train of monkish virtues, from celibacy and fasting to solitude and self-denial. Rather, it seemed to him that a good and fulfilling life should, with proper application and God's blessing, be available to most people. Yet, too often, this was clearly not the case. Among every kind of family that he visited in every kind of place, it was not just the old and the infirm who were most at risk of death or crippling illnesses. On most occasions, especially when contagious diseases were rife, death took its toll without discrimination. After the loss of any of his patients Claver would expect to pray for their family and their soul. But his most difficult prayers, in the cathedral or at a bedside, were probably after the prospect of a good life had been dashed – as when a child was lost. The fact that this was something that he often had to deal with, and had lost his own infant, did not diminish the distress. He would need much more than medical knowledge and skills to comfort and cope with families like the Newcourts.

In June 1689, when Claver was invited by Jerrard and Mary Newcourt of Ivythorn Manor near Street to administer to Elizabeth their daughter, he probably feared the worst as they had already lost their only son. After several visits, it became clear that Elizabeth could not be saved, and she died in mid-October. Claver was now asked to conduct a dissection, which he duly did. This might have helped to bring the parents peace of mind, but it was not something that Claver would normally have undertaken.[15] Yet there were also times when Claver could claim success. Nearby, at Sharpham Park, the former home of the last abbot of Glastonbury, Henry Gould, a judge of the King's Bench, lived with Sarah, his wife, and their young children. Unlike the Newcourts, Claver succeeded in keeping the whole family in good health for years. This was despite the fact that across the Somerset moors, malaria was often rife.[16] He had similar success with another gentry family, at Shapwick, further east across the moors.

By the time Claver made his first visit to the Bull family at Shapwick, just before the death of Grace in January 1689, Henry Bull had already made his will. He was the grandson of William Bull, a wealthy linen draper and three-times mayor of Wells, who had purchased the manor-house and rectory at Shapwick in 1619. In 1660, at the age of twenty-nine, Henry had been elected one of the two MPs for

Wells by the twenty-five members of the city's corporation and, thereafter, several times for the tiny town of Milborne Port, where his brother-in-law John Hunt controlled the seat. More recently, in January 1689, he had been chosen to represent the constituency of Bridgwater where, at least in theory, the electorate consisted of about 400 municipal taxpayers living in the busy port.

Henry, with all his wealth and connections locally and nationally as an MP, barrister and sheriff of the county, was most unlikely to put his life in Claver's hands if he had any doubts about the doctor. He also had a 'dear and entirely beloved' wife, a 'dear and only' surviving son, and two 'beloved' daughters to consider. Elizabeth, the eldest, was 'infirme in body and not having the use and benefit of her speech', so she needed special care. But Henry was just as concerned about the future of Eleanor, his other daughter, who needed regular treatments and, he feared, was also highly vulnerable to the wrong kind of suitor. In his will, he urged that 'whenever she shall think of altering her condition by marryage' she should 'bee very careful in her choice of a sober honest and discreet man'; someone who was not inferior to her in any way in 'a business of soe great weight and moment'. His son, Henry, still under twenty-one, would inherit the estates plus goods worth over £5,000. But £3,000 was to be reserved for Eleanor's marriage portion and £100 for her wedding dress. It may be that Claver was able to identify the source of the squire's sickness from the sweet taste of his urine, and to provide a helpful treatment, for it was not until January 1692 that Henry reportedly died of diabetes. By then, Claver was firmly established as the family's doctor and he would remain so in the years ahead.[17]

With his reputation growing, there were other branches of the Bull family, including several around Wells and Frome, that now called upon Claver for advice. Squire Henry Bull had two sisters whose families were also in need of help. One, Jane, had married Mr Thomas White, a young barrister and the Recorder for Wells corporation. He had managed to get himself elected as one of the MPs for Wells alongside Henry, his brother-in-law, in 1660. Now widowed, from her house in the Liberty and her former home at Shapwick, Jane and her children called upon Claver for support.[18] By 1689, Henry's other sister, Elizabeth, had also lost her husband, Mr Edward Courte of Lillesdon in North Curry. During the course of the year, Claver would visit Elizabeth and her daughters over a dozen times at Shapwick and other places across the county.[19] A little further along the marshy roads of Sedgemoor, he also made trips to attend to the wife and children of Robert Steare, a future mayor of Bridgwater.[20]

With so many new patients, there was less time than in previous years for studying and playing music, or for experimenting with the mixing of new medicines. But Claver was still taking delivery of books that he had ordered when in Bath or London. These included two that reflected his fascination with mechanical innovations. One was a new edition of the polymath John Wilkins' *Mathematical Magick* (1680), examining the principles and possibilities of mechanical inventions such as flying machines and submarines. The other was John White's *Arts Treasury: or, a Profitable and Pleasing Invitation to the Lovers of Ingenuity* (1688); a compendium of household advice on topics such as 'the mystery of dying cloths' and 'Instructions for making Inks' (Claver liked to make his own), as well as 'many extraordinary experiments' on topics such as 'blowing up Houses and Vessels under Water'. He also collected *The Marrow of Historie,* an abridged edition of Sir Walter Raleigh's famous *History of the World* (1614), and a new edition of the study of Latin poetics, *Prosodia in Novam Formam Digesta* (Amsterdam, 1683) by the sixteenth-century Flemish physician, Hendrik de Smet – probably to help him compose an epitaph for a memorial to Grace. But that could wait.

The demand for Claver's services was also growing from old gentry and new wealthy families in the booming woollen manufacturing towns and villages around Shepton Mallet, Frome and Bruton. One of the first visits he made after Grace's death was to see his good friend George Long of Downside, the son of the late Sir Lislebone Long, knighted by Cromwell in 1656, and the owner of estates and coal mines in the region. George had a wife and several young children who all needed treatment, and as he had provided the coach to take Grace's body for burial at Manston, Claver looked after the family for years, always charging a little less than his standard fees.[21]

Inevitably, there were occasions when a visit from Claver did not reassure the patient. On Christmas Eve 1689, he was called to Evercreech, just south of Shepton Mallet, to administer to Mrs Agnes Albin. Her son, the Rev. Henry Albin, author of two published sermons, had been ejected from his ministry in 1660 due to his nonconformity, and was now preaching among the Presbyterian communities. As the family had medical recipes of their own, they may well have resorted to homespun remedies rather than taking professional advice, for Agnes lived until 1695. Yet, within three days of Claver's visit, she was sufficiently alarmed by his diagnosis to have made her will.[22]

A week earlier, on 17th December 1689, Claver had travelled to the manor-house at Witham Friary, a little village near Frome built around a former Carthusian priory, where a branch of the Wyndham family lived. It was his first visit, and one that he would not forget. Thomas Wyndham was known as a stout, short-tempered man. He had been a colonel of the Somerset militia and Tory MP for Wells since 1685. Like the majority of Tories, this meant that he was a reluctant supporter of the Glorious Revolution of 1689, but a strong supporter of the privileges of the Church of England; against Whig calls for greater religious toleration in society, and reforms of the Church that would enable moderate Dissenters to re-join. As a Tory he would also be more sympathetic to the interests of the English squirearchy, as opposed to what appeared to be the Whigs' enthusiasm for foreign Protestants and wars with France (to be paid for by the gentry). Yet Thomas Wyndham showed little interest in the party strife that raged at Westminster, and at the end of November 1689 parliament granted him leave of absence. He used this time to court a 'petite beauty', Elizabeth, the nineteen-year-old daughter and heiress of the very wealthy Henry Pollexfen, MP for Exeter and a former Attorney General. Unfortunately,

Elizabeth preferred another widower, Sir Frances Drake. Unable to cope, Thomas took a blunderbuss and (as one contemporary bluntly noted) 'upon some discontent [he] shott himself' on 16th December. He was buried two weeks later in his village, leaving a grown-up son and two daughters who, among other members of the family, were now in need of medication. Claver's visits must have helped, as in 1690 when Thomas Wyndham's son, Hopton, and his nephew, Sir Edward, were both taken ill, it was to Claver that they turned.[23]

A few weeks after Thomas Wyndham's shocking death, Claver often found himself braving the winter to attend to two branches of the Berkeley family; one at the village of Pylle, six miles south of Wells, and the other at their estates in Bruton, a 'very neate stone built town', thirteen miles south-east. Colonel Edward Berkeley of Pylle, JP and deputy lord lieutenant of the county, was a well-known figure. By 1690, he had been one of the two Tory MPs for Wells for many years, and in the general election of February he was jointly returned again; this time with Hopton, the son of Thomas Wyndham. However, it was as colonel of a victorious regiment of militia that had been stationed at Wells after Monmouth's defeat in 1685 that he was probably best known. After administering to the Colonel's cook-maid (and, later on, his groom), Claver was charged with prescribing for Elizabeth, his wife, and several of their children. Even so, by mid-February 1690, it was clear that an infection was running across both Berkeley families for, at Bruton, Lord and Lady Fitzhardinge were also now in need of treatment.

The head of the Bruton family, Sir Maurice Berkeley, 3rd viscount Fitzhardinge (a peer of the Irish House of Lords), had been one of the MPs for Wells since 1661 before passing the seat to his cousin Colonel Berkeley in 1679. Thereafter, since 1681 the viscount had represented Bath, and in 1689 he had been appointed lord lieutenant of the county. Being sixteen years older than his cousin, and married to Lady Anne, a step-daughter of the earl of Warwick, Sir Maurice was even better known. Having a house in Westminster and being a Fellow of the Royal Society since 1667, he was also something of a courtier. And he was also considerably wealthier than his cousin, having succeeded to the Irish viscountcy at the age of forty in 1668, and to an estate worth £1,500 a year.[24] Yet, by the spring of 1690, he must have known that his condition was not improving, for Claver was now visiting him at least twice a week. Then, suddenly, on 27th May, after visiting his patients at Bruton and at Pylle, all visits ceased.

8

DR MORRIS

As Claver lay in his bed at the old chantry house in the last days of May 1690, he would have known that his chances of survival were not poor – but that they were a long way short of certain. He had been fit and healthy, treating more patients and travelling more than he had ever done before. He was still young: just thirty-one. And he probably knew as much about infectious diseases, and how best to treat them, as almost anybody could. So he bought gloves to protect 'my workers', found a nurse to stay with him and, on Richard Cupper's recommendation, received visits from a Dr Staples. He would not tempt Providence. In keeping with good customs, he paid for bread to be given to the poor, and, with the help of the lawyer David Trym, he made his will.

By the time he had recovered sufficiently to resume his practice it was the end of June. His most recent patient, Viscount Fitzhardinge, had died two weeks earlier, leaving a wife and two married daughters – as well as a mistress and two natural sons who were to be given £500 apiece and land in Ireland.[1] Returning to work on Monday 30th June Claver made a single visit, to see Elizabeth, Colonel Berkeley's wife, at Pylle, who remained seriously ill. The next day he went to the cathedral to attend the funeral of his neighbour Dr Selleck, the eighty-year-old archdeacon of Bath.[2] And on Wednesday 2nd July he returned to administer again to Madam Berkeley. Whatever illness he had contracted at the end of May, just on the evidence of what had happened to his patients, he would have known that he had come quite close to death.

Over the summer, there were plenty of other patients to attend to. Among these were Peggy and Frideswide, two of Robert Creighton's daughters; Sarah Westley during her stay at Bath; Robert Steare and his son at Bridgwater; the eccentric archdeacon Edwyn Sandys in the marketplace; and Henry Bull's most eligible daughter, Eleanor, at Shapwick. Claver enjoyed getting back to work and receiving

DOI: 10.4324/9781003333654-9

the recognition and rewards that work could bring. In the previous year he had worked so hard that he had more than doubled his annual income from 'Advice and Prescriptions' to over £150, and his income was still growing. But this summer he also had a special mission; to oversee the installation of a monument to 'my poore wife' Grace.

The monument was the work of Nicholas Mitchell, a stonemason who lived close to Claver's houses in Crane Court and who had been working on the new St Paul's. His commission was to create a simple but classically-inspired hemicylindrical monument in white marble that could be fixed to the wall of the chancel of St Nicholas's Church at Manston. After securing its carriage to Dorset, Mitchell and several labourers were finally ready in September 'to set it upp'. Fixed with a cherub's head and decorated with flowers, it did not disappoint. The Latin inscription composed by Claver was relatively brief. It spoke simply of Grace being the daughter of a London merchant, of her modesty, kindness and loving nature, her grief at the death of her baby Mary, and her burial six months later at the age of twenty-six, due to exhaustion from a violent disease. But it gave no answer to the nagging question that Claver had embedded in the italic text and that lay at the heart of his continuing sense of loss. Why had God decided that their marriage would only last three years? No amount of elegant Latin could disguise the plain and simple reckoning: '*three years, only three years*'.[3]

In terms of his family life, Claver was not entirely on his own. He still visited Grace's relatives, Aunt Willoughby and Aunt Greene in Wiltshire, and he prescribed for them and their families once or twice each year. And at Manston, he had his mother and father, to whom he remained close. He had lost his brother William in 1675, and a sister, Ruth, in 1683. But now he faced the loss of his second sister, Hannah. She had died shortly after the death of her baby daughter, christened Ruth, in February 1689, leaving her husband Edward Goddard and a four-year-old son, William. As Claver did not trust his brother-in-law (who might well re-marry) to secure young William's future with a good inheritance, he finally decided, after fruitless negotiations, to take his complaint to the Court of Chancery in London. The omens were not good.

Claver was already conversant with the court. In 1687, four years after the death of his sister Ruth, he had taken her husband, Nicholas Shirley, to court in an effort to recover £100 that he believed was due to be returned to his parents as required by the terms of Ruth's marriage settlement. According to Claver, these terms specified that as Ruth was of 'a very weake constitution and might possibly dye in some short tyme after her marriage', £100 of her £500 marriage portion would be repaid if she died within three years. The agreement had been witnessed by John Pope, a physician living at Caundle Marsh, and as Ruth had died well before three years of marriage had elapsed, so Claver had repeatedly asked 'in a friendly manner' for Nicholas Shirley to pay up. Tired of Shirley's 'fraud and artifice', he had eventually taken him to court. In court, however, Shirley claimed to have no memory of any such agreement and had no copy of the marriage contract with which he had allegedly been entrusted. Unless someone could produce the document, he would not pay.[4] So Claver and his parents lost their case. Undaunted, in 1690 he was prepared to proceed again, this time with the more important case against another brother-in-law, Edward Goddard.

In many ways, Claver's complaint against Edward Goddard was very similar to the action he had taken against Nicholas Shirley, who was now a co-defendant. According to Claver, at the time of his second sister's marriage in September 1684, Goddard and Shirley had accepted that, as soon as the marriage had been consummated, Goddard would use Hannah's £500 marriage portion to purchase property as an inheritance for her and any children she might bear. Since then, Hannah had died, leaving a son, William, and Claver had moved to Wells, leaving the Articles of Agreement in the custody of his mother. According to Claver, instead of honouring the Agreement, Goddard and Shirley 'by some undue ways and means and false pretences and insinuations got the Articles out of the custody' of his mother, in order to hide or destroy the document. Moreover, although Goddard was now pretending that he had provided an inheritance for William when he reached the age of twenty-one, in truth, he had only 'lately purchased a small mill of little value and poor repair'. Claver also pointed out that there was an additional clause in the Agreement that meant, in effect, if William died before he came of age, £250 of the marriage portion would need to be re-paid in compensation.

In their joint statement as co-defendants, 'the confederates' as Claver called them, Goddard and Shirley denied taking or destroying any marriage contract and insisted that a good fulling-mill with an adjoining house and meadow had already been purchased for William's future inheritance. The mill was at Sturminster Newton, a few miles from Goddard's home at Stock Gaylard. Since Hannah was still living when it was bought, and she and her father, William Morris, had both accepted that its purchase met the terms of the marriage settlement, there was no case to answer. So the defendants asked the court to order the complainant to pay all costs and charges arising from the action.[5]

Whatever the merits of Claver's complaints against his brothers-in-law, his relationship with them was now poisoned. In his mind, he had fought to uphold the integrity of his sisters' marriage settlements and, most importantly, to protect the interests of his motherless young nephew. Claver's mother and father would have agreed with him: this was surely the right and proper thing to do. But others might believe these disputes exposed Claver as an opportunist, doggedly pursuing his own interest regardless of the damage that would be done. Even if his cause were just, he would know that, win or lose, the Shirleys and the Goddards would not forgive him for the embarrassment of a public hearing. Fortunately, in one respect it hardly mattered, for his reputation as a physician was now so strong, it would not be seriously damaged by these disputes with Dorset relatives.

By the autumn of 1690, Claver was administering to one of the richest men in Somerset, the twenty-three-year-old Sir Edward Wyndham. He had first met Sir Edward at the beginning of the year when he had been called to Witham Friary after the suicide of Sir Edward's lovelorn uncle Thomas. He must have made a good impression at that time, for Sir Edward could afford any physician in London or wherever else he kept a house. He had inherited his father's baronetcy and main estate at Orchard Wyndham on the edge of Exmoor when he was sixteen. In 1685, at the age of eighteen, and with an income of £4,000 a year, it was not difficult to persuade a sufficient number of the 140 taxpaying voters of Ilchester, the run-down old capital of Somerset, to elect him as their MP, even though he was still well under age. Since then, he had been re-elected twice at Ilchester, and married Katherine, the eighteen-year-old daughter of Sir Leveson-Gower, with a dowry of £6,000. He also had a son and had been appointed a JP and deputy lord lieutenant of the county.[6] Fortunately, after his intensive treatment over a period of ten days, plus a bill for twelve guineas, Sir Edward was not disappointed. This meant that Claver was immediately recommended to treat Sir Edward's cousin, Hopton Wyndham, who, with the help of Viscount Weymouth, had just succeeded his father as an MP for Wells. He also treated the viscount's wife, Lady Frances Finch, who had come to Wells with her husband from their great house on the Thynne family's Longleat estates in Wiltshire.[7]

Many of these renowned families owed a large part of their fortunes to the dissolution of the monasteries in the sixteenth century, when they had enriched themselves with lands that had been confiscated from the church. It was a plunder that was not forgotten by the common people, and it was often recited in rhymes like 'Wyndham and Horner, Berkeley and Thynne/When the monks went out, they came in'. Serving such rich and powerful families gave a tremendous boost to Claver's reputation, and it also greatly increased his ability to build his practice on his own terms. The great majority of his patients were not exceptionally rich or privileged, and certainly not titled, though they needed to be able to afford his fees. But, as long as he could collect large sums and expenses from the wealthiest of families, he could afford to reduce the fees he charged elsewhere. And this is what he did. His fees were never strictly set, so he could afford to charge ten shillings to the citizens of Wells, five shillings or less to patients who were poor or had a child, and sometimes make no charge at all.

Among the richest families, there were people who would pay the highest fees even though they were probably living quite beyond their means. And in determining his fee, Claver could take this into account. Eleanor Berkeley, the daughter of Maurice, viscount Fitzhardinge, who had died in June, was a case in point. In the 1670s, she had married Hugh Montgomery, earl of Mount Alexander near Cromer in County Down. He was widely reckoned to be a kind and talented young man but, due to the burden of debts accrued by his predecessors, Hugh's wealth was in serious decline. It was said that his English wife had brought his Lordship very little money and would run him much further into debt. According to the Presbyterian minister at Cromer, she was also 'highlie Episcopall' and keen to return to England. This, together with the civil wars in Ireland over the accession of King William, had brought her back to Bruton.[8] She only paid a guinea for her treatments, but Claver more than made up for this in what he charged elsewhere.

Frances Brooke, formerly Lady Whitmore, was not the wealthiest of Claver's clients, but she was certainly the most celebrated woman that he treated and she paid the highest fees. In the 1660s, along with Margaret, her younger sister, she had been one of the famous 'Windsor Beauties' who had been painted by Sir Peter Lely for Charles II's court. Margaret had married the poet and lawyer Sir John Denham, 'an old limping man' thirty years her senior, before becoming the mistress of James, duke of York. Frances had married Sir Thomas Whitmore MP and had tried to live more modestly. Margaret's conduct as the most conspicuous mistress of the future king was hardly shocking at the time. But when Margaret suddenly died at the age of twenty, having been, so she claimed, poisoned by a cup of hot chocolate that her husband had prepared at the bidding of the duchess of York, a great scandal was unleashed. Immortalised by poets such as Andrew Marvell, the scandal endured for years, even though a post mortem evidently found no trace of the poison alleged by Margaret and others, including Samuel Pepys. And it may well have prompted another poet, John Dryden, to offer comfort to the Whitmores by writing an epitaph that extolled the virtues of Lady Frances. Whatever comfort Claver may have been able to provide, he could not save Frances' life; though he must have spent weeks working on her treatments, for he charged her sixteen guineas.

Before Christmas 1690, he made a final payment of £8 to Nan White in settlement of money that Grace had borrowed, and in January he made a trip to see the festivities and shops of Bristol fair. His purchases were modest: a set of brass scales and weights, a walking cane, a brush for removing lice from clothes, six ox tongues and three pounds of anchovies, plus '6 dozen of Conical-Bottles of my owne invention' for his medicines. Two months later, he made a far more important purchase, paying £11 for a dappled horse from Mr Nicholls at Wrington. He also made a gift of £10 to New Inn Hall at Oxford in preparation for what would be one of the most significant events of his career; his graduation as a *Medicinae Doctor* (MD).

By becoming a 'Doctor of Physic', Claver would attain the highest qualification open to his profession. He would then expect to be addressed as 'Dr Morris' and be treated with the respect and deference due to a gentleman of high professional standing. It was a prospect that he was never likely to resist. He was well qualified for an MD and, with the help of 25 guineas from his parents, he could afford the catalogue of costs. These started with over £56 in fees, and another gift of £10 to New Inn Hall, where he also paid for a meal of 'Scotch-collops, a hash, & 2 dishes of Fowle'. As evidence of his merit, the university required Claver to deliver three public lectures to be read at 1 and 3 o'clock on Monday 29th June 1691, and at 8 o'clock on the following morning.[9] The subject of his talks would be the works of the Ancient Greek philosopher and physician Galen, whose abundant writings still dominated medical education in England.

After his last lecture on the Tuesday, Claver gave three shillings to the congregation and prepared for the official presentation of his degree on Monday 6th July. This was held at Convocation House, the wooden-panelled hall at the heart of the university where parliament had met during outbreaks of plague. Claver hired a scarlet gown (which he adorned with velvet) and bought a doctor's cap as dress for the occasion. He also had additional expenses due to his desire to graduate as a 'Grand Compounder'. This meant that he would be entitled to have a personal procession, led by a trumpeter from Convocation House to New Inn Hall and back again, while the bells of the University Church of St Mary the Virgin were rung in celebration. For Claver, paying 5 guineas to the Faculty for gloves, 16 shillings to the servants, and 11 guineas for wine, sweets and biscuits during the procession was a bargain. By the time he left Oxford on 16th July he had spent over £100 on obtaining his MD. But he was earning over £150 a year as a physician, and the 'MD' would undoubtedly raise his reputation and his income.

The following day he arrived in London where he stayed for several weeks at his newly refurbished house in Crane Court. It was an exceptionally hot summer, parliament was not sitting, and the city was relatively quiet. During his shopping trips, he exchanged his sword for a chased-steel one worth £2, and bought a blunderbuss for a little less. As always on these trips, he bought new clothes, two hats, three wigs (a long one, a campaign one and short one) and books and maps of England, France and Europe. He also visited a jeweller to commission 'a pair of Buttons with my Wife's Hair set in Gold' and 'a Locquet with her Hair and my Daughters', to take home.[10]

9

TWO BISHOPS

Across Europe in 1691, the War of the Grand Alliance against Louis XIV's France showed no sign of abating. The decisive victory of William's Protestant army over James II's largely Catholic forces at the Battle of Aughrim on 12th July 1691 – a year after the Battle of the Boyne – provided some relief in England. There was now hope that after the devastation and loss in Ireland of 100,000 lives from battle, disease and famine, this part of the European conflagration might be over. But in England, with good reason, fears of economic and military exhaustion, and of French invasion and defeat, were growing. Across the kingdom, the religious divisions that William's accession had opened up were as great as they had been since the Civil Wars.

In Somerset, there was an additional source of anxiety that had been simmering for at least two years. On 1st August 1689, Thomas Ken, the bishop of Bath and Wells, 'exceedingly loved in his diocese',[1] had been suspended, along with the archbishop of Canterbury and seven other bishops, for refusing to take the Oath of Allegiance to William and Mary. Having sworn allegiance to James II, Ken's conscience would not allow him to break that holy vow, either for political convenience or out of self-interest. Yet, unlike most of the other bishops and 400 clergy who had also been suspended for failure to take the Oath, Ken dearly wanted to maintain the unity of the Church of England. He had no time for any of the secret Jacobite intrigues of several of his peers, and he urged them to avoid any actions that could inflame divisions. As neither William nor parliament would accept the idea of a 'Regency' (though the concept of a 'vacancy' had no legal, historical or religious precedent), it was inevitable that, along with all the other public office-holders, MPs and clergy who would not take the Oath, the moderate Ken would have to be ejected. At Easter 1691, at the age of fifty-three, his term of office as bishop of Bath and Wells was finally brought to an official end.

DOI: 10.4324/9781003333654-10

Though long anticipated, for the people of Wells the news was shocking. Ken had been appointed in January 1685 as a reward for his service, first as chaplain to Princess Mary at the Hague (where his job had been to protect young Mary's Anglicanism from her husband's boorish Calvinism), and later as chaplain to the royal fleet on a diplomatic mission to Tangier. 'Little Ken', as Charles II fondly called him, had also been a royal chaplain, and although he had occasionally upset the king by speaking plainly and refusing to accommodate Nell Gwyn at his home in Winchester, Charles always forgave him. A few days after his appointment, it was Ken who was called to the bedside of the king, famously banishing another mistress from the scene and calling for the presence of the queen as Charles lay dying.

At the onset of Monmouth's rebellion, Ken was still in London, sitting in the House of Lords, and it was a sure sign of the new king's trust that he was chosen by James II to prepare Monmouth for execution and to accompany him to the scaffold in July 1685. By the time Ken could get to Wells the rebellion was over, though the Bloody Assize was looming. Finding that Judge Jeffreys and the royal court were deaf to his entreaties against the carnage, Ken focused on comforting the prisoners: 'I visited them day and night, and I thank God I supplied them with the necessaries myself as far as I could, and encouraged others to do the same.'[2] James II did not object, and the people of Somerset would not forget.

James respected Ken and thought him 'the best preacher among the Protestants'. But when James re-issued a Declaration of Indulgence in April 1688 – suspending the penal laws against Catholic and Protestant nonconformity to the Church of England, ending the Anglican monopoly of office-holding, and allowing private worship in homes and chapels – a confrontation was inevitable. Having signed a printed petition challenging the king's right to overrule the penal laws, seven bishops (including Ken) were prosecuted for seditious libel. After a brief spell in the Tower, and amidst much public joy, on 30th June 1688 they were acquitted. Invitations were now sent (though not by Ken) for William of Orange to intervene to protect the kingdom from its rightful but Catholic king.

Knowing that he would not take any oath of allegiance to William and Mary that would break the oath that he had sworn to James, Ken left Westminster and the House of Lords for the last time in February 1689 and returned to Wells. Throughout the diocese, he was well known for his generosity, his humility and the simple celibacy of his life, as well as his love of music and poetry, lute-playing and hymn-writing. He had also published a few notable works, including *Directions for Prayer* (1685), which was addressed 'To the poor Inhabitants within the Diocess of Bath and Wells, [by] Thomas their Unworthy Bishop'. Here, as ever, his messages were clear and kind: 'Be sure to teach your Children with all the sweetness and gentleness you can, lest if you should be severe, or should over-task them, Religion should seem to them rather a Burden than a Blessing.'[3]

Above all, Ken was revered for his sympathy towards the poor and needy. It was said that 'On Sundays, he would have twelve poor men and women, to dine with him in his hall [in the palace]; always endeavouring, whilst he fed their bodies, to comfort their spirits by some cheerful discourse'.[4] Seeing so much poverty, he had tried to set up a workhouse in Wells 'to rescue the idle from vicious practice[s] and conversation; and the industrious from the oppression of the tradesmen; who, to use his own expression, did grind the face of the poor, growing rich by their labour, and making them a very scanty allowance for their work'.[5] In this he failed, as he could not find sufficient sponsors. Having given so much of his wealth away, after the sale of all his possessions (aside from books) he had just £700 when he left Wells in 1691. He gave this money to his old Oxford friend Lord Weymouth, who provided him with an apartment at Longleat House and an annuity of £80.[6]

Ken's celibacy and sympathies were not to everybody's liking, especially as they appeared almost saintly by comparison with so many of his peers. But when his successor Dr Richard Kidder, formerly dean of Peterborough, arrived at the bishop's palace for his installation in September 1691, it was not long before almost everyone was yearning for the return of the humble and cheerful 'Little Ken'.

Richard Kidder was born in 1634 into an impoverished family, the eighth of nine children, at East Grinstead, Sussex. After attending Cambridge and being ordained in 1658, he was deprived of his living in 1662 when, on account of his Presbyterian leanings, he refused to accept the Act of Uniformity. After conforming to the Thirty-nine Articles and the new Book of Common Prayer, in 1664 he was appointed rector of Rayne, a 'factious' parish in Essex where he lost all three of his young children to disease. Later, while rector of St Martin's Outwich, a poor parish in London, he lost three more children to smallpox. By the time that William and Mary were crowned in 1689, he had declined several lucrative preferments on the grounds of his own ill health. But he was a highly-respected scholar of Hebrew and the Old Testament, and after his promotion to a royal chaplaincy and the deanery of Peterborough, he was consecrated bishop of Bath and Wells on 30th August 1691.

The artist Mary Beale portrayed the new bishop as having a serious-but-pleasant countenance with a straight nose and dark-brown eyes. But she could not capture either his 'hearty desire to do good' or his dogmatic and self-righteous manner, which verged on paranoia. As Kidder well knew, succeeding to any bishopric that was 'void by deprivation' would not be easy. But, being the 'supplanter' of the much-loved Ken was bound to lead to 'great trouble and envy' if poorly handled. It was for this reason that the promotion had already been declined by the queen's first choice, the archdeacon of Colchester.[7] Though well intentioned, Kidder had neither the authority nor the charm to accomplish all the reforms that he envisaged – unless he could count upon the support of the cathedral's dean and chapter, its governing body.

Under the terms of the royal charter granted by Elizabeth in 1591, the governance of the cathedral was quite clear. The chapter was to consist of 49 canons or prebendaries, each entitled to the income of a particular 'prebend' or estate, ranging enormously in value (by 1691) from a few pounds to the 'Golden Prebend' of Wiveliscombe worth about £500 a year. The chapter was to be presided over by a royally-appointed dean, and supported by five senior and three lesser dignitaries. Between six and eight of all the canons were required to spend at least three months each year in residence at Wells, for which a 'canonical house' in the Liberty would be provided. The dean was not required to be in residence, but several of his fellow dignitaries were. Together, these residential canons were to be known as 'the dean and chapter' and they were to be wholly responsible for the 'rule, management and government' of the church.[8]

To facilitate the pre-Reformation chapter's work, in the thirteenth century a grand octagonal chamber, the Chapter House, with large windows on all sides and one central column supporting a vast fan-vaulted ceiling, had been built on the north side of the cathedral. Placed above the Undercroft, where vestments and other treasures were secured, the chamber could be reached by climbing a famous flight of steps that would later also lead to the enclosed footbridge of the Chain Gate and the Vicars' Close. Around the walls of the chamber there were 50 stalls with decorated canopies for all the prebends (plus one for the bishop), and this is where they met.[9]

During the seventeenth century, the prebends could still all meet by taking their seats in the grand old Chapter House. But as most prebends now lived in towns and villages across the diocese, and the business of the chapter was (in accordance with the Elizabethan charter) now almost entirely in the hands of the residential canons, there was little need for everyone to convene. To conduct the cathedral's business, it was simply more convenient for the residential canons and their assistants, men like William Westley, to meet for a few hours every week in warmer rooms of the cathedral, or even in their private homes.

Ken had not tried to break into, or break up, this close-knit ruling group in which the members, for all their differences, had at least one common interest – to preserve their wealth. In addition to whatever income each canon received from their private estates, their prebendaries, and any other offices and benefices they held, they shared an interest in maintaining the value of the allowances they received for residence, and the dividends from the rents, fees and other revenues paid into the chapter's common fund. From their allowances, each residential dignitary could expect to receive, on average, a supplementary income of at least £120 per year, and a non-dignitary resident just £10 less. In theory, up to £20 of this income was dependent upon meeting the requirements for periods of residence, during which time the canons were expected to maintain church attendance, offer hospitality and provide relief to the poor. The interpretation of these rules could sometimes lead to disagreements, but self-interest ensured that most disputes were swiftly settled.[10]

Kidder did not meet the dean and chapter in September 1691, because after his installation he returned immediately to London in order to take the Oath of Allegiance and his seat in the House of Lords. However, his correspondence with the chapter over the winter would have convinced him, by the time he returned to Wells with his wife and daughters in May 1692, that there would be severe challenges ahead. Essentially, he would have to deal with the five principal office-holders (quinque personae) of the dean and chapter:

- The dean, Dr Ralph Bathurst, was head of the chapter with overall responsibility for its work and the discipline of its members. After his ordination in 1644, he had studied medicine, becoming a physician and obtaining his MD at Oxford in 1654. Generous and hospitable, he became a founder of the Royal Society in 1663, president of Trinity College Oxford in 1664, and dean of Bath and Wells in 1670. Dedicated to his work at Trinity, after 1690 he was rarely, if ever, at the Deanery, and was in his seventies when Kidder was appointed. He was going deaf and blind.
- The precentor, Dr Robert Creighton, was in charge of music, choral services and the liturgy. The son of a former bishop of Bath and Wells, Creighton had been a professor of Greek at Cambridge and a chaplain to Charles II. He was a canon of Wells and the rector of Ashbrittle in Somerset before his appointment as precentor in 1674. Living with his children at the Tower House near Vicars' Close, he was only fifty-four in 1691. Strong-minded and ambitious, he was renowned for his preaching and writings against all Protestant Dissenters from the Church of England and their sympathisers.
- The chancellor, Andrew Paschall was responsible for schools, the reading of lessons and sermons. A graduate of Cambridge University, he became a preacher there in 1658. He was appointed rector of Chedzoy in 1662, from where he witnessed the battle of Sedgemoor. Though a staunch Anglican, he was inexperienced, having only been appointed chancellor in 1689 and a prebend in the following year. In 1691, he was still waiting to become a canon in residence.
- The treasurer, Dr Richard Busby, was responsible for the cathedral's valuables and the provision of candles and any other materials needed for church services. He had been appointed headmaster of Westminster School in 1639, and treasurer of Bath and Wells in 1660. At the time of Kidder's installation, he was eighty-five and had lost the ability to preach. As a 'residential canon', he had a house in the Liberty but he was deeply committed to his work at Westminster and, aside from one week in the 1670s, he was never in residence at Wells.
- The archdeacon of Wells, Edwyn Sandys was responsible for the cure of souls in most of the 383 parishes of the diocese. He was also the rector of two parishes near Yeovil, a prebend of the cathedral, and had been appointed archdeacon in 1683 at the age of thirty-nine. A new house had been built for him in the marketplace, but after Kidder's installation (the legitimacy of which he questioned), he preferred to live at his rectory in Yeovilton.

From Kidder's point of view, the prospect of obtaining any kind of help from these men must have seemed remote. Under the Elizabethan charter, the dean was not required to be in residence, though he had a good home at the deanery on the cathedral green if he chose to use it. In his absence, the sixty-six-year-old subdean Dr William Levinz MD, professor of Greek and president of St John's College, Oxford, and the rector of a parish there, had been Bathurst's deputy since 1679. Although he was a prebend of Bath and Wells and possessed a canon's house, by 1691 he was no more 'in residence' than his dear old friend, the dean. Nor was there any better prospect of Kidder finding support from among the two other lesser dignitaries – the archdeacons of Bath and Taunton – or from the great majority of minor office-holders, as their positions were almost entirely dependent upon the patronage of their seniors.

In addition to those dignitaries whose canonical houses came with their high offices, there were usually one or two other houses in the Liberty that could be granted to other canons. As these homes were largely in the gift of the dean and chapter, it was most unlikely that they would be given to anyone who championed the new bishop's cause. The most recent grants, in 1689 and 1690, had been to Thomas Brickenden and Thomas Cheyney after they had made the customary contributions to the chapter funds and paid over £7 to each of the other seven residential canons. Brickenden, a fellow of New College, Oxford, and vicar of Corton Denham and the churchless parsonage of Sock Dennis, had been personally recommended by James II on account of his 'piety, loyalty and sufferings'. Dr Cheyney, a fellow of St Mary's College, Winchester, and rector of Bawdrip near Bridgwater, had been bishop Ken's most favoured chaplain.[11]

Although Kidder 'often repented' of his decision to accept what he soon regarded as the poisoned chalice of the bishopric of Bath and Wells, on his return from London in May 1692 he was determined to do his duty 'in the place which the providence of God had set me'. Yet, as soon as he arrived in Wells he suffered such a 'violent fit of the gowt' he feared he was 'in danger of my lyfe'. Dr Morris was now the most distinguished physician in the city, so he was swiftly called upon, and on the 23rd and 24th of May, he made his first visits to the palace.[12]

As a proud new doctor of Medicine, Claver was keen to show his extensive skill in diagnosis and prescription. Treating the most holy (and possibly the most self-important) individual in the county, he would also want to make a good personal impression. For gout, there were plenty of homespun remedies to consider, such as a local one that required the making of an ointment based upon the boiling of eight pounds of unsalted butter with a pottle of black snails, a dozen unwashed herbs, a porringer of cow dung and fresh horse dung, all mixed with frankincense and nutmeg before being strained and clarified for application. There were also innumerable highly-recommended professional cures and palliatives for all kinds of gout. Claver would rule out treatments that were based upon animal ingredients, such as the warming of a patient's feet in the paunch of a freshly slaughtered ox; or the placing of a suet of goat, spiced with saffron, on a patient's knees; or the rubbing of legs with oil made from the cooking of a fox, preferably of middle age; or the drinking of a cordial concocted from the boiled bodies of the fattest snakes (though, in May, this recipe was well in season). And he probably ruled out the 'infallible remedy' of the archdeacon of London; the daily consumption of a pint of fresh urine from a cow.

As there appeared to be no need for chemical preparations, it was more likely that Claver would have relied on traditional herbal remedies. So he probably made a poultice based upon the leaves of arsmart or water-pepper that had been roasted between two tiles, or made a soup from tansy roots.[13] Whatever the treatment, it concluded happily. Within a week, on Trinity Sunday, Kidder was well enough to conduct his first ordinations as a bishop, though he was still so weak he needed to be carried on a couch to do this in his private chapel at the palace. From Claver's point of view, this first encounter with the bishop had been a great success.

10

WICKED PRACTICES

On 28th June 1692, Claver was called back to the bishop's palace. In the preceding weeks, he would have heard from friends and patients that the new bishop had set out his stall, and that he was not a man of compromise. So much bad blood would now be spilt between Kidder and his flock, it was inevitable that Claver would be drawn into the disputes and even find himself at the centre of an especially bitter quarrel. It had all started innocuously enough. Like any other bishop, Kidder had a fundamental duty to support the faith and welfare of the parishioners and clergy of his diocese, and to ensure that church property, finances and records were well kept. So he had every right to inspect any part of his domain and to order the correction of whatever failures or abuses he might find. Ken had done this in his first year of office, setting out the questions he would ask the churchwardens of each parish, and considering their written answers before travelling to conduct his 'visitation'. In his Articles of Visitation and Enquiry,[1] Ken listed seven headings under which he would ask questions, addressing his 'Concerns' about:

1. The Churches, with their ornaments and furniture.
   Is the church in good repair, with a stone font, decent carpet, pulpit and communion table with white linen-cloth and chalice? Is there an authorised version of the Bible and a copy of the Book of Common Prayer? Are the parish registers well kept?
2. The Churchyard, with the houses, glebes and tithes belonging to the church.
   Are the church lands, parsonage and other properties in good condition, and church rates collected?
3. The Ministers.
   How often are the ministers and curates (their deputies) in residence? Do they preach each Sunday, adhere strictly to the authorised services, and wear white surplices? Do they baptise infants properly, and promptly if at risk of death?

DOI: 10.4324/9781003333654-11

Do they teach the catechism to parish children, and visit sick persons? Do they always publish marriage banns, and are they 'of sober life and conversation'?

4. The Parishioners.
   Is there any adultery, incest, drunkenness or blasphemy among the parishioners, or 'filthy talkers, or sowers of sedition or faction among their neighbours'? Do any parishioners cohabit or refuse to pay church-rates?
5. The Parish Clerks and Sextons.
   Is the clerk at least twenty-one, and does he lead an honest life and do his duty: keeping the church clean, attending services and 'ringing the bell before divine service, and when any person is passing out of this life'?
6. The Schoolmasters, Schools, Physicians, Chirurgeons, and Midwives.
   Are there any unlicensed schools, and does anyone practise physic, surgery or midwifery without a licence?
7. The Churchwardens and Sidesmen.
   Are the churchwardens properly appointed and doing their duties: maintaining the church, providing fine bread and wine for communion, collecting church rates and keeping honest accounts?

Such concerns about the Church were a commonplace throughout the country. Like the society it supported, the Church was a hierarchy with great power, wealth and privilege at the top, followed by various groups among the 'middling orders', and terminating with what, from the vantage of the higher ranks, appeared to be great swathes of endemic poverty, ignorance and sin at the common base. All kinds of inequality and patriarchal authority sustained this structure. The Church taught that inequality and patriarchy were simply and irrevocably ordained by God when He gave Adam authority over Eve and their children. And if there were any doubt about what happened when this divinely ordered hierarchy was usurped, it seemed that the evidence of life under Cromwell's dreadful republic (when the world was turned upside-down, with no bishops and no king) was more than a sufficient answer.

Nobody doubted that Ken was deeply concerned about the poverty and ignorance he witnessed, and the deplorable condition of many of the lower clergy and their churches. And Kidder was no less sincere in his concerns – especially in saving souls. But his religious convictions and his character led him in quite a different direction to his predecessor. After recovering from his gout in June, he chose the ancient cloth-working and mining town of Axbridge, near Cheddar on the Mendips, for his first visitation, and soon published his demands.

In the first part of *The Charge of Richard, Lord Bishop of Bath and Wells, to the Clergy of his Diocese, at his Primary Visitation begun at Axebridge, June 2, 1692*, Kidder demanded that his clergy and their families set blameless examples of a Christian life: 'There is no man so vile as a profane Minister of Religion; He is of all the most abject, the most self-condemned, and destitute of plea, and liable to the heavyest plagues of another life.' He told the clergy of their duty to teach by weekly preaching and catechising, and to administer the sacraments, especially the Lord's Supper which was 'notoriously neglected'. And he reminded them that they should visit the sick, take care of the poor, promote peace among their flocks, and 'overcome them with kindness if it be possible'.[2]

The second part of his address was shorter. It included exhortations that greater care should be taken to ensure that anyone recommended for ordination or confirmation was entirely worthy; that funeral sermons should not overpraise the dead (thereby giving a false sense of security to the living); and that Protestant Dissenters from the Church of England should be treated with humanity. There was, however, an uncompromising message here. First, Kidder reminded his clergy of their oath to keep residence among their flock, and that only their bishop could relieve them of this obligation. Secondly, he spoke of the great scandal of clergy holding several offices or livings (plurality) and often, unlike Jesus, 'choosing to live in a better aire, or among more fashionable persons'. Thirdly, he warned the clergy that he would suspend them if they conducted marriages without banns or licenses, or without the consent of parents. For it was his view that ministers who conducted clandestine marriages for money, were worse than common highwaymen in the pain and damage that they caused. The profanity of these ministers' offences, he insisted, was so much greater than the highwaymen's, they were actually more deserving of execution.[3]

As soon as he had completed this visitation, 'which was no small labour', Kidder returned to the palace, believing that 'my gowt was then so violent that there was little hope of my lyfe'.[4] Once more, Claver was called upon for help. Two weeks later, on 14th July, and thanking God, Kidder was sufficiently recovered to proceed with the battle that had been looming ever since his consecration: a visitation of the cathedral church itself, and of the college of its vicars choral. With his life in so much danger, he could not afford to neglect his duty, come what may.

The dean and chapter answered their bishop's 'Articles of Enquiry', in Latin and under oath. But their answers were so evasive, in Kidder's view, he was forced to press them for fuller and clearer responses in a second round. To questions about their periods of residence, they replied 'that they do their duties personally or by their lawful Curates'. When asked about their provision of hospitality during their residences, they replied that they were all in residence except Dr Busby (treasurer) and Dr Levinz (subdean), though they later admitted that Mr Sandys (archdeacon) was also absent. When pushed, they would only name two prebends who had not fulfilled their preaching obligations, and they would not name a single choral vicar who had neglected any of his duties, though they reported that a few of the vicars were 'sometimes absent from Divine Service'. In answer to a question about the condition of the canonical houses, the first response had been that they were in good repair, but a second answer conceded that two had been 'thrown down and ruined'.[5]

The battle with the vicars choral was no less bruising. Like the dean and chapter, the vicars had been granted a new royal charter in 1591, establishing between fourteen and twenty of them as a self-governing community, entitled to raise income from holding and leasing properties as a corporation. Under the charter, the vicars were expected to live next to the cathedral in the Medieval Vicars' Close, a terraced street that had been built especially for them with its forty-two small houses, a chapel, shared facilities and dining hall. For all their duties – singing, attending services and deputising for the canons – they would each receive at least £3 a year. And although they were to be managed by the dean and chapter, they were also accountable to the bishop, who was their official 'visitor'.

When Kidder met the vicars (there were only ten of them in 1692), he found their responses to his questions no better than those of the dean and chapter. Among the college's abuses, it was clear that the vicars were not all diligently attending services (though they said they were), or closing the gates of their Close at night. Above all, and against the strict requirements of their charter, it was clear that most of the vicars were living in places around the town, and that they had leased their designated houses in the Close for personal gain.[6]

Determined to put an end to these 'wicked practices [that] cry to Heaven for Vengeance', Kidder attended a meeting of the chapter in late August. After much debate, it was agreed that a calendar recording each canon's residence should be publicly displayed, and that each canon would swear to the veracity of any allowances he claimed. Similarly, for the vicars choral, a record would be kept of every absence from divine service, and those who failed to provide a satisfactory reason for non-attendance would be punished. Both sides had compromised, or so they thought. But, as everybody knew, it would probably take years of new episcopal appointments before the bishop could count on a significant number of the chapter for support. Until then, he could expect 'very ill usage from these men', though he told himself 'could I have winked at their evil practices, I might have lived at peace with them' – a most unlikely prospect, given his low-church sympathies and inexhaustible self-righteousness.[7]

Believing that the bishop had 'attempted some encroachment upon their privileges', the chapter were now more determined 'to make a noble stand'.[8] They also suspected that this assault upon the customs and corruptions of the Church of England was not motivated by a love and respect for its faith and institutions, but by a sinister attempt to undermine it from within. An obvious example was that, just before his 'agreement' with the chapter on 24th August 1692, Kidder had ordained a 'phanatic' former Dissenting preacher, John Gardiner, and appointed him as rector of the parish of Hinton St George, the Poulett family seat. The fact that this had been done with the approval of the Archbishop of Canterbury only made the matter worse. For it could be seen as proof not only of Kidder's conniving methods, but also of a nationwide conspiracy designed to advance the Dissenters' cause against the true interests of the Church.[9] There was now, therefore, every prospect of a running battle between Kidder and the chapter; one that would be fought throughout the city and the diocese for years to come.

11

A TURNING POINT

For Claver, the battle between the bishop and the dean and chapter placed him in a quandary: most of the senior clergy were his patients. Of the five high dignitaries, the dean and the treasurer were invariably absent. But the precentor, archdeacon and chancellor were patients. So too were the residential canons Henry Dutton, Thomas Brickenden and Thomas Cheyney, as well as William Westley and Richard Healy, the legal officer. So, by 1692 Claver was the family doctor for almost every working member of the dean and chapter. It would not be easy to maintain their trust if his intimate knowledge of their private lives (of the kind that only doctors and nurses knew) should ever be leaked to an adversary such as the bishop. On the other hand, in terms of Claver's reputation and career, the opportunity to administer to the bishop himself was no small honour.

The fact that Kidder was far more sympathetic than Claver to the plight of Protestant Dissenters need not have been a problem, at least as far as Claver was concerned. He was used to administering to patients with beliefs and opinions that were not his own. Among his most conspicuous friends were the Strodes of Downside near Shepton Mallet, a family with exceptionally strong republican and Presbyterian roots. In 1684, squire Edward Strode had taken the dean and chapter to court over rights to the rectory of Long Sutton, leading to a furious reaction by the chapter over Dissenters who 'foment designs' against the church and state, and 'despise her lawes and professe themselves her enemies'. The clerics were so incensed, they passed a new ruling: no leases would be given or renewed to anyone who would not take the Anglican communion.[1] Nor was this the height of Strode's offence.

At the start of the rebellion in 1685, 'Ned' Strode had made a great show of giving 100 guineas to the duke of Monmouth, and even sheltered him for a night after his defeat at Sedgemoor. Though pardoned, Ned was regularly summoned

DOI: 10.4324/9781003333654-12

and fined at the quarter sessions for refusing to take the Oaths of Allegiance and Supremacy; making a third refusal in the summer of 1692. That was when Ned, as guardian of the young minor, John, 4th baron of Poulett, invited Kidder to appoint a 'phanatic' Dissenter to the vicarage of Hinton St George. Although Ned's eldest surviving son had already left England in search of greater religious freedom, Claver would continue to treat Ned's other children; including his eldest daughter, Elizabeth, who would exceed even her father in her support for the Dissenters' cause.[2]

If the doctor–patient relationship of Claver and Kidder were to flounder, it would be due more to differences of character than to matters of belief. Kidder was twenty-five years older and no lover of the West Country, or of his home in Wells. This did not endear him to most of the people he was meant to guide and serve. But while Claver was just as strong-minded and determined as the bishop, he was far more sociable and pleasure-seeking – enjoying music, dancing, dining, drinking, shopping, making and spending money, plays and fairs, and probably other indulgences that the puritanical Kidder would consider human weaknesses or worse. Both men could be proud and overbearing, but whereas Claver found it easy to make and keep his friends, Kidder struggled. The bishop had working relationships with a small number of like-minded clergy and scholars with whom he corresponded, and he excelled in preaching – though his sermons were not to everybody's taste.[3] But for most people, Claver was simply much the better company, and a very loyal friend.

Although Claver still missed his wife and daughter, at the age of thirty-three he did not intend to lead a solitary life. On hearing that Princess Anne and her husband, Prince George of Denmark, had come to Bath for their health and relaxation, he followed them to the city in the summer of 1692. It was a bad time for the country as a whole. An Anglo-Dutch fleet had managed to prevent a French invasion in late May, but in June, the strongest fortress in the Spanish Netherlands, Namur, had fallen to the French with the loss of 4,000 men. Then, on 3rd August 1692, 8,000 of the English, Scottish, Dutch and German troops that made up the allied army under William's command, were killed or wounded as they were badly defeated at the battle of Steenkirk. At home, fears of plots and conspiracies abounded, and the Jacobite intrigues at Court had also created a rift between Queen Mary and her half-sister Anne.

Princess Anne also had problems of her own. At the age of twenty-nine, she had already suffered two miscarriages, and recently buried her seventh new-born baby. But she was a popular princess and a major boost for Bath's rising reputation as a health spa. So the mayor and aldermen made a great fuss of her, waiting on her daily – much to the annoyance of Queen Mary.[4] Claver would enjoy the excitement of the princess's visit, and especially the music, dancing and promenading that were making the little city such a fashionable resort. At Bath, he would meet new faces and prescribe for notable people such as the poet Matthew Prior and the diplomat Sir Philip Meadows, whose daughter required treatment.

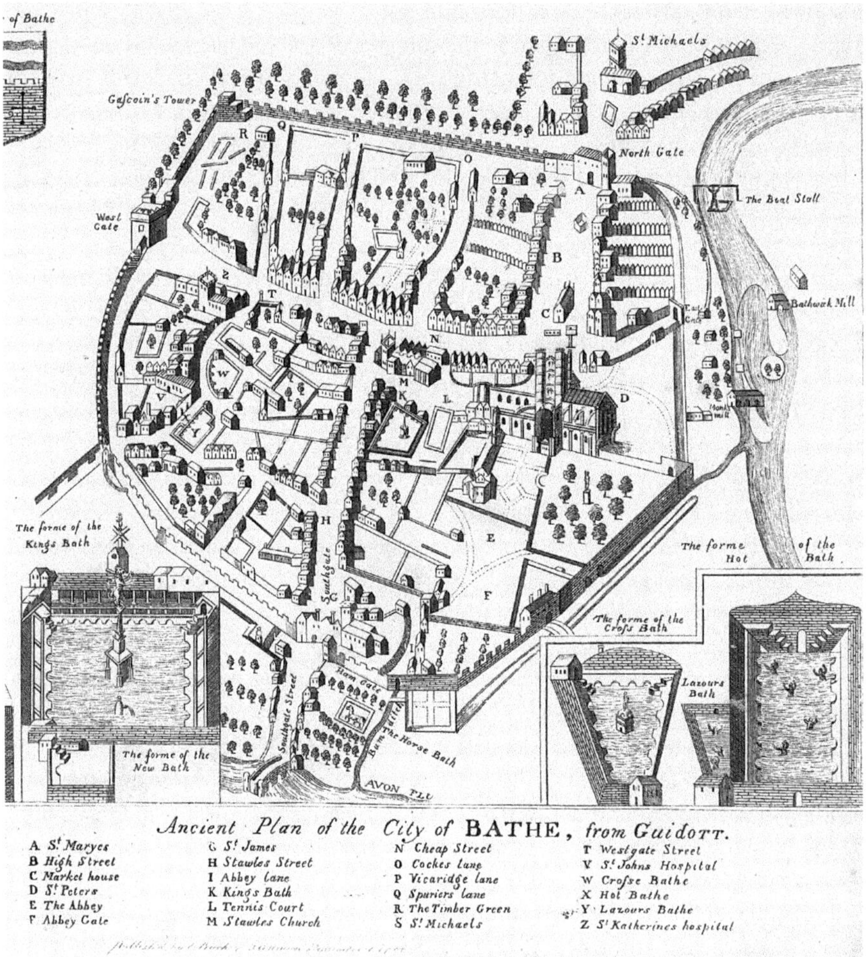

FIGURE 7 A Map of Bath, c.1706
This *Ancient Plan of the City of Bathe*, first published in 1706, is based on Thomas Guidott's *Thermis Britannicis* (1691)

As well as providing visitors with an endless supply of brackish mineral water for drinking or for bathing in its thermal baths, the city offered every other kind of service both for those visitors who were genuinely sick or for those just fashionably concerned about their health. No less important, in its summer-to-autumn season, the place was becoming one of the nation's favourite haunts 'for gaming and for whoring', and it was already becoming the most famous place to find a wife or husband. As one wit wrote, the city was truly 'a Valley of Pleasure, yet a sink of Iniquity'.[5] So this was not the kind of city that its bishop, Kidder, would enjoy. But, for Claver and other members of society who had time and money to spend on their health and leisure, it was becoming irresistible.

In Wells, Claver was managing to maintain his physician's income of £140 a year, of which £40 was accounted for in food and household items. There were also other necessary expenses, such as rent and taxes, the stabling of his horses, and the wages for his live-in servants, Sarah Mogg and Richard Prince, who each earned £3 a year. More costly were his shopping trips, and especially his expensive tastes in wigs, clothes, boots and shoes. But as he enjoyed an additional income from the lease of his fields at Felton and his properties in London, he was not in debt or needing to reign in his spending. He was, however, planning to move house.

In many ways, the move to a medieval gabled manor-house with grounds and garden ('De Salis', 17 The Liberty) was quite straightforward. It was only a hundred yards across the road from his present home in the Liberty. The manor-house was a little cheaper; just £10 a year, instead of the £13 that he had been paying Mrs Evans for the chantry house. And this simple move from where he had lived with Grace, and briefly with their baby daughter, might also help to lift his spirits. Yet the move also signalled something else: Claver's deepening association with members of the dean and chapter, and especially the precentor Robert Creighton.

Unlike the privately-owned old chantry house, the gabled manor was owned by the dean and chapter and normally leased to lay people, rather than to clergy. But at the end of its lease in 1689, when Ken was bishop, the dean and chapter had decided to reserve the manor exclusively for use as a canon's residence. The change of plan was probably due to Creighton, who wanted to provide his son with a home in the Liberty that would later enable him to become a residential canon. But even by 1693, his son was still a student at Cambridge and would not graduate with his MA until 1699. So, having secured the change of use and a new lease for the gabled manor, it made good sense for Creighton to sub-let it to Claver, his friend and doctor.[6] It was a handy arrangement as Creighton's widowed sister, Catherine Poulett, still lived in the house next door. And it also signalled very clearly that the city's most eminent physician was now well within the precentor's extraordinary sphere of influence.

By the time Claver had moved into the manor-house at the end of May 1693, Bishop Kidder had returned to Wells. He had left for London in the previous autumn to attend the re-opening of parliament in November and to deliver a sermon before the king and queen at Whitehall on the following day. Though no-one had been killed on 5th November 1605, Kidder declaimed, as expected, that 'never was there a greater instance of Barbarity and Unmercifulness' than the Gunpowder Plot, and in the evening a mob duly burnt an effigy of the pope to complete the annual ritual.[7] After staying in London for the winter, he delivered another sermon to the king and queen on 12th March. On this occasion his subject was Christ's Sermon on the Mount, in which he found that Christ's command to 'Love thine enemies' was excellent advice for Christians, but not practised by the Jews who were always 'Enemies to those of another Nation and Religion'.[8]

However well he was received in London, in Wells there was more than enough antagonism to keep Kidder busy throughout the summer. This time he could claim a measure of success. After a confrontation with Creighton over the ordination of another 'fanatical' former Dissenter, Nicholas Mallarhé, Creighton was finally persuaded to submit, though Cheyney continued to object. And when the seventy-year-old canon Henry Dutton died in May, Kidder eventually managed to get the chancellor, Andrew Paschall, a canon's residence. Yet, set against these little victories, all the fundamental objections to Kidder's rule remained. After accepting an invitation to dine with the mayor of Bridgwater, he felt that he was 'horribly abused and represented as a phanatic for dining with those they [his enemies] reputed' to be Dissenters.[9] So, while completing and preparing his long *Commentary on the Five Books of Moses* (1694) for publication, he was probably relieved to return to London for the re-opening of parliament in November 1693, though the public mood was no better there.

The facts were simple. By the end of 1693, the French Mediterranean fleet had destroyed or captured over ninety Dutch and English merchant vessels in a convoy off the coast of Portugal. King William's army had been routed at Landen, with 12,000 killed and 2,000 captured by the French. The strain of the war on public finances had led to the introduction of an annual 20 per cent tax on the value of all land and public salaries. And, due to a combination of the crimes of forgery and coin-clipping (for which hundreds of people were being hanged) and the melting of silver for sale abroad, the value of the country's currency was being seriously debased. Even the value of the humble farthing was falling, due to the corrosion of the tin from which most of the small coins were made. Wells was not the only place where there had been a 'great disturbance' and punishment of the poor, 'occasioned by the bakers, shopkeepers and others refusing of the farthings within the city'.[10]

In the summer of 1693 Claver settled into his new home with very little expense or bother, and he managed to stay on good terms with Kidder. He had been invited to the palace to administer to a guest, and twice in June to prescribe for the younger of the bishop's two surviving children, his six-year-old daughter, Ann.[11] But the summer also marked a turning point in Claver's life when he was called upon to treat a new patient at Ditcheat, a small village lying between Shepton Mallet and Bruton. Edmund Dawe, lord of the grand new manor-house and patron of the equally imposing church, had called on Claver to treat the husband of his eldest daughter, Elizabeth.

Robert Jeanes, a young gentleman from a respectable local family, had married Elizabeth Dawe at St Mary le Bone, London, in June 1689, when he was twenty-six. He lived in London, serving the barristers of the Middle Temple, but his family owned pockets of land in several parishes adjoining Ditcheat. Treating him at the manor-house in the summer of 1693 Claver got to know Edmund Dawe, his wife Anne and their sons and daughters very well; especially their married daughter, Elizabeth Jeanes, for whom he also administered in the autumn and regarded as a beauty. A year later, when he returned to the manor to treat Edmund Dawe, his son-in-law Robert Jeanes was dangerously sick and ready to make his will. On 24th November 1694, at the age of thirty-one, he died, leaving no children but a 'deare tender loveing and affectionate wife', the beautiful Elizabeth, a widow at the age of twenty-six.[12]

12

SECRET MARRIAGE & COURTSHIP

In the summer of 1694, Bishop Kidder returned to Wells and resumed his running battles with the dean and chapter. He fought them over the charging of administrative fees, only reaching an agreement a day before the dispute was due to be tried at the assize in Wells.[1] He fought them over the appointment of a vicar for the town of Chard, and over the suspension of the vicar of St Mary Magdalen, Taunton, who had toasted the health of the exiled James II at a tavern in the town. But of the 'great many troubles' that beset Kidder in 1694, the most intractable concerned his relationship with the archdeacon of Wells, Edwyn Sandys, who could not even bring himself to acknowledge Kidder as the rightful bishop.

Sandys was well known as a difficult man, though he was a dear friend of Bishop Ken and also, according to Kidder, a defiant Jacobite. However much the archdeacon failed to do his duties, Kidder found it impossible to shame him; and having decided to suspend him, Kidder was humiliated when this punishment was overturned. So, residing at his rectory near Yeovil, Archdeacon Sandys and his wife and friends continued to snub the bishop with impunity, much to Kidder's fury.[2] Nor was this the least of his troubles, for in 1694 Kidder was embarking upon what would become another insidious dispute. It was no less painful for having little to do with politics or religion. This was a falling-out with Claver Morris, and it was personal.

From Claver's point of view, his most pressing problem in 1694 was not the loss of Kidder as a patient, though the bishop still suffered badly from attacks of gout. Rather, it concerned his best friend and apothecary-partner Richard Cupper, and the reputation for good medical practices that they had built together. Cupper's son, Richard, a bachelor, was twenty-six and working as an apothecary with his father from their shop in the marketplace.[3] Here and around the county there were rumours that he had become a father and had secretly been married. The former

DOI: 10.4324/9781003333654-13

charge would cast a shadow over his reputation, but it would not be ruinous: it was not uncommon for young men to father children outside marriage. The mother always carried by far the greater burden of shame and punishment, even if the father contributed to the infant's upkeep, either willingly or through the sanctions of the parish. But, with no prospect of divorce, the consequences of a clandestine marriage were potentially calamitous, depending on the circumstances and the character of the couple.

To quash the rumours and clear his name, Richard Cupper took his case to the consistory court. Presided over by the bishop's chancellor, the court ruled over a wide range of ecclesiastical and civil matters, from church discipline and taxes to defamation and matrimonial affairs, with a clerk recording the evidence of each witness called. Often held in the comfort of a local inn, a tricky case might run for months and lead to revelations that went far beyond the original concern. So Richard Cupper and his father must have hoped that the proceedings would be short and sweet, though their hopes were dashed as soon as Mrs Aylesbury, wife of the Reverend William Aylesbury, began her labyrinthine tale.[4]

According to Mrs Aylesbury, she was in bed with her husband at their home in Cloford, a tiny village between Frome and Shepton Mallet, when, late one Sunday night in April 1694, she heard a knocking at the door. The couple outside said they wanted to be married, so she invited them inside. They introduced themselves as Richard Cupper, an apothecary from Wells, and Frances Lovett, 'in a Gentile dress', and they said they were desperate to get married because Richard was going to Ireland the following day. So the four of them went upstairs, and there 'by ye moon light' they were duly married with the use of a mourning-ring that Mrs Aylesbury happened to be wearing. On returning downstairs the couple demanded a marriage certificate, and when Richard Cupper tried to read it by the light of the fire, he dislodged his periwig revealing the 'redish colour' of his hair. He begged the Aylesburys to keep the marriage secret until midsummer and paid them five shillings.

Under examination Mrs Aylesbury had much more to say, about a later visit from Richard Cupper's angry father, and how three young men had forced her and her husband to sign a recantation of the event; though, being illiterate, she could not say what any of the writing meant. It also emerged from dozens of other witnesses that Frances had previously given birth to a baby that had died; that she had pretended to be married to Richard once before; that Richard was terrified his father would find out; and that his father had allegedly beaten Frances with a stick.[5] Being 'old Mr Cuppers particular friend', Claver was called upon to intercede, but he could only discover that the younger Cupper 'did utterly disavow' the match. Several credible witnesses, such as the midwife Margaret Symes, confirmed the accounts that Frances, her mother (Gladys) and her sister (Elizabeth) gave, but in graphic statements other witnesses claimed the whole affair was just a ruse by the Lovetts 'designed to get money' from the Cuppers. So Frances' reputation was called into question: sometimes quite bluntly, as when Ann Davis told how Frances

Lovett and one Edward Webb (a convicted thief) had been such 'busy bedfellows' they might well have had a child; and sometimes with a little more discretion, as when a local innkeeper noted that 'since she came to woman's estate, Frances had but an ordinary reputation in the city'.

Unfortunately for Frances, the reputation of the Reverend William Aylesbury did not help her cause. The son of a clergyman who had been a Clubman in the Civil Wars, William had not been to university but had been declared a 'Literate' in 1667 and thus fit for ordination as a priest. In 1682 he had been expelled from his rectory due to his legendary drinking and swearing and, since then, had scratched a living from marrying couples without banns or licenses, though he had been disciplined for this misconduct too.[6] He lived in such poverty with his wife, allegedly a 'drunken sottish woman', that when Elizabeth Lovett visited them to verify her sister's marriage, she left a shilling for the relief of their poor children. To make matters worse, it was claimed by several witnesses, including Richard A'Court, one of young Richard Cupper's friends, that the Aylesburys had been mistaken about the groom's identity, and had laughed when they learned of their mistake and signed the recantation that was now before the court. It was even alleged that Mrs Aylesbury had said that it was not Richard Cupper but a man with 'dark or black haire' and 'a face like an owle' who had married Frances on that moonlit night.

Far from becoming clearer as more witnesses gave evidence, the case became ever more bewildering the longer it ran. The marriage certificate had disappeared, and even simple facts, such as the time of the marriage service, could not be determined easily, because the Aylesburys were too poor to own a clock. Even so, it was the solemn duty of ecclesiastical courts to uphold the sanctity of marriage, however strange or regrettable the circumstances of the match might be. Indeed Bishop Kidder had demanded that every marriage should be treated as a 'sacred institution', as close to a sacrament as it was possible to get.[7] So Richard Cupper and his father (who had just become a member of the Mercers' Company) had taken a mighty gamble in bringing their appeal to court. The presiding judge, William Hughes, was one of Claver's closest friends, but this could not be expected to count for much, if anything at all. For Hughes answered solely to the bishop, and he could not afford to infuriate his patron by annulling any marriage without good cause. When Hughes announced that he had found in Cupper's favour, it was probably the fairest judgement he could reach.[8]

A few years later, Cupper's reputation was called into question once again, when a bastardy order was issued against him in the courts. Then, acting on new information, just before the quarter sessions ended, the judges changed their minds. They rescinded their order and, in its place, issued a new one against Richard A'Court, the 'gentleman' who had supported Cupper's claim that his identity had been mistaken by the Aylesburys. A'Court had a history of bad behaviour, and another bastardy order would be issued against him in the years to come.[9] Whatever the truth about Richard Cupper's conduct and his relationship with Frances, however, after the court ruling in 1694, he was a single man again.

Claver was single too and was also about to become embroiled in a dispute, though in 1694 he had no time or mind for courting. By the time he arrived at London in January 1695, another harsh winter had set in. The Thames had frozen over for five weeks and an outbreak of smallpox had 'increased exceedingly, and was very mortal'.[10] On 28th December it had taken the life of Queen Mary, at just thirty-two. A devout supporter of the Church of England, she had been married to William at the age of fifteen, and he and most of the nation were now in mourning. Only Jacobites, like those in Bristol, would not forgive her for usurping the throne of her Catholic father James II.[11] Earlier, in October, Claver's old friend and neighbour, the widow Catherine Poulett, had also died, having taken out a new forty-year lease from the dean and chapter on her house, which she left with the rest of her estate entirely to her brother, the precentor Robert Creighton.[12] And at Manston in November, Claver had overseen the laying of a black marble tombstone, carried by sea and land from London, to commemorate the life of Grace. He was still calling her 'my wife' when he paid for the restoration of her portrait in his house.

The snow and ice that lay on London's streets did not deter Claver from his love of shopping. In addition to new wine glasses and every other kind of glass (a lamp glass, a mustard glass, a weather glass, a diamond-cut bottle) which he bought on almost every trip, on this occasion it was pictures that especially took his interest: a still life, a crucifixion scene, a portrait of Cardinal Wolsey, a landscape, and a depiction of Salomé dancing. There were more practical items too: pocket scales and weights, buckles for shoes, buttons for sleeves, and much more. He attended to his investments and properties in the city which were looked after by a Mr Heber, and even saw a few new patients while he was in town. These included the wealthy Mrs Dorothy Cocks of Gloucester, Mrs Arnold of London, and Robert Dillon, 6th earl of Roscommon, who paid £6 for treatments. No trip would be complete without the purchase of new books, so he was pleased to return to Wells with a copy of Richard Sault's 'A New Treatise of the Algebra'. This was newly published as a fifty-page annex to William Leybourn's *Pleasure with Profit: Consisting of Recreations of Diverse Kinds* (1694); a great compendium of mathematical puzzles that appealed to his insatiable curiosity about scientific experiments and inventions.

When Queen Mary's lavish funeral was held with music by Henry Purcell at Westminster Abbey on 5th March, Claver was in Ditcheat attending to its lord of the manor, Edmund Dawe. It was always a sad but very important part of his duty to make an honest assessment of a patient's chances of recovery so that they could make whatever preparations they felt were necessary in the event of death, not least with regard to their estate. Edmund's condition was clearly serious for, despite Claver's administrations, on 20th March he made his will and he was dead within a month. At Ditcheat, his funeral was an important moment marking the accession of Edmond, the eldest son, as head of the family and village. Edmond's brothers, Thomas and Charles, were well provided for, with estates of their own, and his sisters, Elizabeth and Anne, were each bequeathed a generous sum. Anne was still only twenty, so a marriage portion of £1,000 was reserved for her, or £40 a year. As for Elizabeth, she had already inherited land from her late husband Robert Jeanes, but her father still left her all his property nearby in West Bradley and Baltonsborough which he valued at £1,200.[13] It was a very generous gift to a widowed daughter, and it meant that she could afford to remain a widow.

During May and June, Claver spent days riding back and forth to Bath, mainly looking after the Wyndhams as well as several members of the family's Dunraven branch from Wales. At the end of June, the Wyndhams also lost the head of their family when the exceptionally wealthy Sir Edward died quite suddenly at the age of twenty-eight.[14] Although Claver had not been treating Sir Edward before he died, this was someone whose death would have had a considerable impact. And during the summer, he was also feeling the heat of a very personal dispute with Kidder and his family, with whom he had corresponded but not treated for two years.

According to the bishop, the dispute began quite simply with his teenage daughter Susanna developing a crush on Claver and becoming 'so very sick upon it' he was fearful for her life. Flattered by the attention, Claver might have exploited the situation, encouraging Susanna to promise marriage to him, against the wishes of her parents. According to Kidder, Claver told Susanna in a letter (echoing the views of the former vicar of Chelsea, Adam Littleton) you have 'as much right to a disposall of yourself as anyone. Human kind have all equall priviledges and may justly take them'. This was credible, though Kidder also maintained that Claver now cast base reflections upon Susanna's parents. Later, after the bishop had most reluctantly given his consent and offered a marriage settlement, Kidder claimed that Claver 'endeavoured to skrew him higher', demanding that any settlement for Susanna should be equal to that for her younger sister, Ann. This was something that Kidder 'absolutely refused' on the grounds that 'he would not oblige himselfe to do as much for a child that chose for herselfe, as for one that in that affair [of marriage] should be governed by him [the father]'. Claver's response was, allegedly, that although he had turned down much higher sums from other families, with regard to marrying Susanna 'he would take her without one farthing'.

After a meeting at which Kidder explained to Claver that Susanna had changed her mind and no longer loved him due to his 'frequent invectives against her parents', his alleged lies and his attempt to bribe her with £100 to procure an ecclesiastical promotion for a friend, any semblance of cordiality came to an end. Blaming Kidder's 'fraud and wickedness' for Susanna's change of feelings, Claver now allegedly spoke only of revenge and spitefully disparaged Susanna's reputation among potential suitors. Though Kidder believed himself (as in all of his disputes) to be 'perfectly innocent as to the whole matter', and willing to 'take the Holy Sacrament upon it', the picture that he painted of Claver was quite out of character, for although the doctor was strong minded and determined, he had no spite. Such behaviour was neither in his heart nor interest. But he was not blameless.

Susanna, aged sixteen, was fully entitled to change her mind; not least legally, as there was no pre-marriage contract. Above all, she needed to protect her reputation. Yet her needs seemed to have had little bearing on the behaviour of the protagonists. Having involved their friends, with Kidder even consulting the dean of St Paul's cathedral in the course of the dispute, both men were now so publicly humiliated by this unseemly scandal, they were unwilling to back down. For Kidder, there was the additional anxiety of his health. In February he had made his will, treating his daughters *almost* equitably, except that Susanna would have her £1,500 marriage portion reduced by £500 if she chose a husband of whom her mother disapproved. Yet, Kidder could never quite decide if the 'perfidious' Dr Morris had ever been truly committed to the match, or had just toyed with it; maybe to gather information as a member of Creighton's circle or simply to cause distress. What made Kidder question Claver's sincerity was that it was reliably reported that, 'as for the business of Marriage', Claver was 'at ease, and well content with a single life'.[15]

By the autumn of 1695, Kidder was so deeply embroiled in other disputes he was in no mood to devote any more time to resolving his family's affairs. To advance his own authority, he was quite prepared to use his extensive powers of patronage to promote people that he liked, as in his appointment of the German-born scholar Dr Anthony Horneck to a prebendary in 1694. But he was also determined to correct what he considered to be the profound abuses of the cathedral's governance. So, he struck at the heart of the dean and chapter's power – their ability to decide who was 'elected' to a canonical residence, thereby joining what he regarded as their deceitful and self-serving club.

Following the death of Dr Busby, the eighty-eight-year-old treasurer of the cathedral and headmaster of Westminster, the dean and chapter had swiftly and furtively arranged for the election (by themselves) of Thomas Lessey to the only available canonical house in Wells. This would thwart the ability of the newly appointed treasurer Ralph Barker, the former archbishop of Canterbury's chaplain and Bishop Kidder's choice, to take up residence. Unlike Barker, Thomas Lessey was not even one of the cathedral's dignitaries, but he was married to a daughter of another residential canon, Thomas Brickenden, whose election Kidder also questioned.

Trawling through every twist and turn in the dean and chapter's Elizabethan charter, Kidder found plenty of Latin evidence to support his contention that the dean and chapter, and their unofficial leader Dr Creighton, were corrupt. In Kidder's view, they broke their oaths and statutes in order 'to get their kindred and relations into the Church preferment'. From the dean and chapter's point of view, they were merely following precedent and acting upon Elizabeth's sincere intention that 'to preserve their own peace and happiness', they were 'invested with a power of Admitting Members whom they Judged to be agreeable to them, and of excluding such as they Judged to be disagreeable'. When they ignored Kidder's declaration that Lessey's election to a canonical house was null and void, Kidder escalated the case by calling upon the most distinguished lawyer in the land for help. However, the Lord Keeper of the Great Seal, John Somers, was not impressed and 'advised him to be quiet'.[16]

Undaunted by this setback, Kidder knew that he had a better opportunity to defeat his enemies as it was three years since his first Visitation of the cathedral, so another one was due. The key issues were the same as in 1692, but for all his interrogations of the dean and chapter, and his hair-splitting objections to their answers and evasions, he could not land a decisive blow. This time, despite meetings in the great Chapter House throughout August and September, and even a personal visit to Dr Creighton's home, there was not even the semblance of an agreement. Rather, the animosity deepened as Kidder felt that 'Men may trifle with their Bishop, but God will not be mocked'.[17]

Although Claver would have heard from Creighton all about the dean and chapter's side of these proceedings, he was not personally involved. He had plenty of existing patients to look after, as well as new ones such as Lady Katherine Lowther, the sister of Viscount Weymouth, who was taking the waters at Bath. Alongside all the gossip about Claver, the bishop's daughter, young Richard Cupper and the dean and chapter, the city had more important matters to consider when an outbreak of smallpox took several lives during October 1695.[18] Fortunately, it was almost over by the time that parliamentary elections were held on 7th November, and it was no surprise to anyone when Colonel Edward Berkeley of Pylle and the wealthy lawyer William Coward of Wells were re-elected.

At the elections, having the support of a well-known West Country family was an important factor in ensuring a candidate's success. While there were major differences between the Whigs and Tories, the most pressing issue for all candidates was who exactly had the right to vote among the various masters, burgesses and freemen of the city. This meant that the electorate might be anywhere between 25 (the mayor and 24 members of the corporation) and 150 (the freemen of the city), depending on who did the counting. What was not in doubt, however, was that all of the city's women as well as the great majority of its men were not entitled to vote. This did not mean they had no public voice, and sometimes they demanded to be heard. Parliamentary elections were usually regarded as raucous occasions in which canny voters could often solicit drinks and treats from candidates, and the political outcomes were often of little local significance other than to the standing and influence of rival families. But anything that touched upon religious beliefs and animosities was quite another matter. A week after the parliamentary elections, almost everyone would have had a strong opinion about the prospect of a Quaker coming to preach in centre of the city.

13

WILLIAM PENN

On Friday, 15th November 1695, it was not just any member of the Religious Society of Friends who wanted a public platform in a backwater of the town. William Penn, founder of Pennsylvania and the most famous living Quaker, had arrived to preach. He had been touring towns and villages across the West Country for weeks; teaching and holding meetings with Friends, largely without incident. But preaching under licence at a private house or barn in a Mendip village like Chew Magna, or at a place like Street that had a notable Quaker community, or even at the town hall of a busy port like Bridgwater with its traditions of Protestant Dissent, was quite a different matter from 'Declaring the Truth' in the very heart of Wells. Here, in the marketplace, Penn would be a stone's throw from the greatest church (a 'steeple-house' to Friends) in the diocese, and within spitting distance of its highest-ranking clergy (the 'hireling priests'). There was no need to hold a meeting of local Friends for, as far as anyone could tell, there had never been a single Quaker living in the city. Excluding Bristol, there were only a few hundred Quakers in the county overall, most living in manufacturing towns where Dissent was strong, like Taunton, Bruton and Shepton Mallet. So, the whole point of the visit was, in Penn's own words, 'to break up that Dark Citty of wells, where a meeting never was to that day, a Bishops sea[t]'.[1]

The original plan was to hold a meeting at a private house in the marketplace. To obtain permission, one of Penn's colleagues, John Whiting, a Quaker from Long Sutton near Bristol, went to see the bishop. It was fortunate that Kidder was at home, as he would normally have been in London for the opening of parliament had he been in better health. After asking a couple of questions, Kidder gave the meeting his assent, and a grant was issued by the clerk of the marketplace, which was under the bishop's jurisdiction. In the event, however, after being pressured by public opinion and the supporters of Colonel Berkeley MP, the market clerk refused to let the Quakers into the designated house.[2]

DOI: 10.4324/9781003333654-14

Under the Toleration Act of 1689, entitled 'An Act for Exempting their Majestyes Protestant Subjects dissenting from the Church of England from the Penalties of certain Lawes', most Protestant groups were allowed to hold their own religious services if they first obtained licences for their meeting places. This new freedom of worship did not alter the fact that Dissenters, like Catholics and Jews, were still banned from holding public offices and attending English universities. But as a growing number of moderate Dissenters began to circumvent the law by what most Anglicans regarded as the despicable practice of 'occasional conformity' (taking Anglican communion just once a year to qualify for office-holding), it seemed to most Anglicans that their monopoly on municipal and national power (including membership of parliament) was under threat. Across the country, under a Calvinist king about 1200 licenses for meeting houses had been issued within the first year of the Act. Many new chapels were now being built and licensed. This appeared to offer further proof that Protestant Dissent was on the rise at the expense of the established Church.

So, Berkeley's followers would not be alone in wondering why a city such as Wells would want to provide a bunch of extremists, such as Quakers, with any kind of platform for their seemingly heretical and subversive views; let alone at a place that was so close to the cathedral and the entrance to the bishop's palace. For most Anglicans, and even moderate Dissenters, there were so many dreadful things about the Quakers' customs – their refusal to wear wigs and doff their hats, to swear oaths (even of Allegiance), to bear arms and pay church taxes, and their socially disrespectful habits of speech (saying 'thee' and 'thou', instead of 'you'), their sitting on tubs, and the conical hats of their women – it was difficult to know which were the most objectionable.[3] To most Anglicans, the Quakers' perverse belief in the equality of all men (though Quakers in Pennsylvania kept slaves), their hostility to all clergy and religious ceremony, and the strangeness of their ways of worship were no less shocking. Yet, the Friends were so used to abuse and persecution wherever they went, they were most unlikely to give up.

Having been refused a house, they managed to persuade the landlord of the Crown, where they were lodging, to give them a large room with a balcony from which they could address the crowd gathering in the marketplace below. And to ensure the legality of the assembly, John Whiting went to the palace to request a new certificate. Again, Kidder received him in a friendly manner and said that he would grant a new certificate if it were needed. So, from the balcony of the grand old coaching inn, Penn preached to a crowd of two or three thousand until, just as he was 'committing the People to god', a constable arrived and scrambled over a table to reach the balcony with a warrant for his arrest. The constable permitted Penn to bring his preaching to a close, before leading him across the marketplace to meet the mayor.

The warrant was issued by the mayor, Matthew Baron, and a former mayor, William Salmon, who the Friends regarded as 'a peevish old Presbyterian'. It demanded that Penn be arrested to answer the charge of having 'riotously and unlawfully assembled' to preach 'in a House not licensed according to the Act of Parliament'.[4] Yet, after a brief examination by the mayors and the attorney William Hughes, Penn was soon released. Working his way through the rejoicing crowds, he returned to the balcony to tell his listeners to depart, and then went for dinner at the Crown. A little later, having been invited by William and Sarah Westley to their house on the other side of the marketplace, he went and noted that 'there the man said he witnessed the truth of wt was sayd, & his wife [was] assenting & very kinde'.[5] Since the Westleys were both from very respectable Anglican families, and William himself was clerk to the dean and chapter, this was no small measure of success.

On 15th November, Claver was not in town to witness Penn's performance or to discuss it with the Westleys. And he was still away in London when Penn and colleagues returned a few weeks later to find that the landlord of the Crown had been threatened with a fine for hosting the previous meeting. So Whiting went to the bishop again, obtained the certificate he needed, and eventually tracked down Matthew Baron to show it to him and complain about the illegal treatment and harassment the Quakers had received. He did not mince his words, for 'The Mayor (Poor Man) stood like one speechless'.[6]

As it was Penn's view that the city was 'a-thirsting for another meeting', it was agreed that a house should be hired and a licence obtained for future gatherings so that 'the blessed truth may be published in the Citty of Wells'. It was also agreed that as the next Quarterly Meeting of the Somerset Friends would be held at the Crown, this would require a further licence. So, Whiting went to the bishop once more, and after a discussion about oaths and swearing in which the bishop was very 'mild and moderate', they parted on such good terms that the bishop walked John Whiting to the Palace Gate to bless him. When the Meeting took place in March 1696, there was no harassment and little business. The main topic of discussion among the thirty-seven representatives was the 'rude & Clamorous' claim of Thomas Hymens of Bridgwater that he had a right to marry Hannah Champion, a widow from the village of Meare near Glastonbury. The Friends had heard this tiresome claim before, and they would hear it yet again, though they all pronounced that 'Thomas Hymens is utterly wrong'. But, as far as Wells was concerned, the Friends could now honestly proclaim that 'the Standard of Truth was set up in that town'.[7]

When Claver returned to Wells just before Christmas 1695, his dispute with Kidder continued, notwithstanding attempts at mediation. Financially, however, Claver was doing rather well.[8] Income from his medical practice was earning him about £150 a year, and his expenses remained largely unchanged. His mother had sent him £100 with a request that he should return £10 a year to her, should she ever need it, and his move to the gabled manor was saving him a few more pounds a year. On the other hand, he was now paying a new tax under the Marriage Act of 1695. This levied annual charges (according to wealth and status) on all marriages, births, burials, bachelors over twenty-five, and childless widowers.

The aim of the Marriage Act was to help pay for the war with France, and although the Bank of England had been created in 1694 to fund the national debt, new taxes were essential. Most money would be raised from the standard charges levied upon almost everyone except those receiving alms; four shillings for a burial, two shillings for a birth, and two shillings and sixpence for a wedding. But the only charge that affected Claver was the tax on childless widowers. For doctors of Divinity, Law or Medicine this was twenty-six shillings every year – twice as much as the levy on a canon or archdeacon. The sum made no financial difference to Claver, but these payments would have served as a sad reminder of the wife and child that he had lost.

In 1696 Richard Cupper's case had barely been settled in the bishop's court before there was further trouble on the far side of the cathedral green where Gladys Lovett and her daughters lived. This time Elizabeth Lovett (the elder daughter) was called as a witness in the case of Frances Taylor versus Sarah Hippesley (sic.), whose families kept shops directly opposite each other in Sadler Street. According to Frances Taylor, at the beginning of Lent in 1695, three of her children (as well as other witnesses) had heard Sarah Hippesley repeatedly call her an 'old Bawd' and accuse her of keeping a bawdy house. In an attempt to preserve her reputation, Frances was now seeking damages for defamation; a common cause of litigation in the bishop's court. In Sarah's defence, it was agreed that when she opened her shop on the morning of Shrove Tuesday, she saw that 'a stinking chamber pot' had been thrown all over her front door, and that a pair of horns had been hung on the wall above. Everyone agreed that the contents of 'a stinking vessel of excrement' had been deposited in this way, but the Taylors claimed that they were innocent of the offence. The family rivalries remained unresolved but, in this instance, it was assumed that Sarah's anger and accusations had been misplaced.[9]

While Kidder would not have concerned himself with such mundane cases in his court, his patience with Edwyn Sandys was running out. Having suspended the archdeacon for failure to conduct ordinations, Kidder summoned him to appear at the consistory court. It must have come as a surprise when Sandys actually attended, if only to attest that he had previously been sick. Kidder did not believe it, but felt that he had to accept this diplomatic-but-deceitful explanation. A month later he regretted his decision when, in his role as a Justice of the Peace, he received depositions from the parish officers of Puddimore and Yeovilton complaining that their rector, Sandys, was omitting all prayers and blessings that were meant to be said on behalf of William, the king. It was a sorry situation, for as one of the churchwardens pointed out, 'he [Sandys] taketh little care of his parishioners, though he enjoy two livings to the value of £260 per annum at a mile distance from each other'.[10]

During the summer, Claver made short trips to Bath to attend to patients such as young Edmund Dawe and Colonel Berkeley who were staying to take the waters. There were also patients there with whom he could share his love of music; men like Sir John Fust and his wife from Hill Court in Gloucestershire, for whom he procured an oboe for a pound – as well as a rather smarter one for himself, with ivory joints and tips.[11] At Bath, he bought new horses and took a trip to Chipping Sodbury in the Cotswolds where, for centuries, there had been a 'mop fair' for hiring servants and farm-labourers. The town was most famous for having 'the greatest cheese market in all that part of England'; something that would certainly have appealed to Claver's taste for all the finest foods.[12] He was now courting Elizabeth, the twenty-eight-year-old widow of Robert Jeanes and daughter of the late squire of Ditcheat, Edmund Dawe. Like Claver, her first marriage had only lasted a few years, and she had not been blessed with children. But two years had passed since the loss of her husband and, like Claver, she must have thought that it was time to marry again.

At the bishop's palace, the news of Claver's courtship of Elizabeth Jeanes was the final straw. Regardless of Susanna's feelings, by preferring a local widow, it seemed to Kidder that the self-important and deceitful Dr Morris had now emphatically demeaned him, the Lord Bishop of Bath and Wells, a figure of national import and esteem. Such disrespect would never be forgiven. But among Claver's colleagues there was cause for celebration. The Dawes were a fine old gentry family; they knew Claver very well, and they were not short of money, influence or friends. Some of Claver's friends probably felt that, as it was seven years since Grace's death, it was high time for him to re-marry. There was no need for a big wedding between a widow and a widower with no step-children to consider, so a simple wedding would suffice. And after borrowing thirty guineas in cash from Richard Healy, for expenses, at the end of 1696 Elizabeth and Claver were quietly married in the village of Ditcheat. Elizabeth then moved to live with Claver at the manor-house he was renting in the Liberty. There, on 9th January 1697, he paid the tax of five pounds, two shillings and sixpence for his marriage; no doubt believing this would be the best money that he would ever spend.[13]

PART TWO

1697–1718

14

BABY BETTY

By the end of the spring 1697 Elizabeth was expecting her first child. It was widely recognised that 'it is very hard to know a false conception from a true until four moneths be past', and for all his medical education and experience, Claver knew no better. Many people thought that the best guide to such matters was probably *The Midwives Book: or the Whole Art of Midwifery Discovered* (1671), which listed fourteen 'signs that woman is conceived with Child', some of which were based upon observation and experience, and others drawn from ancient medical beliefs and superstitions. So, when Jane Sharp, 'a practitioner in the Art of Midwifery above thirty years', addressed 'the Midwives of England' in her plain-speaking book designed to reduce 'the many Miseries Women endure in the Hands of unskilful Midwives', her advice was worth considering. She recited, questioned and even occasionally corrected the received wisdoms of most physicians, derived primarily from the works of Hippocrates, Aristotle and Galen.

Sharp began with a frank exposition of the generative parts of men and women, founded upon the conviction that 'we women have no more cause to be angry, or be ashamed of what Nature hath given us than men have; we cannot be without ours no more than they can want theirs'. She then warned about the dangers of 'moles or moon-calfs', miscarriages and monstrous births, before explaining that 'if a woman's courses be stopt, and the Veins under her lowest Eyelid swell', this was a sure sign of conception in the first two months. Thereafter, a simple test would be to place a needle in the woman's urine; 'it will be full of red spots if she have conceived, or otherwise it will be black or dark brown'. But there were plenty of other tests to try, such as the local advice to 'take a new laid egg, lay it in the woman's water and if she be with child there will come upon the egg, as it were, a white line or sand'.

It was a little easier, at least in theory, to determine the baby's sex, for it was very well established that girls were produced by seed from the left-hand testicle and lay on the left side of the womb, while boys came from and lay on the right-hand side.

DOI: 10.4324/9781003333654-16

Again, there was a simple test: put 'drops of breast Milk into a Bason of water, if it swim on the top it is a Boy, if it sink in round drops judge the contrary'. There were plenty of local measures too, such as 'Take the milk of a woman when she is quick and put it in a redwort leaf, and bind it up close. Lay it in the embers while you may goe halfe a mile, then open it, if it be curded, it is a male, if not a female'.[1]

While Elizabeth was wondering about her chances of carrying her baby to full term, Claver was busy making plans.[2] Until his marriage to Elizabeth, the only land he owned, aside from the houses in Crane Court, was a small estate at Felton, fifteen miles away across the Mendips, which he leased for £24 a year. But with the land that Elizabeth had inherited from her late husband, Claver now found that there were many rents to be collected from tenants in the villages of West Pennard, Pilton and Ditcheat. At West Pennard there was an estate of nineteen acres that he let for £14, but most tenants only rented two or three acres for a few pounds every year. There were also several debts still owing to Robert Jeanes that Claver gradually collected, amounting to over £100.[3] But by far the greater part of Elizabeth's wealth (now Claver's) came from the legacy of her father, who had left her all his property in the villages of West Bradley and Baltonsborough near Glastonbury which he estimated to be worth £1,200.

The town of Glastonbury was 'a ragged poor place', according to one traveller in 1698. But, being the legendary cradle of Christianity in England, it still attracted pilgrims to its holy sites. It was here, in the first century AD, that Joseph of Arimathea was believed to have buried the Holy Grail and to have thrust his staff into the ground from which the sacred Glastonbury Thorn had grown. Later, it became the

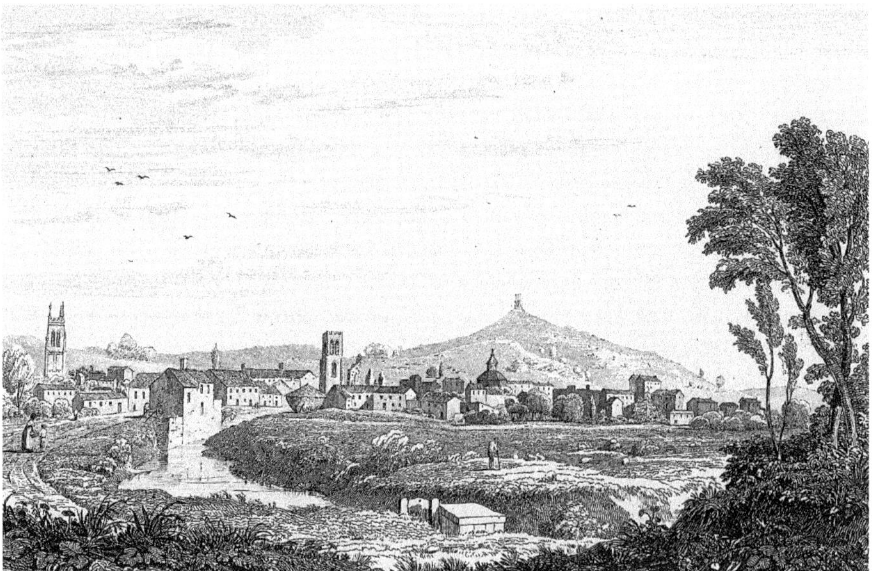

FIGURE 8 A View of Glastonbury
This view from the south-west shows the Tor and the River Brue

legendary burial place of King Arthur and his wife, and in 1539 it was the place where the last abbot of the oldest monastery in England had refused to surrender to the king. He was hanged at the medieval tower on the top of Glastonbury Tor, his head exhibited on the Abbey gates, and his quarters sent to Wells.[4]

Looking out from Glastonbury Tor, Claver could see all the land that he had recently acquired. In this panorama of small cottages, ploughed fields, pastures, woodlands and small lakes, most of the largest buildings were the churches, as there were no great manor-houses here. But the fields were fertile, especially for dairy farming, and sufficiently profitable for Edmund Dawe to have wanted to purchase the manor-house and sixty acres at West Bradley in 1691. As with Robert Jeanes's legacy, apart from one plot of twenty-two acres, the West Bradley lands were often leased in holdings of one or two acres for a few pounds every year. So, Claver was keen to draw up larger and longer leases whenever the opportunities arose. Before long, at West Bradley he had leased out a house with orchards and sixteen acres for £12 a year; let two houses with meadows and pastures for £34; and for £14 had bought a couple of good acres from his friend, the yeoman Henry Bull, who, being illiterate and unable to sign the contract, made a mark against his name.[5] Claver was also as busy as ever with his patients, and watching closely the progress of his wife. By September 1697, however, his thoughts were also turning to two new ventures.

First, there was the prospect of enclosing (privatising) some of the common lands at Baltonsborough; an idea that he was considering with several of the local gentry. It was an ambitious proposition from which it should be possible both to make a lot of money and to improve the productivity and the health of farming families. But it was fraught with difficulty. The open fields over which villagers often held some ancient rights – usually to grow crops, graze animals and collect firewood – could sometimes be divided and 'enclosed' by local agreements for the benefit of all. But the whole process of consolidating landholdings, compensating villagers for their loss of rights, and hedging or ditching all the properties to be enclosed, was a complex and often-inflammatory business.

In Tudor times, when arable fields were turned to pasture in order to increase profits from the grazing of sheep for wool, enclosure sometimes led to the impoverishment of entire communities and the desertion of their villages. A century later, in the 1640s and '50s, the Court of Chancery had approved several enclosures of the moors of Somerset. These included the enclosure of 180 acres (home to 432 'beasts') of Church Moor in Baltonsborough, and part of the commons at West Pennard which, though 'time out of mind used as arable lands', had been converted into meadows. There had also been more recent attempts to improve the drainage of the moors of Avalon which were often flooded. This was due to the mouths of their rivers being blocked by the sand and silt deposited by the exceptionally high tides of the Severn estuary. Plans for enclosure and better drainage, therefore, often went hand in hand. A decade later, Claver was sworn-in as a Commissioner for Sewers for Somerset, no doubt partly to promote his enclosure venture. But despite much talk, there had been no major improvement to the drainage of the moors since the Restoration.[6]

Undaunted by the difficulties, Claver took encouragement from recent developments. In March 1699, a Bill for 'opening the ancient Roynes [ditches] and Watercourses in *Sedgemore*, in the County of *Somerset*, for rendering the said Moor more healthful and profitable to the Inhabitants' was read for a third time in the Commons and was passed in April after amendments in the Lords.[7] So, Claver and his friends were not alone in thinking that there would be new opportunities to enclose the common lands. By the end of the year he had enlarged his stake in Baltonsborough by paying a local gentleman, Henry Foxwell, for the whole of his family's estate. This only amounted to £100 in cash, because the estate was heavily encumbered by two mortgages, one of which had been given to Elizabeth as part of her father's legacy. Together, these debts amounted to £522; a sum that Claver spelt out in his neatest handwriting as he drew up the agreement in October.[8] This might be a good investment for the future, but for someone who was inexperienced in law or land-dealing, it was certainly a gamble.

The second venture that Claver had in mind was a much surer business. He would buy the seven-chimneyed old house of his next-door neighbour, the place where the Pouletts had lived until Catherine had died in 1695 shortly after taking out a new forty-year lease from the dean and chapter and bequeathing everything to her brother, Robert Creighton. On 4th October 1697, Claver agreed with Henry Layng, Creighton's son-in-law, that at Christmas he would purchase the house, garden, stable and orchard, together with the oak panelling and furniture, tapestries and pictures, all for £125. The plan was not to live there for very long, but eventually to knock the building down and replace it with something better. So, straightaway with this in mind, at West Pennard trees were felled, timbers sawed and carpenters employed (at a shilling a day) to prepare for two years' seasoning of good wood. When Christmas came, Claver found that he needed to borrow £100 from his mother in order to complete the purchase of the house, 'to be repaid with what speed can conveniently be made'. But his personal happiness now outweighed any concerns he might have had about the loan.[9]

On Saturday 4th December 1697, two days after great celebrations marking the long-awaited peace with France,[10] Elizabeth gave birth to a baby girl. Her midwife and a small group of women who oversaw the birth – men were normally kept well away – agreed the baby appeared to be quite healthy. But it was most important now that all precaution be taken to protect the mother and child from infection. As everybody knew, and Jane Sharp explained, due to Eve's tasting of the forbidden fruit, 'the accidents and hazards that women lye under when they bring their Children into the world are not few', for 'it was that curse that *God* laid upon our sex to bring forth in sorrow.' It was also generally believed that 'if the child be ill, the Nurses milk is commonly the cause of it'. Among the poor, who expected to breast-feed their babies, this was rarely any problem. But among the rich, as Jane Sharp argued, women often 'pretend weakness when they have no cause for it, because they have not so much love for their own, as Dumb creatures have'.

Although 'the usual way for rich people' was 'to put forth their children to nurse', in Sharp's view this was 'a remedy that needs a remedy' because the practice 'changeth the natural disposition of the child, and oftentimes exposeth the infant to many hazards'. She advised that, if a wet-nurse were essential, great care should be taken to ensure that the woman was not 'crooked, or squint-eyed, nor with a misshapen nose or body, or with black ill-favoured teeth, or with stinking breath'. It was also important in Sharp's view that 'a female child must suck the breast of a nurse that had a girl the last child she had, and a boy must suck her that lately had a boy'.[11] But not all medics were of this opinion.

When Betty was one week old, she was christened in the cathedral. The Book of Common Prayer did not require a baby's mother to attend, as she was often still recovering, and even fathers only played a minor role. But in the Church of England the sacrament of baptism was of immense importance as it provided the foundation for a Christian life. It was also of great social value, bringing the baby's parents and godparents, family and friends, and often a whole parish, together in prayer and celebration. After the ceremony there would be plenty of music, dancing and much drinking in the Liberty. To ensure his regular stock of wines did not run dry, Claver had purchased an additional thirty-six pints of sherry and sixteen pints of brandy, as well as a three-year-old fifty-eight-pound cheddar cheese and twelve dozen tobacco-pipes. And in the morning and for the rest of the month, he was either too befuddled or just too busy showing off his baby to remember he had a daily record of patients' prescriptions to maintain; a record that, until Betty's baptism, he had kept without interruption or omission since 1686.

15

BAD OMENS

It was customary for new mothers, if they did not have to work, to stay in bed for several weeks after giving birth, and after this period of 'lying-in' to attend a thanksgiving or 'churching' service. By the 1690s, the churching ritual had become as much about holding a social gathering in which the survival of the mother could be celebrated with her female friends, as it was about an older religious observance and the saying of a special prayer. But as the ritual owed its origins to Jewish customs of purification as well as Catholic traditions, it was detested by most Puritans. In particular, they objected to what they saw as the abominable superstition of mothers wearing a white veil.[1] So, in January 1698, when Elizabeth chose to wear one as she walked to the cathedral with her friends, there could be little doubt that she was making a clear statement about both her female status and her faith.

In this ritual, the role of Claver and other men was simple; to provide support. So, he arranged for Joshua Lasher, a choral vicar, to take the service, gave two shillings to the poor and bought a further, but smaller, supply of wine. He had designed a special candlestick 'contriv'd to keep ye child's milk warm at night' and a bib weighing five and a half ounces in solid silver, though it soon required some redesign. Before the end of January, he also bought Betty a rug for her cradle, and a coat and head-caps embroidered with flowers made in white, green and crimson silks. For Elizabeth, there was a new quilt and opulent new bedding made with sixty-six yards of gold-coloured Avignon silk, thirty-six yards of crimson and green camlet and seventeen yards of printed calico, costing over £30, plus another £3 for satin cushions. For himself he bought new nightshirts, cravats, winter boots and a set of silver stud-buttons for the flap on his new breeches. There were also fresh furnishings and repairs needed at the newly purchased house and garden before any of the family, their two maids and man-servant could move in.[2]

Though it took six days to move everything from the gabled manor-house to the newly purchased house next door, by the spring Claver and the whole household

DOI: 10.4324/9781003333654-17

were well settled into their new home. Claver had a stroke of luck too. With 'a guinea ventured in a lottery', he had won a newly-translated copy of Nicolas Fontaine's *History of the Old and New Testament* (1697), a richly illustrated book with over two hundred copper-plates and maps. He had also recently bought John Dryden's translation of *The Satires of Juvenal and Persius* (1693) and Thomas Creech's *The Odes, Satyrs and Epistles of Horace* (1688), which were full of humanity, wit and poetic beauty. Perhaps with Kidder's sympathy for Dissenters in mind, he also bought two books defending the Church of England from Puritan and Presbyterian assaults; Richard Hooker's *Of the Lawes of Ecclesiastical Polity* (first published in 1594) and John Sage's *The Fundamental Charter of Presbytery* (first published in 1695). A few months later, he bought *The Works of the Honourable Robert Boyle, Esq.* (1699); a new four-volume abridgement of the great scientist's experiments in chemistry and physics. In addition, he bought an old copy of Pliny's colossal *Natural History,* including the philosopher's thoughts on medicine, drugs and magic, first published in English in 1601, though there was a much rarer Venetian edition in the cathedral library.[3]

Of all the books that Claver bought for study or as gifts, the most important was the first book of Andrea Palladio's seminal *The Four Books of Architecture* (Venice, 1570) which had been translated from a French edition into English and published several times in London since 1663. The first book consisted of Palladio's account of the five orders of Greek and Roman architecture and of all the building materials and methods of construction that were needed for matching the walls, pedestals, galleries, entrances, halls, floors, staircases, roofs and chimneys. To complete the look, even the 'rules to be observed in making doors and windows' needed to be obeyed. This neoclassical style, echoing the magnificence of ancient Rome, had not swept all vernacular styles aside but, being international, studied, fashionable and expensive, it exuded the wealth and self-confidence of many Englishmen in an age of imperial expansion.

For Claver, the strict geometry, mathematics and mechanics required for classical architecture were his meat and drink: he had an eye for detail in the design and appearance of everything, from the buckles on his shoes to the binding of his books. So when he read Palladio's opening statement that 'Three things in a Building (as saith Vitruvius) ought to be considered, without which it will not deserve commendation: those are usefulness or accommodation, lastingness and handsomeness', he was in his element.[4] A more cautious person might have considered the costs and embarrassment of failure. But, for Claver, the opportunity to show off a building of his own design was irresistible. There were other self-taught architects who were excelling, Sir Christopher Wren among them, so it seemed that experience was not essential. And with the cathedral in close proximity, there would be no shortage of master masons, good builders and glaziers who could do the work that he envisaged. But no work could begin in 1699 while Claver and his family were still living in the house and preparing for a far more important occasion. At the beginning of the year, it appeared that Elizabeth, now thirty-one, was pregnant with their second child.

Claver's cheer at the prospect of another baby was tempered in January by the news of his father's death at the age of seventy-five. Having come from an ordinary family, William Morris's studies at Oxford had been interrupted by the Civil Wars when he became a standard-bearer in the royal cavalry and, after the Restoration, a priest. He had enjoyed a good living at Manston, though it was largely from his wife's family that he had accumulated the surpluses that were used to support his son's academic studies and career. Six years before William's death a stroke had left him partially paralysed. Nevertheless, he continued as rector of St Nicholas and was buried by the altar there on 13th January 1699. It was ten years since he had buried his daughter-in-law Grace and granddaughter Mary in the same place. For Claver and his mother, who had lost all her other children, this was hard to bear.

William's gravestone made no mention of his family and stressed his learning (though there was no record that he had ever been awarded an MA), and his pride in fighting for Charles I. His will, however, showed something of the hurt that he still harboured over the actions of his sons-in-law, Nicholas Shirley and Edward Goddard, as he pointedly left them a shilling each. Thereafter, £10 was to be set aside for his grandson William Goddard when he came of age; Claver was to have all his books and gold coins; and everything else (about 56 guineas) was left to his widow Hannah. Claver's relationship with his mother had always been very close, and now, with the death of his father, it was even stronger.[5]

In scholarly circles, as well as popular opinion, there were long-held beliefs in premonitions of misfortunes, especially regarding death. When spring arrived in 1699 after an exceptionally wet winter, a great storm drove a fifty-six-foot whale a long way up the Thames. This had also happened to a whale in 1658, when the event was seen as a portent of Oliver Cromwell's end. Then, as soon as summer came in 1699, the weather turned exceptionally dry and hot, with 'a great drought' lasting for three months. This was the last thing that anybody needed after 'seven lean years' of poor harvests and high prices in most parts of the country.[6] In Scotland, where there had been almost a decade of cold weather, conditions were much worse: failure of yet another harvest would now lead to starvation and depopulation. And in the autumn, due to lunar and solar eclipses across Britain, 'many [people] were frightened by the predictions of astrologers', including one William Knight, a self-proclaimed 'Student in Astrology, Physick [Medicine], and Chirurgery [Surgery]'. Among his dire warnings was the prediction that this season would be a time of 'barrenness of the Earth, and barrenness among Women, many Miscarriages, and abortive Births'.[7] There were political forebodings too.

In London, the government was still wrestling with the fundamental problem left by the Peace of Ryswick in 1697, which had ostensibly brought an end to nine years of war with France. In the treaty, 'the most Christian King' Louis XIV had made what appeared to be a great concession in recognising the Calvinist William as 'King of Great Britain *by the grace of God*'. Louis had also agreed to a 'perpetual peace and friendship' between the warring families '*and their successors*', and had given '*his royal word*' that he would not aid any of William's enemies in the future. But no-one believed a word of it, or at least that any peace would last for long.

The problem was simple: how to prevent the entire Spanish empire from being acquired by France after the death of the sickly king of Spain, Carlos II, thus making the House of Bourbon near-invincible. The solution, it was hoped, lay in secret Partition Treaties signed by all the major European powers, including France. But if Carlos II left a will leaving the Spanish empire to Louis XIV's grandson, and Louis accepted this (as he would), another war would be inevitable.[8]

Bad omens aside, in Wells, Claver was busy with his medical practice and planning his new ventures. In August, there was also cause for celebration (and relief, considering the scandal of the alleged secret marriage) when Richard Cupper junior married Grace Ford at West Quantoxhead on the Somerset coast. In August everything was prepared for Elizabeth's delivery. The birth of Betty in December 1697 had proceeded smoothly, with Elizabeth recovering well enough to have her 'churching' celebration just a few weeks later. This time, as Elizabeth struggled, she tried to put her baby's life before her own; but it was in vain. Before the end of the day on Thursday, 17th August 1699, both were dead.

As a member of a gentry family, a Dawe by birth, Elizabeth's passing could not be treated as a private matter. There was much to prepare. Before the funeral on 20th August, twenty silk and paper escutcheons (standards bearing the family coat of arms) would need to be made and flown over the hearse that would carry Elizabeth's body from Wells to Ditcheat. Claver would need to specify the design and decoration of the hearse and coffin. Fifteen gold mourning-rings were ordered and engraved for family and friends, and over 150 pairs of 'double Shammy', 'London Sheep', 'Yeovil Lamb' and 'White Kid-Leather' gloves prepared for other mourners according to their age and status. Claver and his man, and Betty and her nurse-maid, had to be fitted with new mourning clothes and shoes, and four hatbands made for Elizabeth's three brothers and the coachman. By the time everything was ready for the service (at a cost of £62, including servants' wages, and the making of bread for the Ditcheat poor), Claver was in need of rest. After the service, twenty-four pints of sherry and eighty pints of claret warmed with sugar and spice were given to the guests.[9] Aside from Elizabeth's immediate family and Claver's mother who had come from Manston, the principal helpers were the pall-bearers, all of whom were Claver's friends.[10] And he called upon another helper, Anthony Walkeley, a choral vicar, to play the organ.[11]

In Claver's mind, 'the dismal solemnity' of burying his 'tenderly affectionate and entirely Beloved wife' in the Dawe vault under the south transept of St Mary Magdalene's was not something that would fade with time. When Grace had died in 1689, he had railed against the fact that she had been taken from him, for no reason that he could fathom, just three years after their wedding. Now, he was burying his second wife before they had been married even for that short length of time. His belief that Elizabeth had sacrificed her life in the hope of saving their unborn daughter was clearly stated on the memorial tablet that he erected at Ditcheat six years later.

The large wall-monument, containing a Latin inscription on black marble in an ivory-and-red-veined marble frame, decorated with small flowers and cherubs, was not a nodding gesture to the memory of a wife. Claver commissioned it for £30 from 'the ingenious' John Harvey, a stonemason and architect who was just completing the building of the first grand Pump Room at Bath at the request of the city's flamboyant new Master of Ceremonies, Richard 'Beau' Nash. So, Claver fully intended his commission to be a striking commemoration, and it was. In a semi-circular enclosure above the main tablet there was a white marble bust of a classically dressed woman in a likeness of Elizabeth, with a lock of hair resting on her breast. Below the main tablet, a coat of arms proudly displayed Claver's three red lions *couchant guardant,* impaling Elizabeth's three white cross-crosslets on a sable background. Perhaps thinking of Betty's needs in years to come, six years later he oversaw repairs to a large window beside the monument, which cast light upon the vault below.[12]

Within days of Elizabeth's funeral, Claver moved his whole household out of the wretched house he owned and into the vacant canonical residence next door. He had only lived in the house he owned for less than two years, since he had bought it from the Creightons at the end of 1697. Now, as this was the place where Elizabeth and her baby had died so tragically, it did not deserve to stand. So, on 3rd September 1699, just two weeks after their deaths, he instructed his builders to pull the whole place down.[13]

16

A NEW HOME

Following Palladio's advice, Claver wanted his new house at the top of the East Liberty to be a masterpiece. On entering from the street, the house, faced with ashlar stone, appeared to be three storeys high, as the lower-ground-floor's mullioned windows could be seen a few feet above the level of the small front garden. A visitor would walk along blue flagstones and up fourteen steps to the front door within a porch that rose the full height of the house, set in a moulded architrave with a pediment and frieze of acanthus leaves. On each side of the door, at both the upper-ground and first-floor levels, there were two large sash windows with decorative mouldings, as well as a window above the door itself. Ten years later, after the bricking up of nine windows to reduce liability for tax, there were still another twenty-nine windows on which tax was due. This was to be a light as well as a meticulously symmetrical and well-proportioned home, and there were also two circular windows on either side of the porch. At the top, a modillion cornice with brackets ran around the house, incorporating the eaves guttering in the roof.

DOI: 10.4324/9781003333654-18

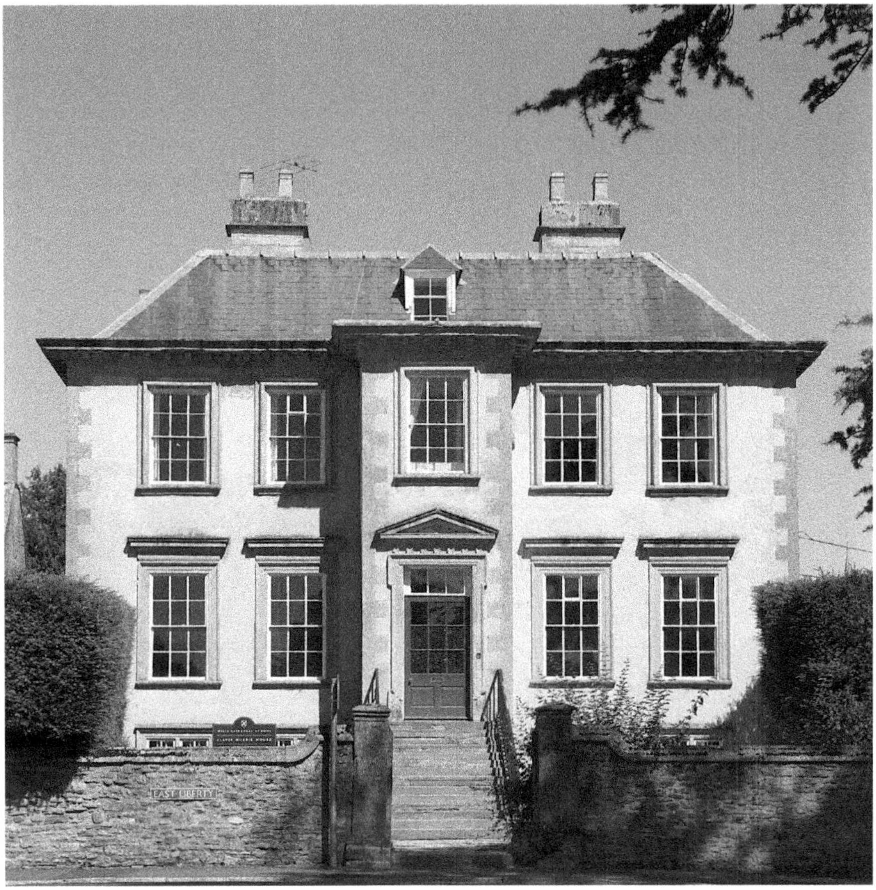

FIGURE 9 Claver Morris's new house, *c.*1700

Inside, a staircase with turned balustrades and moulded handrail led to large rooms with grand fireplaces, bolection-moulded panelled doors and highly decorative architraves and cornices.[1] Here, the aim was not just to create a luxurious interior that would delight the eye with its classical taste, but also to create a home in which there was plenty of space to entertain guests. This was primarily a private residence, but Claver's sociability, and the needs of his medical practice, meant that visitors and patients could be expected any time.

As the building work progressed, Claver made a trip to London to buy new furnishings and tableware, including: a large mirror for the great parlour; a japanned table; a folding walnut-veneered dressing-table for the brewhouse chamber; and two dozen plates which he purchased from John Prince (a pewterer in Pall Mall) which he had engraved with his coat of arms. He had added to his picture gallery a 'prospect of Greenwich', a 'Picture of Fame, a most beautiful piece, by Ray', and a still-life painting of 'a dead Pheasant hanging against a Deal Board' bought at an auction at the George in the High Street. He also bought several Dutch drawings, portraits of Democritus and Heroclitus, and a portrait of 'King Charles the 1st in an oval Frame'. The re-walled garden and orchard at the back of the house were no less important to the whole domain, and both needed to be laid out in a semi-formal style. The garden was large enough to plant eight fir, seven cherry and three cypress tress to complement the Italianate appearance of the house. Behind the garden, the orchard was planted with fifty fruit trees: eighteen golden-pippins, and several pears, peaches, nectarines, apricots and plums, as well as black-cherry trees for brandy. Claver was delighted with the planting by Mr Baker, a gardener from Salisbury, who charged £3 for everything and was happy with a shilling tip.[2]

To pay for the new house and garden, Claver still had £390 from 'Grace's Orphans Money' deposited in the Bank of England, and on a trip to London in 1701 he sold the larger of the two houses in Crane Court for £630. This meant that in 1702 when he drew up the accounts for what would now always be known as 'Dr Claver Morris's house', he still had savings. After accounting for every farthing, the total cost of the new home amounted to just over £807, of which £407 was for materials, and £400 for labour.[3]

Looking to the future, when he had bought the old Poulett house in 1697, Claver had also purchased a stable and coach-house at the side of the old gabled manor-house (De Salis, 17 The Liberty) to the north next-door, plus a tiny plot of land between the back of the coach-house and the home of his friend and helper, George Orchard. And while knocking down the Poulett house and marking out the boundaries of his new domain, he could not resist the temptation to widen his own grounds by taking a strip of land from the canonical residence to the south in which he was living while his new home was being built. As long as nobody in the dean and chapter spotted the appropriation, Claver foresaw no problem. But if the dean and chapter ever learned about it, they would certainly be aggrieved. Fortunately for Claver, when his house was finished and he requested a new forty-year lease for the land in 1702, no-one recalled (or told of) the intrusion. So, a new lease was granted for the usual rent of sixteen shillings and eight pence a year. But that was no security against the possibility of discovery in the future.[4]

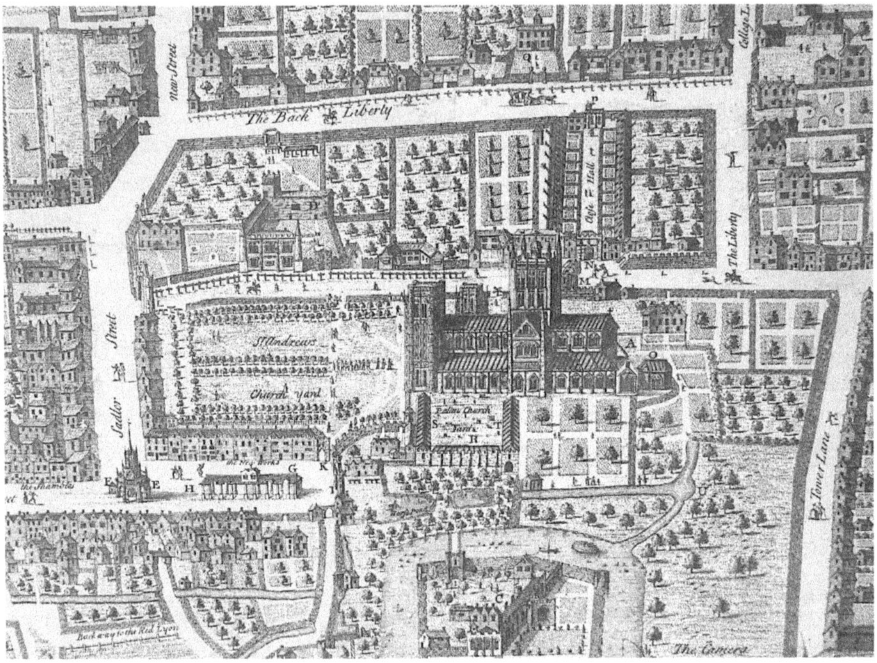

FIGURE 10 Detail from a map of Wells, 1735
Claver Morris's house is shown at the top-right of the Liberty. It looks down 'Back Liberty', past the chantry-college buildings on the right, and the top of Vicars' Close ('Close Hall') on the left. South of the cathedral, the city's mineral springs ('U') flow into the moat around the bishop's palace ('C'). The Conduit ('F'), High Cross ('E'), and Assize Hall ('G') can be seen in the Market Place ('H')

While on his trip to London in February and March 1701, shortly after he had moved into his new home, Claver purchased twenty new books on medicine, anatomy, history, mathematics, politics, philosophy and religion. He also bought the expensive new folio edition of Daniel Le Clerk's two-volume *The Great Historical, Geographical, Genealogical and Poetical Dictionary* (1701), and the first book of John Playford's *Orpheus Britannicus. A Collection of all the Choicest Songs for One, Two, and Three Voices, compos'd by Mr. Henry Purcell* (1698) from his shop in Fleet Street, together with 'The Art of Descant, or Composing Musick in Parts' by Thomas Campion, the third book of *An Introduction to the Skill of Musick* (12th edn, 1694).

In London, he also chose the tailors to make his new clothes, including a silk gown in green, trimmed with silver lace, and a Mantero-silk brocaded waistcoat from shops in Ludgate. These clothes would match the new half-skirted saddle, stitched and wrought with silver, and the silver-lace cloth bags that were made to house his pistols. As always, he would not return to Wells without presents, so in addition to 'a Brass Fountain Pen' for himself, he bought six more 'to give away'. For his mother he bought a 'very large' umbrella that cost six shillings, and a pair of spectacles in a fish-skin case. No less important and twice the cost were the toys for Betty: a little ivory picture-box, a humming top, a box of comic pictures on a roll, eight brass medals, three wax-figures in their glass-topped boxes, and 'a Wax Baby [doll] with an Invention to make it Cry, & to turn it's Eyes' – a contraption that would certainly have fascinated Claver, though it may well have terrified his daughter.[5]

By the time Claver's new house was built his family had been reduced to three: his mother, Betty and himself. Without her husband to look after, Hannah was now free to come up from Manston to help with the care of her granddaughter. With no other family dependants or responsibilities, Claver could spend any savings he had accumulated on whatever luxuries he chose; for, in his mind, there was no question that life was always for the living, not the dead. It was not long after acquiring the stables and coach-house at the side of the old gabled manor-house, that he decided to put them to good use. He only paid ten guineas for a carriage, but it cost another six to fit it out with scarlet fabrics and gold lace. The sturdy coach-horses were an even greater and continuing expense, but on a visit to the May Fair at Amesbury, a few miles from Stonehenge, he found the two black horses that he wanted at a cost of thirty-three guineas. One of them had '2 White Feet' and the other had 'a Starr in his Forehead', and he named them Duke and Buck. If anyone doubted the doctor's wealth and status now, his ownership of a coach and horses was proof enough.[6]

Not everyone was delighted by worldly accomplishments that were so conspicuously displayed, or even felt any sympathy for Claver over the death of his wife and new-born child. At the bishop's palace, Kidder was still angry as he nursed his own seriously debilitating gout. But most of his attention was now focused on 'the many causles [causeless] troubles and injuries don me by Harry Bridges Esq.', one of Claver's acquaintances in Wells, though not a friend.

Harry Bridges was the eldest-surviving son of the wealthy old royalist squire Sir Thomas. He owned the manors of Keynsham (between Bath and Bristol), Rodney Stoke (between Wells and Cheddar), and other properties across the county and also in Covent Garden. When Kidder first fell out with him in 1698, Harry was in his early fifties, a well-educated and well-travelled gentleman who spoke several European languages and served as a Justice of the Peace. He had been married to Lady Diana Holles, daughter of the 2nd earl of Clare, but she and their daughter had long since left him.[7] So Harry had come to Wells where he had several interests, including ownership of the Saracen's Head in New Street, not far from Claver's home, and a large house in Chamberlain Street where he lived with Thomas Muttlebury and his children, the richest man in the street, holder of the manor of Wookey just outside the city, and a well-known Roman Catholic.[8]

Harry Bridges was not a Catholic, but he was certainly sympathetic to the plight of James II, though this was not the main cause of his dispute with Kidder. It had begun in 1698 over the parish of Chew Magna on the Mendips where the vicar had been censured for negligence. Harry recommended a replacement cleric and promised to repair the rectory, but when a curate was not appointed and the vicarage was not restored, Kidder lost patience and ordered the squire's arrest. Harry was incensed, but worse was to follow. Following a tip-off from his chancellor, William Hughes, that an unmarried woman, Ann Dunn, had given birth to a boy at Harry's house in New Street, and that they were still living there 'to the great scandal of honest people', Kidder had Ann arrested and kept in custody until she could be tried in his consistory court.[9]

Harry put up bail to keep Ann out of prison, but when she came to the bishop's court she denied having any children. The midwife Margaret Symes and others testified that Ann had indeed been delivered of a son, and that she now lived at the house of John Balsh in Chamberlain Street.[10] Through her lawyer, Ann was forced to own her child. Yet this was not good enough for Kidder, who insisted that 'she must own it herself in open Court'. In November 1698, he excommunicated the 'very famous whore', mindful of the 'enormity' of her offence. Believing this to be exceptionally vindictive, Harry took the case to the Archbishop of Canterbury's Court of Arches, held in London, but he then failed to provide any legal representation at the hearing, so the case was soon returned to Wells. He also wrote to the archbishop of Canterbury, who offered to hear both sides of the case. This would prove impossible as Kidder's gout was so severe that he was unable to travel for a period of six months. It was then that Kidder decided to sue Harry for *Scandalum Magnatum* (the defamation of eminent persons; a law used largely to protect the interests of peers of the realm) at the King's Bench, the highest criminal court in England.

Sir Thomas Bridges, in his eighties, took a dim view of his son's behaviour, as he did of bastardy in principle, so he set up a trust to ensure that his illegitimate grandson, James, could never inherit the family estates.[11] And just before the trial at the Guildhall in June 1700, he offered to pay Kidder's costs if he would be willing to drop the case. Kidder said that he would, on the condition that Harry signed an apology and presented it in person to the archbishop or the lord mayor of London. Rejecting this, Harry petitioned to be tried by a special jury, composed exclusively of titled or wealthy citizens, and this wish was granted by the Lord Chief Justice. But after the jury had been sworn and Harry had objected to the inclusion of two London merchants, his counsel suddenly told the judge that their client was 'ready to own his fault' and pay all costs. Thus, in open court, Harry was forced to admit that 'he had don his Lordship wrong; was sorry for it; Begged his pardon; and promised to behave himself dutifully' hereafter.[12]

Kidder revelled in his victory and immediately paid for a notice to be placed in the *Flying Post,* a Whig newspaper, to publicise the 'mortification' of his adversary. For those commentators such as the Somerset-born Whig journalist John

Oldmixon, who were in sympathy with Kidder's religious and political convictions, there was an ironic lesson here; that a Tory country squire such as Harry Bridges, a great 'attester of the divine right of Bishops', was 'otherwise of such [low] morals as not fit for sober History!' Less partial observers recalled, however, that Harry had mockingly portrayed the bishop not only as a religious fanatic but also as spiteful and ridiculous; a man who was so mean he actually 'sold carrots and milk at the pallace' in Wells.[13]

Although Harry and Kidder tried to have each other struck off as magistrates, it was Kidder who succeeded when he showed the Lord Keeper in London that Bridges had been convicted at an assize court in Taunton of speaking ill-words against the king. Kidder also succeeded in having Ann Dunn re-arrested and incarcerated for several months in the county prison at Ilchester. It was later alleged that Harry bribed the jailer and brought 'his excommunicated whore' back to Wells, 'in defyance to the law of God and man'. Yet, after issuing writs to recover his legal costs, and seeing Harry dodging every one of them, in February 1701 Kidder's strategy finally backfired. Having received intelligence that Harry was going to be travelling to Bristol, the plan was for two of the bishop's servants to arrest him on the Mendips, which they tried to do. But during the scuffle that arose, a pistol held by one of the servants accidentally went off, wounding Harry in the arm. Kidder paid John Taylor, an apothecary-surgeon in Wells, to treat the minor injury, and Harry settled part of the costs with which he had been charged. But he also sent a note to the vicar of St Cuthbert's asking him to give public thanks to Almighty God for delivering him from an attempted assassination.[14]

Harry now did everything he could to damage Kidder's reputation, spreading stories about him in the House of Commons, ostentatiously snubbing him at services in the cathedral, and trying repeatedly to have his servants convicted of assault. Far from enjoying his legal victory, Kidder felt that he had become 'the talk of all the Coffee houses in London, as well as in the Country', and not in a good way. Harry also encouraged a High Church friend, the pamphleteer Samuel Hill, vicar of Kilmington and a prebend of the Cathedral, to traduce Kidder's standing in the church, publishing papers claiming that the bishop was in favour of ordaining Presbyterians and was using his high position to undermine the lower clergy's rights. So it was no surprise that when Hill managed to get himself elected as schoolmaster of the free grammar school (King's) at Bruton, an appointment worth £80 a year, Kidder refused to grant him a license on the grounds that he already had a living and a prebendary worth £150 a year, and that he would not be able to meet the demands of another full-time post. The twelve governors of the school were so divided that even after the Lord Keeper had decided that Kidder should lead a new commission to investigate the problem, several of the governors tried, unsuccessfully, to have three of Kidder's adversaries, Edwyn Sandys, Harry Bridges and Claver Morris, appointed to the commission. Yet when the commissioners finally met at Bruton in March 1702, it gradually emerged that under the terms of the school's Tudor charter, they did not have the power to remove Hill from his post.[15]

While these 'scandalous' disputes between Kidder and some of the most privileged members of his diocese were in full swing, Claver was looking after Betty and his mother and building his new house. For the mayors of Bath and Wells there were more pressing problems. At Bath during the summer season, it was feared that the city was being overrun by 'poor and indigent people' who soon ran out of money and 'cannot return home because of their poverty unless they are whipt'; a punishment that the mayor believed 'very inhumane to poor creatures'. And at Wells, fearing that the city was being overrun by pedlars and dishonest market-traders, the mayor ordered his constables 'to search out and apprehend all men and women' who were strangers or who were selling ale without a licence, as well as the usual slew of night-walkers and drunkards.[16] These were serious and persistent problems for small communities, but they were dwarfed by the prospect of another round of savage wars with France.

In July 1700, the last of Princess Anne's children, her eleven-year-old son the duke of Gloucester, died. She had been married and devoted to the congenial Prince George of Denmark since 1683, and after seventeen pregnancies and no surviving children, she was broken-hearted that she would have no more. As king William also had no children, in terms of the bloodline, the heir to the throne would be Anne's half-brother, James, the infant whose birth to Mary of Modena in 1688 had sparked the Glorious Revolution. The infant James's accession had been outlawed, along with all other Catholic heirs, by the Bill of Rights in 1689. Yet nobody could be sure what would happen – who and how many people might support him – if James renounced his Catholicism and tried to reclaim his father's throne, with or without the support of Louis XIV. In September 1700, Carlos II died bequeathing, as expected, the whole of the Spanish empire to Louis XIV's grandson. And a year later, the ousted king James II died; a prince who, in the eyes of most Englishmen, 'after a short and unprosperous reign' had 'indiscreetly attempted to bring in Popery and make himselfe absolute in imitation of the French'.[17] France immediately recognised his son as 'James III', the rightful king of England, Scotland and Ireland.

To preserve a Protestant succession, Parliament had passed the Act of Settlement in June 1701, which meant, after Anne, the crowns of England and Ireland (but not of Scotland, a separate kingdom) would go to a granddaughter of James I, the seventy-year-old Sophia, electress of Hanover and her Protestant children. She was not a Catholic, and that was crucial. But the prospect of a Lutheran duchess-dowager from a minor German principality inheriting and ruling Britain and its growing empire did not fill most people with enthusiasm. A few months after the Act of Settlement, William signed a new treaty with the Dutch Republic and the Holy Roman Emperor, to form another Grand Alliance to combat the French. By then, however, a new war in the Spanish Netherlands had broken out. So, it was no surprise that when William died at Kensington Palace in March 1702, his death did not plunge the whole country into mourning. Though he had died of pneumonia, it had been brought on by a riding accident in which he had fallen from his horse at Hampton Court after it had stumbled on a molehill. The Jacobite supporters of 'James III', the 'Pretender' to the throne, needed to be cautious, but everybody knew what it meant when they raised a toast 'To the little gentleman in black velvet.'

17

WEDDING BELLS

A popular rhyme about the royal family had been coined shortly after the Glorious Revolution of 1689:

> King William thinks all,
> Queen Mary talks all,
> Prince George drinks all,
> And Princess Anne eats all.

Anne became queen in 1702 at the age of thirty-seven. Short in height and overweight, she was attractive, charming, sensible, dutiful and sincerely committed to the Church of England. Unlike her sister Mary, she had a husband, George, who was happy to be her royal consort. So, it was no surprise she was popular, or that she was greeted with adulation by the crowds that gathered at Westminster to see her dressed in her crimson velvet robes, ermine and lace, and with a circlet of gold on her head as she appeared in the procession for her coronation on St George's Day, 23rd April 1702. Having received snubs to her royal status during William and Mary's reign, she was now a great stickler for ceremony and court etiquette, so it was unfortunate that she could not walk to the Abbey due to an attack of gout. Yet it hardly mattered, for being carried in an open chair under a canopy of yellow velvet borne by sixteen barons, she still made a good impression. And she made an even better one in her first address when, echoing the words of her great predecessor Queen Elizabeth, she overcame her natural shyness to say very clearly and melodiously to everyone's delight, 'I know my heart to be entirely English'.[1]

Two weeks later, the new 'Queen of England, Scotland, Ireland and France' made the official declaration: her kingdoms were now at war with Spain and France. It was a popular decision, supported by Anne's most talented and trusted friends and servants, 'the duumvirate' of Lord Godolphin the Lord Treasurer, and

DOI: 10.4324/9781003333654-19

John Churchill, duke of Marlborough, the Captain-General. Another friend and favourite, Sarah Churchill, duchess of Marlborough and Mistress of the Robe, was the most senior lady and skilful politician in the royal household. Supported by the Speaker of the House of Commons, the consummate political operator Robert Harley, this was an exceptionally able team.

At first, the most serious challenge to the government came from the landslide Tory victory in the general election of July. Riding a wave of popular support for Anne, High Church Tory members of the Commons were keen to outlaw the 'abominable hypocrisy' of occasional conformity by which Dissenters could qualify for public offices by taking Anglican communion just once a year, and then return to their Dissenters' meeting house or 'barn'. Such a proscription would not help to unite the Protestant nation at a time of war, and as the government resisted these Tory efforts, so the cry of 'the Church in Danger' grew louder every year.

The war also became another source of great division. In October 1702, morale was high after an Anglo-Dutch fleet won a famous battle by defeating the entire French fleet escorting Spanish treasure ships at Vigo Bay in Spain. But as further decisive victories proved elusive, support for the continuation of the war began to wane. Aside from the carnage of the conflict, the cost was high, even when battles were being won. In addition, the regular loss of English ships to privateers seriously disrupted trade. The Allies' armies and the English payments that supported them were increasing at an alarming rate. Scandals about the prosecution of the war were rife and, as taxes rose, people saw no point in prolonging a conflict in which the safety of the queen and country were not obviously at stake.

In the summer of 1702, it was feared that Prince George's life was in danger due to his chronic asthma. A trip to take the mineral waters at Bath was arranged, and in August the royal couple set out with a train of ministers, courtiers and servants on a progress to the spa, passing through crowds of well-wishers at Oxford and Cirencester on the way. At Lansdown, on the edge of Bath, they were greeted by members of the corporation, a group dancers and hundreds of young boys and girls 'richly attired, many of them like Amazons, with Bows and Arrows, and others with gilt Sceptres'.[2]

Anne's popularity was so high that the corporation of Bristol, England's largest and most prosperous provincial city, which had spent a fortune celebrating the coronation, immediately requested a royal visit. The city was just a dozen miles from Bath, but on 3rd September the roads were so treacherous for the party of thirteen coaches, each drawn by six horses, that a direct route proved impossible. So, Anne only stayed a few hours, just long enough to enjoy the tremendous pageantry provided by a city tour and an enormous dinner held in her honour, before journeying back to Bath. By the time she returned to London, via Marlborough, she had made such a strong impression in the West Country, it would always hold her in great affection. She had also helped her much-loved husband, as it was reckoned his recovery was due to his drinking of Bath's mineral waters.[3]

That summer, Bishop Kidder had also come to Bath to preserve his health, though he did not stay to meet the queen. Perhaps fearing the worst, he was now busy writing his autobiography; an exceptionally self-righteous account of all the battles he had fought, largely against the wicked clergy and citizens of Wells. In this bitter tale, he did not name his wife or children, for it was only with regard to his own reputation that he hoped to set the record straight, whenever these writings might be published after his death.[4] But, by 1702, anyone who knew him as the bishop of Bath and Wells had already made up their mind about his life and character.

In the autumn of 1702, Claver was also writing, neatly setting out the terms of the new leases that he wanted to agree with the illiterate tenant-farmer Henry Bull and his son, for new pastures at West Bradley. Although there were legal disputes over Claver's holdings in the parish, the Bulls agreed a rent of £99 for a two-year period, with Claver's mother as a witness.[5] It was now three years since Elizabeth had died in childbirth, and in that time Claver had also lost some friends. These included Sarah Westley, the 'very kind' wife of William, who, in honour of his wife, had bought a fire engine for the city to be kept under the stairs of the council's chambers in the marketplace. David Trym, the 'wheedling' legal officer to the mayor and corporation who had helped Claver with his will, had also died. So had the troublesome old squire Ned Strode of Downside who left an endowment for the building of houses for 'four poor old men, professing the Protestant religion' in Shepton Mallet.[6] In spite of these bereavements, most things were going well as alongside the treatment of his patients, Claver was managing his estates and playing the sonatas of Albinoni, Bassani, Corelli, Finger, Novell and other composers. He would also enjoy developing Betty's musical abilities, for which he purchased Purcell's *A Choice Collection of Lessons for the Harpsichord* (1st edn, London, 1696), and he always found some private time to read and study.

For a sum of twenty-five shillings, he subscribed to a copy of the first illustrated English encyclopaedia, *Lexicon Technicum: or, an Universal English Dictionary of Arts and Sciences,* by the clergyman John Harris. As befitting a massive work in which Isaac Newton, already reckoned the greatest living scientist, was one of the contributors, the book was 'very Full and Particular in the Mathematicks, because 'tis the only Solid Foundation on which a Useful Enquiry into Nature and all Physical Learning, can possibly be built.' It also contained an unrivalled scholarly effort to define every English word from 'Abacot' to 'Zymosis', which Claver would have relished. Among nearly a thousand other subscribers throughout the country, Wells was exceptionally well represented with over a dozen supporters, as well as its former bishop, Thomas Ken. But when Claver opened the book to peruse the 'List of Subscribers' he would not have been pleased to see his name presented as 'Claudius Morris, M.D. of the City of Wells'.[7]

The second book that he purchased in 1703, *The Craft and Frauds of Physick Expos'd* (1702), would have provided much greater satisfaction. Its author, Dr Robert Pitt FRS, a senior member of the Royal College of Physicians, was on a mission to defend the College's decision, after forty years' debate, to open a dispensary in London to provide free medicines for the poor. While only a few of the

College's 130 members objected, the great majority of the 1000 or more members of the Society of Apothecaries believed that the decision had 'no Charitable design' but was simply an attempt 'to ruine the Apothecaries trade', as they had a monopoly on the sale of all medicines in the city. Putting a break upon the tremendous growth of apothecaries, especially those shopkeepers who peddled medical advice and expensive treatments, was not an unimportant consideration for the College. But Pitt and his supporters had no doubt that a dispensary offering free advice and medicines at no more than 'their Intrinsic value' (normally a penny) would serve 'the Public Good'.[8]

Reading Pitt's declarations – that 'the Sick have been inhumanely opprest by many useless, nauseous and hurtful Medicines, to procure great Profit by the sale of Physick'; that 'the best Medicines have been deny'd you, because they will easily be discovered to be very cheap'; that 'the greatest part of the most efficacious [medicines] grow in our own Gardens' – would have pleased Claver and his colleagues. But Pitt went further, explaining how various ingredients advocated by apothecaries – based on precious metals and stones, animal horns and bones, pearls, mummies, snake skins and swallows' nests – were expensive but 'of no virtue in Medicine'. He also tried to explain the nature of common illnesses and their treatments. None of this would detract from the work of physicians such as Claver who would have been delighted to read about the importance Pitt attached to Chemistry. 'Being practis'd by Gentlemen of Honour, and Physicians of Integrity, [the science of Chemistry] expos'd the impudent Presumptions, and the fraudulent Exactions of all the Chymical Impostors' among quacks and apothecaries.[9]

With a well-established reputation as one of the best physicians in the West Country, an income sufficient to run a coach and horses, a fashionable new house and friends aplenty, it might have appeared that Claver did not want for much. At the age of forty-three, he had been widowed twice, having enjoyed just six years of married life. But he had not given up on the prospect of another match, and after acquiring a new pair of black breeches and a new lining for his green embroidered waistcoat, on 10th May 1703, he set out for a coaching inn at Crewkerne, an ancient town on the road between Exeter and London, where he asked Molly Bragge to be his wife.

Molly, aged thirty-seven, was the eldest daughter of Major William Bragge of Sadborow Hall in Thorncombe, a large village which, for reasons that no-one could reliably recall, was a part of Devon, though the village itself was surrounded by Dorset parishes and ten miles from Lyme Regis on the Dorset coast. Until the dissolution of the monasteries, Sadborow had been one of the manors of Forde Abbey, now a private residence recently inherited by Francis Gwyn MP, and it was from the Bragge family's success as merchants in the local woollen industries that they had acquired the funds to purchase most of Sadborow manor in 1576. So, Mary Bragge, or Molly as she was always known, came from a well-established landed family and was possessed of a very substantial marriage portion of £3,000, should she ever decide to marry.

Although Claver had met Molly's mother years before, briefly prescribing for her at Wells in 1686, she had died in 1693 leaving her husband Major Bragge and five surviving children. Since then, Molly's sister Anne had married and had children with John Leigh of Newport on the Isle of Wight, and her thirty-year-old sister Elizabeth had remained single. But in 1702 another sister, Margaret, had died and was buried with her still-born daughter only a year after her marriage to John Prowse, a gentleman of Compton Bishop near Axbridge. And just before Christmas in 1702, Molly, Anne and Elizabeth had also lost their only brother William, who had left a widow, Edith, and four children.[10]

As a family, the three sisters, their sixty-three-year-old father and their nieces and nephews were very close, so Molly's decision to leave her father and Elizabeth in the family home at Sadborow Hall in order to marry a physician who lived forty miles away would not have passed without a great deal of debate. As a customary act of courtship, on 10th August 1703, three months after their engagement, Claver brought a collection of gold coins (worth a little over £46) to Sadborow to give to Molly, and three weeks later, on 31st August, in St Mary's Church at Thorncombe they were married by the young High Church vicar there, Thomas Cook, to whom Claver also gave a piece of gold.[11]

Apart from Mrs Davies of Crewkerne, there were no special guests invited to the wedding. Molly's father, her sister Elizabeth, and her father's steward were witnesses. Alongside Claver's coachman and the head gardener there were a dozen other household servants to whom Claver gave £3. Molly stayed at Sadborow until Claver returned with his new coach and horses on 18th September to bring her home to Wells. They were in no hurry. With a train of Major Bragge's coach and horses, several of his servants and Molly's sister, the couple stopped at the Red Lion at Somerton. The landlords, the Fishers, were Claver's patients, so it was no surprise that they treated Claver and Molly to an entertainment led by fiddlers. The wedding party then spent two nights with Sir Henry and Lady Sarah Gould at Sharpham Park. From here it was ten miles to the Liberty, and on 25th September they 'both came home to Wells'. It was not a quiet occasion, for on their way the couple were met by about a hundred well-wishers on horseback, and as they entered the city the bells of both St Cuthbert's and the cathedral were ringing out in celebration.[12]

18
THE GREAT STORM

After Major Bragge's horses had been rested at the Christopher inn, his coach was returned to Sadborow, and a month later a horse with a pillion saddle was hired to carry Molly's sister Elizabeth back home. Molly also rode pillion with Claver on a trip to Compton Bishop near Axbridge, where her sister Margaret had been buried after dying in childbirth less than a year before. Margaret's husband, John Prowse, lord of the manor, had succeeded his father, inheriting the family's estates at the age of twelve in 1688, and since then Claver had been the family's doctor, looking after John, his mother and his two sisters.

When Molly and Claver visited the Prowses in 1703, the recently widowed John was only twenty-seven, but he had already shown himself to be something of a gentleman when, at the age of twenty, he had defended the reputation of a young woman who was being repeatedly abused. As well as visiting Margaret's grave, there was business to attend to. Claver was preparing to put up security for his marriage; the manor of West Bradley, its cottages and about 60 acres of land, as well as the 50 acres of his estate at Felton on the Mendips. But these business interests did not detract from the couple's growing friendship with John Prowse, and Claver was quite determined to find him a new wife.[1]

In mid-August 1703, Queen Anne (for her gout) and Prince George (for his asthma) returned to Bath and, to the delight of the city's corporation and traders, they stayed until October. However, Claver and Molly were still too busy settling into their new home to join the throng of visitors to Bath. Claver's mother, Hannah, was still living with them, helping to care for Betty, who was now nearly six years old. But Hannah's help as a grandmother was no longer so essential, as it was clear that Molly was going to love and care for Claver's daughter as if she were her own. In the garden, Claver had planted autumn fruits, and in November, before the weather changed, he took a dish to pick and eat the 'very ripe Raspberrys' with

DOI: 10.4324/9781003333654-20

Betty and his mother.[2] But this was a calm before the storm, for after weeks of driving rain, on Friday 26th November a storm broke through the night, 'the like not known in the memory of man'.[3]

Across the south of England, thousands of people lost their lives, and the physical damage was immense as the tempest tore up trees (4,000 oaks in the New Forest alone), wrecked buildings and sunk ships. It even destroyed landmarks like the Eddystone Lighthouse on the Plymouth coast, killing Henry Winstanley, its creator, along with his workmen. At Bristol and over the Somerset Levels the hurricane winds and high tides drove seawater into the streets and warehouses of the city, and drowned thousands of sheep and other animals across the moors. According to a farmer, the tempest was so strong in Somerset that, even lying flat on the ground and holding on to stones, 'I had hard matter to save myself from being lifted up from the earth by the vast winds'.[4] Inevitably, it was not long before people were proclaiming that the storm was 'a Judgement of GOD on this Nation'.[5] Even the most diligent chronicler of the event, the Dissenter and Londoner Daniel Defoe, thought that the loss of the royal navy's ships was a punishment for its poor performance against the French and Spanish fleets in the first year of the new war.

Defoe himself was about to be recruited by Robert Harley, Speaker of the House of Commons, as a secret agent for the government. But in 1703 he was best known to the public as the author of an anonymous pamphlet, *The Shortest-Way with the Dissenters* (1702), in which he impersonated the views of High Church firebrands like the clergyman Dr Henry Sacheverell who not only objected to the hypocrisy of occasional conformity but to the very tolerance of Dissenters and their meeting houses. Thinking that he could employ heavy irony to expose the inflammatory rhetoric of such zealots, Defoe proposed that it was time 'to pull up this heretical Weed of Sedition, that has so long disturb'd the Peace of our Church'. He conceded that 'Tis Cruelty to kill a Snake or a Toad in cold Blood, but the Poison of their [Dissenters'] Nature makes it a Charity to our Neighbours, to destroy those Creatures'. So, they should be sent to the gallows or sold as galley slaves. Unfortunately, no-one was amused and, after dodging arrest, Defoe was imprisoned, pilloried and bankrupt.[6]

Although he had been convicted of seditious libel and his *Shortest-Way* had certainly misfired, in a flash of journalistic genius a week after the great storm, Defoe placed an advertisement in the *London Gazette,* promising to publish 'an exact and faithful collection' of what had happened up and down the country on that dreadful night, if 'gentlemen' would send their honest accounts to his publisher in London. Among over sixty letters that he published (all but three of them from men), several were sent from Somerset, and the most important of these came from Edith Conyers, the widow of a Bristol wine merchant who now lived in Wells. Edith was neither wealthy nor distinguished, but she was probably the most impartial public witness to the fate of the most prominent victims of the storm.[7]

According to Edith, at the palace in Wells, the bishop and his lady were 'killed by the Fall of two Chimney Stacks, which fell on the Roof, and drove it in upon my Lord's Bed, forced it quite through the Flower [floor] down into the Hall, and buried them both in the Rubbish'. She added: 'tis supposed my Lord was getting up, for he was found some Distance from my Lady, who was found in her Bed; but my Lord had his Morning Gown on, so that tis supposed he was coming from the Bed just as it [the chimney] fell'. Around the city, other chimneys had collapsed, two small houses had been flattened, an abundance of apple and elm trees had been rooted up, and wheat and hay stacks blown away. According to Edith, however, there was 'no other Accident as to Death in this Town or near it'. The fact that 'no one either in the palace, or in the whole town, beside them, had any hurt', made it all the more astonishing to the former bishop Thomas Ken; especially as it happened on 'the very day of the Cloth Fair' in the city, 'when all the country were spectators of the deplorable calamity, and soon spread the sad story'.[8]

Such an improbable event astonished the whole nation, and required an explanation. For those who supported Kidder's convictions it was simply a tragic accident for Wells to lose 'a Grave and Excellent Divine, who had presided over that Diocess [of Bath and Wells] with great Honour, Clemency, and Piety'.[9] But this was not the majority opinion. An Oxford correspondent bluntly wrote that the bishop was 'found with his Brains dash'd out'; a view that at least one other correspondent shared. At the 'Conclusion' of his book *The Storm* (1704), Defoe explained that to preserve their authenticity, he had not changed the 'country' or 'homely Stile' of the letters he had received for publication by 'dressing them in other words'. There was, however, one letter that he could not print. This was from a gentleman at Somerton who had heard that, rather than accept the demands of the lower clergy, Kidder had said '*he had rather have his Brains knock'd out'*. For Defoe, the fact that this correspondent took 'the Disaster for a Judgment of God' was less important than the fact that he had 'filled his Letter with some Reflexions indecent [about the bishop]'. Even this was insufficient grounds for its suppression, but as the correspondent had not signed his name, Defoe felt that it was not right to 'leave a Charge on the Name of that Unfortunate Gentleman [Kidder]' who, 'being dead could not answer, and we alive could not prove [it].'[10]

While Kidder's life, and the providential nature of his death, would always be contested, in terms of his own aims for his leadership of Bath and Wells there was no great legacy. For all his sympathetic treatment of Dissenters, including Quakers, most members of his diocese were probably less tolerant of them now than they had been at the start of William's reign, when Kidder was appointed. This was due largely to the growing fears of Anglicans that the Church was being undermined by 'false brethren' from within; fears that Kidder's character and behaviour as a bishop did nothing to allay. More specifically, his tireless efforts to check the 'traditional privileges' – or, as he saw it, the 'corruption and abuses' – of the dean and chapter left no lasting mark.

Kidder could only watch as the grip of Robert Creighton, the music-loving and Presbyterian-hating precentor, grew even stronger with the assistance of his children. By 1704, Creighton's son was vicar of Combe St Nicholas near Chard.

His eldest daughter, Katherine, was married to the Irishman Henry Layng, subdean of the cathedral and the nephew of Dean Bathurst, a man for whom Kidder had a particular contempt. Creighton's second daughter, Margaret ('Peggy'), was married to John Pope, the vicar of St Cuthbert's. And his youngest daughter, Frances, was married to Marshall Brydges, a residential canon and chancellor of the bishop's court. Claver had been the doctor to all of these children, as well as to their aunt Catherine Poulett, so it was no surprise that after they were married, they remained his friends and patients.

A few months before Kidder's death, in 1703 his *bête noire* Ralph Bathurst, the dean of Bath and Wells for over thirty years, had added a seventh codicil to a will that he had been writing for five years. At the age of eighty-three, he was now 'stark-blind, deaf and memory-lost', according to one acquaintance. In his will he said that he had 'not made it the labour of my life to live great or dye wealthy', and had already spent over £2,000 on building a new chapel for Trinity College Oxford. But he was determined that scores of friends and servants and the poor would benefit from his estate. So, among his legacies, £100 was left to Wells almshouses; books and money were bequeathed to the libraries of the cathedral and the choral vicars; and fifteen-shilling rings were left for his friends in the Liberty, including Claver Morris.[11] Similarly, when a former mayor of Wells, Archibald Harper, an old clothworker, died in 1713, he bequeathed his dwelling house and part of its garden in Chamberlain Street, plus £500, to set up a charitable trust for 'five poor and decayed wool-combers of the city'.[12]

By contrast, Kidder had always regretted his decision to accept the bishopric of Bath and Wells, and never felt valued or at home in either city. So it was unsurprising that his legacy was negligible. There were no buildings to mark his presence or any other signs of generosity, and just a perfunctory £10 was left in his will 'to the poor of Wells', though thousands were bequeathed to each of his two daughters, who both left the city immediately.[13] Most of the inhabitants of Wells, or the diocese, had not cared for Kidder in his lifetime, and comparing his legacies with those of men like Bathurst and Harper, it was unlikely that anyone would change their mind now that he was dead.

At Anne's Court, where there had been a plan to transfer Kidder to the less prestigious diocese of Carlisle, it was no surprise that within weeks of Kidder's death the queen had chosen Dr George Hooper, a royal chaplain, a firm Anglican and a man she knew and trusted, as his successor. She had only appointed Hooper as bishop of St Asaph in the summer of 1703, and at first he declined the new offer on the grounds that he believed his lifelong friend Thomas Ken should be restored to Bath and Wells. The queen agreed but, being 'disabled by rheumatic and colick pains', Ken felt unable to return to pastoral duties, though he was delighted that his former diocese would not have to suffer another 'Latitudinarian Traditour [traitor]' like Kidder, and he strongly urged Hooper to accept. At £1,400 a year, the bishopric of Bath and Wells was worth more than twice that of St Asaph's, and was also of a higher status, so Hooper required no further encouragement.[14]

In Wells, the dean and chapter did not hesitate to accept Anne's 'permission to choose' Hooper, and by January 1704 the matter was settled to everyone's delight, especially as Anne had also granted a pension of £200 a year to Ken. After Hooper's enthronement by proxy on 3rd April 1703, the citizens of Wells were eager to know what their new bishop would be like. Opinion was mixed. His former headmaster at Westminster and treasurer of Wells cathedral, Dr Busby, reckoned that when George was just a boy he was 'the least favoured in features of any [boy] in the School, [but] he will be the most extraordinary of any of them', for the breadth of his learning was astonishing. Gilbert Burnet, the low-church Whig writer and bishop of Salisbury who was out of favour under Anne, regarded Hooper as 'a man of Learning and good conduct', who was also 'reserved, crafty and ambitious'.[15] It was undoubtedly true that Hooper was a good scholar, an exceptional mathematician and a master of Arabic, but it was also true that similarly great academic abilities had not endeared his predecessor Kidder to the dean and chapter. Far more important to his chances of success was his reputation as a High-Church Anglican; someone who genuinely believed the cry of 'The Church in Danger', and was quite prepared to say so. Having a respectable and sociable family that felt at home in Wells would also help.

On arrival in Wells at the age of sixty-three, George Hooper had been married for twenty-five years to Abigail, the forty-eight-year-old daughter of a wealthy cavalier and brewer from Lambeth. Together they had had seven daughters and two sons, most of whom had died in infancy. Hooper had also lost his siblings although he had a nephew, Edmund, who also came to live at Wells. So, by the time the Hooper family arrived at the re-roofed palace in September 1704, there were only two surviving daughters; Abigail aged nineteen, and Rebecca who was ten years younger, plus their uncle Charles Guilford who resided in the Liberty.

It was a good time for Hooper to set about restoring the fractured relationship between the bishop and the dean and chapter for, following the death of Bathurst, a new dean, Dr William Grahme, a Clerk of the Closet to Queen Anne, had been appointed in the summer. Although Grahme briefly took up residence in Wells, his general absence and lack of interest in the diocese meant that Hooper would have a much freer hand in his dealings with the chapter than might otherwise have been the case. There were other good omens too. Queen Anne's Bounty, a popular scheme for relieving the poverty of the Church of England's lower clergy had also been approved, raising the spirits of the clergy as a whole. And on 2nd August 1704, under the command of the duke of Marlborough and Prince Eugene of Savoy, over 50,000 British, Dutch and Imperial troops had won an extraordinary victory at Blenheim on the banks of the Danube in southern Germany. The Allies had lost about 13,000 men, but over twice as many French and Bavarian soldiers had been killed or captured; the Austrian empire had been saved; and the heaviest defeat had been inflicted upon Louis XIV's army, wrecking the myth of its invincibility. In England, Anne rewarded Marlborough with a deer park in Oxfordshire, where Blenheim Palace would be built for about £250,000; a cost that would inevitably raise questions and complaints. But, meanwhile, stories and celebrations of the army's victory would lift the country's spirit and confidence for several years.

While Claver looked forward to the prospect of forming a good relationship with the new bishop and his family (something that was soon accomplished as Lady Hooper and her brother called upon him for advice), by the summer of 1704 he too had cause for celebration as Molly was expecting her first child. In anticipation, he had bought four gallons of Spanish wine, and Mary was born on 6th January 1705 and baptised in the cathedral twelve days later. For the christening, bottles of claret, four gallons of brandy, six pints of sweet white wine from the Canary Islands, and ten pints of strong 'October' beer were also needed, though the party spirit would last for weeks as friends arrived from far and wide to wish the family well. Betty was now eight years old and attending Grace Pierce's day-school in Wells for sixpence a week. But Claver was more interested in her musical education than her sewing; henceforward, she would also be learning the violin for two guineas, and taking singing lessons for another guinea, every year.[16]

Having baby Mary, young Betty and a new household of maids and servants to manage, Molly was busier than she had ever been as the eldest daughter of Major Bragge at Sadborow Hall. And Claver was also planning the biggest investment of his life at this time. In 1704 he had purchased the lease on land at Dulcote, just a mile south of Wells.[17] Now he wanted to buy 110 acres of very fertile land on the coastal plains near Weston-super-Mare, twenty miles from Wells. Ebdon Farm was owned by Ashe Wyndham, 'a young gentleman of very considerable estate' who was rumoured to be 'the richest commoner in the country', though he was also reckoned to have become 'a downright atheist, a commonwealthsman [republican], and an Italian in his morals' due to his time abroad. For Claver, such a character would not have been endearing, but Ashe came from the Norfolk branch of the Wyndham family, and this was purely a business venture even if Claver's friendship with the Wyndhams of Somerset had helped to seal the deal. Having paid Ashe Wyndham £1,470 for the land, he could now expect an income of £80 a year from Joseph Cook, the husbandman who already leased and worked the farm.[18]

For all his work as a physician, Claver was now a landed gentleman – and quite a wealthy one. By February 1705, all of the £3,000 of Molly's marriage portion had been paid by Major Bragge in cash or kind, enabling Claver to pay £947 for a farm at Sand Park, near Wedmore, and £1,050 for Perridge Farm in Pilton. He could also afford to build a new brewhouse for £40, loan hundreds of pounds to local families, including the Dawes of Ditcheat, and to help his servant, Jane Walker, 'she being poor', to clear her debts.[19] So it was befitting that he commissioned the London goldsmith Jeremiah Marlow to engrave the seal of his new coat-of-arms (his red lions and the Bragge's red bulls) onto a carnelian-stone ring.[20]. However busy he was with his new estates, he would always find time for friends, though sometimes he may have wished he had stayed at home. On a Saturday evening during May 1706, while enjoying one of his customary trips to read the London newspapers at the Mitre tavern in Sadler Street, he was among half a dozen locals in the parlour, including the apothecary Charles Baron and the haberdasher John Browne, when there was an altercation between two lawyers he knew well, Robert Quirke and Francis Day. Quirke believed that Day had repeatedly insulted him by calling him 'an old knave'. With everyone watching, Claver, acting as the peacemaker, tried his best 'to divert ye discourse'. But it was to no avail; Quirke clearly felt sufficiently aggrieved to take the matter further by suing Day for defamation.[21]

Though of no significance, 'the libel' at the Mitre was a telling reminder that in Wells there were always rivalries and scores to settle, no matter how trivial they seemed. Six months earlier, before the annual celebrations on 5th November 1705, Claver was himself aggrieved when the city's corporation 'put to the vote of this house whether Claver Morris Dr in Physick should have leave of this house to be admitted into any company or society belonging to this city, in order to make him free[man] thereof'. At this meeting, his friend Ben Taylor, an innkeeper, was admitted to the Stocking-makers' Company, and two other friends, John Prowse of Axbridge, and William Berkeley (the younger brother of the MP for Wells) were admitted to the more prestigious Company of Mercers. In these cases, there was no need for any vote: Taylor was from a well-known local family, and Prowse and Berkeley were old gentry. But Claver's application was rejected. After twenty years in residence he was still a newcomer, with no deep family roots or ties to call upon. So in 1706, he still had plenty of work to do in terms of cultivating friends and favours if he were ever to become a freeman of the city he loved.[22]

19

THE TOLLING BELL

Alongside his thriving medical practice, Claver still found time to keep abreast of new ideas, and the surest way of doing this was to keep his reading up-to-date. In the field of medicine, Dr Thomas Sydenham, a Puritan physician from Dorset who had died in 1689, was already considered 'the English Hippocrates'. Famous for his insistence upon the careful examination of patients and for his hostility to any over-dependence upon academic theories, Sydenham believed that you might as well send a man to the University of Oxford to learn shoe-making as to learn how to practise medicine. Though he championed the use of laudanum (tincture of opium) to relieve suffering, he also believed that 'the arrival of a good clown exercises a more beneficial influence on the health of a town than of twenty asses laden with drugs'. Such a practical approach clearly appealed to Claver, who bought the third edition of Sydenham's *Opera Universa* in 1705.

He also bought two works by another highly regarded young English physician, Dr Richard Mead, who had trained at the universities of Utrecht and Leiden and who was trying to apply Newtonian principles of observation and the use of mathematics to medical problems. By 1705, Mead's *Mechanical Account of Poisons* (1702), on snake venom, and his *De Imperio Solis ac Lunae in Corpora Humana* (1704), exploring the influence of the sun and moon on the diseases of the human body (including thoughts on the causes of the high tides and floods of the Great Storm), had already attracted much attention. Yet Claver also purchased books by less famous authors; works such as James Harvey's *Praesagium Medicum: or the Prognostick Signs of Acute Diseases* (1706) and T. Hicks's *A Compleat Treatise of Urines, Shewing the Right Method of Urinal Prognostication* (1703), which reflected his desire to learn about the latest methods of diagnosis.

This interest in the acquisition of knowledge through the meticulous observation of nature and the use of mathematics for measurement (as opposed to the uncritical following of traditional beliefs) was driving the rise of modern science,

DOI: 10.4324/9781003333654-21

and it was central to Claver's studies. Works such as the 1704 translation of Georgio Baglivi's *The Practice of Physick, Reduc'd to the Ancient Way of Observations* (Rome, 1698) were based upon the belief that 'to form a right Judgement of Diseases is a very difficult Matter' that could only be achieved by close examination of the patient and the exercise of scepticism towards conventional thinking. Similarly, Claver was keen to acquire the 1704 translation of the French chemist Louis Lémery's work *A Treatise of Foods* (Paris, 1702), which examined the best sort of foods for medicinal use and the effects that they produced. The well-illustrated folio translation of the German surgeon Matthias Purmann's *Chirurgia Curiosa: or, the Newest and most Curious Observations and Operations in the Whole Art of Chirurgery [Surgery]* (1706) was another text that proposed new practices, though many, such as the recommendation to use mercury-based ointments and pills for the treatment of syphilis, remained unchanged.

Reflecting his wider interests, Claver bought new books on history and mathematics, including the long-awaited three volumes of Clarendon's *History of the Rebellion and Civil Wars in England* (1702–1704), the 700-page *Supplement* (1705) to Le Clerk's two-volume *Dictionary*, which he had purchased in 1701, and a copy of Edward Cocker's *Decimal Arithmetic* (3rd edn, 1703). In matters of religion he was still looking to the past, buying George Stanhope's translation of *Pious Breathings: Being the Meditations of St Augustine* (2nd edn, 1704) and a new edition of the Catholic writer John Austin's *Devotions in the Ancient Way* (1st edn, 1668), a collection of psalms, hymns and prayers for everyday use which had recently been adapted for Protestant worship, and which Claver bought as a gift for his new father-in-law, Major Bragge.[1]

From all his learning and years of practice, Claver knew that if he were to observe someone with 'an Inflammatory Fever, accompanied by an Eruption or breaking out of small red Spots, like Flea-bites, that by degrees increase, and ripening like little Boils, grow full of Matter', he was facing trouble. And if the patient was suffering from 'a great Heat, a swift and labouring Pulse, pain in the Back, Vomiting, Sickness and Head-ache', he needed to act quickly. The problem was that, despite its prevalence, there was very little agreement about the best way to treat the dreaded smallpox; as the death of Queen Mary in 1694 had shown. The great physician Sydenham believed that the disease had a lower mortality among the poor, precisely because they could not afford the expensive treatments of the rich, such as bloodletting and multiple prescriptions. Consequently, he refused to confine any patient to bed until the fourth day of their illness, and thereafter recommended a 'cool regimen', as opposed to the traditional 'warm' regime based upon a heated room, loads of blankets and hot drinks. Some authorities, such as Gideon Harvey, agreed that bloodletting was more likely to kill than cure, but most believed that everything depended upon the condition of the patient as the disease progressed.[2]

According to Sir Richard Blackmore, one of the queen's physicians whose 'Method of Cure' mixed elements of both the 'cool' and 'warm' regimes, at the first sign of the disease it was essential to 'let blood to a considerable Quantity' (about a pint) and to administer a vomit twelve hours later. At the second stage, when the patient was having difficulty breathing and suffering from a swollen throat and a face full of growing pustules, it was time for laudanum and bloodletting from the veins under the tongue. Thereafter, as he frankly admitted, there was nothing more that anyone could do but let Nature take her course. In this, the final stage of the disease, 'the most Malignant Confluent Kind will hear no Reason, but puts all Methods and Medicines out of Countenance; and in these deplorable Instances the Physician will shew his Judgment and Honesty by declaring that the Case is above the Reach of Skill and Remedies, and inconsistent with Hopes of Recovery'.[3] If these patients survived, probably with pock-marked faces, and possibly with blindness or severe disfigurements, there was the consolation that, having been infected once, they were almost certainly now immune for life.

Claver was quite used to facing difficult decisions about how best to treat his patients – that was the job of a physician. But when the lives of both his daughters, as well as his man-servant and apprentice-boy, were at stake, he was confronted with the kind of choices that no father or physician would ever want to make. So, he must have feared the worst when nine-year-old Betty and baby Mary contracted smallpox in December 1706, even though Mary's mother found a live-in nurse to tend to them and the servants for three months. Over the critical period of the first three weeks as the smallpox ran its course through each person and Claver did what he thought best, he probably prayed as much as he prescribed. Betty survived but, on 18th December, three weeks before her second birthday, Mary succumbed to the disease. Immediately, to mark her death and to ward off any evil spirits, the heavy sound of the cathedral's biggest bell, the 'Harewell', could be heard across the city for an hour.

Claver's first wife, Grace, had been buried on a freezing day at Manston in January 1689, six months after the death of their baby. At Manston, they were laid together in the most sacred place, under the altar, where Claver's father and mother would offer prayers. His second wife, Elizabeth, had been buried a decade later with her still-born daughter in August 1699, in the family crypt at Ditcheat. Since then, Claver had erected notable monuments in both churches. As Mary had been baptised in the cathedral, that is where they wished her to be interred. But, first, a messenger was sent to bring Mr Ivyleafe from Wedmore, ten miles west of Wells, to paint a posthumous portrait of her; a small coffin needed to be assembled and lined; and mourning clothes, gloves and scarves made for the family and nurse Tanner.

By convention, after every death a passing bell would be rung nine times for a man, six times for a woman and three times for a child, followed by a short pause before a chime was rung for each full year of the departed's life. It was a sequence that could be repeated for however long the bereaved family desired and how much they were prepared to pay. At noon on 23rd December, the day of Mary's funeral, with three strikes for a child, and one strike for her single full year of life, the Great Harewell of the cathedral rang out the simple message for three hours. It did not take long for the funeral procession to make its way from the East Liberty, around the corner of St Andrew Street, under the Chain Gate footbridge, and into the north porch of the cathedral. Next to the porch door, there were sculptures of a wolf retrieving the head of St Edmund the Martyr after his beheading, and a figure holding a banner reading 'INTRA IN GAVDIVM DOMINI TVI', 'Enter thou into the joy of the Lord'. A grave, walled and plastered over six feet deep, had been prepared in the Lady Chapel, directly behind the high altar of the Choir, in the open space between the slender marble pillars where people would often walk and congregate before a service. In the fourteenth century, the Chapel itself was built as an addition to the east end of the cathedral, where daily mass was sung. But it was as spacious as a modest parish church, and its five large stained-glass windows and star-vaulted ceiling were legendary. With the accompaniment of music from the small organ of the Chapel, this was as good a place as anywhere to lay Mary to rest.[4]

'The Order for the Burial of the Dead' from the Book of Common Prayer was meant to help all mourners come to terms with death and to uphold their faith: 'in the midst of Life we are in Death'; 'The Lord gave, and the Lord hath taken away'. But it could not say anything directly about the meaning of Mary's particular life and death. For this, the cathedral itself might have helped. Its presence explained why Claver had first come to Wells, and it was the place where he had prayed almost every week for twenty years. Most poignantly, this was where Mary had been baptised, at the Saxon font where babies had been christened for a thousand years. From the great West Front of the cathedral to the smell of the chained books in the cathedral Library, Claver knew each part of this medieval wonder intimately. Close observation was in his nature and training, so there was little that he would ever miss or pass without a thought. He knew that all the stained-glass windows, like the famous Jesse window depicting the genealogy of Jesus, were packed with stories from the Bible, and there were hundreds of inscriptions on the walls and floors, on the tombs of former bishops and in the chapels, all bearing witness to a Christian life and the grief of death. But there was little here that spoke about the death of a baby daughter, and even less to a ten-year-old sister about her loss.

In his *Directions for Prayer,* Bishop Ken had urged all parents 'Be sure to teach your Children with all the sweetness and gentleness you can', so that religion would always seem a blessing, not a burden. This was a sentiment that Claver and Molly shared. Just as Claver was keen for Betty to love singing, dancing and playing music, he wanted her to love the cathedral too; not as a historic space in which everything sounded different, or as a place where strange rules and rituals were observed by men who often preached for what could seem like days, but as somewhere that she, like her father, would always feel that she belonged. So, in the north transept, Claver would have enjoyed showing Betty the amazing astronomical clock; a fourteenth-century model of the Christian universe showing the motion of the sun and the phases of the moon (with Phoebe the moon-goddess) as they revolved around the earth. Above the colourful clock-face there was a stage-set carousel on which four jousting horsemen span around, two in each direction, when the hours were struck. Their cue for action was the ringing of small bells at the hands and heels of a curious life-size figure, known locally as Jack Blandiver, who was sitting high-up, minding his own business in a sentry-box on a wall nearby. On the carousel, one of the poor horsemen would be knocked down every time that he appeared, at least on every hour for over three hundred years. Even so, he still lived in hope, always sitting up each time behind the scenes, before re-appearing to receive another blow.[5]

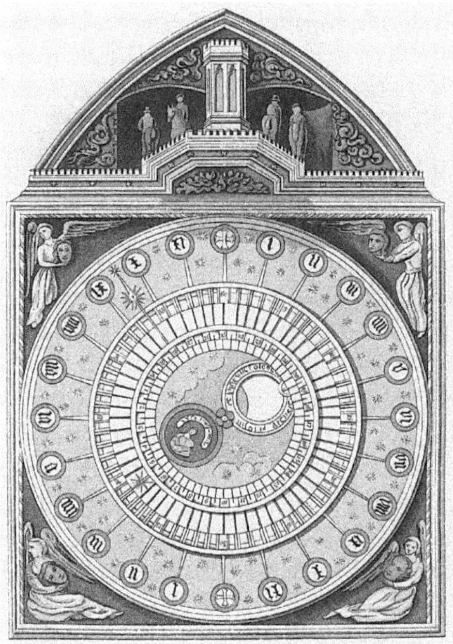

FIGURE 11 The astronomical clock

In the Choir, where Claver attended matins at six o'clock several times a week, there were over sixty stalls for prebends and other clergy whose seats were fitted with misericords (oak ledges) to provide support when standing during hours of prayer. On most misericords there was a meticulous sculpture of a familiar creature. Most required no explanation, for the delight lay in the simplicity and character of the depiction: a sleeping dog; a cat playing the fiddle; a ewe suckling a lamb; a fox preaching to four geese, one of which had fallen asleep. But many of the sculptures raised questions about their meaning: a mermaid suckling a lion; a monkey with a squirrel on a lead; a bearded man on lion's legs. There were similar stories and mysteries depicted on the capital stones at the top of columns around the whole cathedral. Near the astronomical clock, four capitals told the story of what happened to two men who had stolen grapes. Above the Saxon font there were sculptures of a man grimacing with toothache; a farmer pursuing a fox with a goose in its mouth; and a woman pulling a thorn out of her foot.[6] But these were curious things for Betty and Claver to explore on other days.

After the funeral service, a stone slab was laid over Mary's grave, on which the dates of her birth and death would be engraved under a coat of arms combining Claver's three lions and the Bragge family's three bulls. A Latin couplet completed the inscription, and it spoke of the grief at suddenly losing such a bright and hopeful child. When everyone was ready, the great bell tolled again. It would soon be melted down to be re-cast, as it was too susceptible to cracks, but on the afternoon of Mary's funeral it rang for at least another hour while the mourners made their way to Claver's house for dinner, and as much claret and sherry as they could drink.[7]

In 1707 Claver also lost two of his oldest friends. The first, at the age of sixty-three, was Colonel Edward Berkeley of Pylle, whose family he had been treating for nearly twenty years. Edward left Elizabeth, his wife, the £500 due from her marriage settlement, and everything he thought she might still need: jewellery, a coach and horse, two saddle horses, six of his best cows and six of the best plough-oxen. He left £1,400 and lands worth £118 a year in trust for his youngest son William. The rest of the estate went to his twenty-six-year-old eldest son Maurice, already MP for Wells. But these legacies were not the only things on his mind. He felt the need to 'earnestly request' in his final wishes 'that after I am gone there may not only be Peace but an entire Friendship and Kindness between 'em [his wife and children] which will procure God's Blessing'.[8] The second friend that Claver lost was old Richard Cupper who died leaving his apothecary's shop to his son, who was soon admitted into the Mercers' Company in place of his father and was also made a constable.[9] A decade earlier, Claver had helped the son to clear his name from allegations of a clandestine marriage. Having been married to Grace Ford for seven years, and now approaching forty, Richard was sufficiently settled and experienced to take over the important and lucrative business of preparing medicines according to Claver's orders. For Claver would not risk his reputation on an apothecary who was anything less than excellent and loyal to a fault.

The loss of these good friends hurt, but Claver was pleased that after two years of urging John Prowse, the thirty-year-old squire from Axbridge, to court Abigail, the twenty-two year-old daughter of Bishop Hooper, his labours as a match-maker had finally borne fruit.[10] Claver and Molly had been friends with John ever since the death of his first wife, Molly's sister, in 1702. Since the arrival of Hooper in 1704, Claver and Molly had also become friendly with the bishop and his family. Claver visited the palace as their doctor and even bought two of Hooper's books: one on the false claims of the Roman Catholic church to infallibility; and the other on the meaning of Lent, though these were not texts that he would normally have rushed to read. By the autumn John and Abigail were married and expecting their first child. By the standards of most gentry families, the couple were wealthy, and soon after their son Thomas was born, in May 1708 John was elected by the freeholders of Somerset to represent the county as one of its MPs; an election that was not contested but was well supported by his father-in-law, the bishop.[11] So, after the bitter disputes with Kidder, by 1708 it must have seemed that Claver and Molly were not only going to live in peace with the bishop's palace but that the Hooper, Prowse and Morris families would become the best of friends.

Within the Morris family the most pressing decision to be made in 1708 concerned the future of Betty's education. She had been attending Mrs Heath's day-school in the city, and been having extra lessons on how to sew and how to play the violin, but this would not ensure that she became a fully accomplished lady. Yet, how exactly this might be achieved was largely a matter of opinion and tradition. In seeking out the best advice it was natural for Claver to turn to books before making up his mind, so he bought a copy of *Instructions for the Education of a Daughter* (2nd edn, 1708). Written by François Fénelon, the archbishop of Cambrai, since its first publication in 1687 the book had been a great success, leading to Fénelon's appointment as a tutor to Louis XIV's grandson. It had been translated by the former dean of Worcester, George Hickes, so its pedigree was impeccable.

Although Fénelon held quite conservative views about the nature of women, he believed that 'there is nothing more neglected, than the Education of a Daughter', not only to support the happiness and moral welfare of any particular family, but for the benefit of society as a whole. When properly educated, a woman could exercise her vital role in raising children and managing the household, and this was by far the best defence against the rise of luxury, vanity and immorality in society. According to Fénelon, there was no need to make girls 'ridiculous, by making them learned', for 'it is not their Business either to govern the State, or to make War'.[12] Nor did girls need to learn any modern languages, other than French, as these were generally corrupting. Yet the range of learning recommended by Fénelon was much broader than that traditionally expected of a girl. It included Latin, reading, writing, mathematics, history, music and needlework, as well as instruction in religion. Moreover, according to Fénelon, as girls were more naturally responsive, sensitive and inquisitive than boys, there was no need for most of the coercive methods and punishments commonly deployed in educating boys.

These views would have found a ready home in Claver's mind and probably in Molly's too, for, in Betty's eyes, Molly was her 'best friend' as well as 'mother'. So, by the spring of 1708, ten-year-old Betty was enrolled at Mrs Deer's boarding-school at Salisbury, for £12 a year. Here, there were separate teachers for writing, dancing, learning the violin, French and other subjects, all requiring an entrance fee of ten shillings. A former chorister and choral vicar of Wells, Anthony Walkeley, had been appointed organist of Salisbury cathedral in 1700 (when Claver had attended a St Cecilia's day concert in the city), and he was one of Claver's friends. Thus, Betty would be given extra lessons from this young composer and musician. Even so, it was a hard decision to leave Betty at the school, and to encourage everyone to take good care of her he gave tips (of various sizes) to all the staff: Mrs Watts 'the teacher who dresses her'; 'the cook maid'; 'the maid she likes best' (who received the biggest tip); and 'the other maid'. For Betty's pocket money, he left thirteen shillings with Mrs Deer, and gave Betty herself a guinea and half a crown. There was no doubt that in Wells, Betty would be missed, though Claver would write to her regularly, and also to Mrs Deer. At the boarding-school, there was at least a little comfort for Betty: her father paid Mrs Deer to provide her with sixpence-worth of fruit each week; this was the most costly item of her education, other than her accommodation.[13]

With Betty away, Claver had more time for studies of his own, and his purchases and his collection of books from shops in London, Sherborne, Bath and Wells, was growing.[14] He acquired:

- Bundles of new music, including 'Bassani's Sonata in D'; 'Sets of Airs'; Daniel Purcell's *The Judgement of Paris* (1701); *Songs in the New Opera call'd Thomyris,* arranged by Pepusch (1707) as well as the *Symphonies or Instrumental Parts* for the work (1707); and Tibaldi's *Sonatas or Chamber Aires* (1708).
- Practical books: *Dictionarium Rusticum* (2 vols, 1704) by Nathan Bailey, an illustrated guide to gardening, husbandry and 'All Sorts of Country Affairs'; an edition of *The Vermin-killer* (1st edn, 1680), 'a Compleat and Necessary Family-book' showing the best way to destroy a host of unwanted creatures, from frogs and fleas to wasps and weasels; a copy of the schoolmaster, Elisha Coles' *The Newest, Plainest and Shortest Shorthand* (1st edn, 1674); and the Tory astrologer, George Parker's *Ephemeris*, an almanac for 1707.
- Medical texts: Dr James Drake's *Anthropologia Nova; or New System of Anatomy* (2 vols, 1707); a translation of the French obstetrician Paul Portal's *The Compleat Practice of Men and Women Midwives* (1705), based on the discussion of eighty-one case studies of problems encountered in labour; and Sir John Floyer's *Psychrolousia, or The History of Cold Bathing* (2nd edn, 1706), which extolled the benefits of cold bathing and recommended 'the wonderful effects of the Bath-Water, drunk hot from the Pump' at the new Pump Room in Bath.
- Four books on mathematics, one each by William Jones, William Leybourn and John Ward, and a second-hand copy of Isaac Newton's pioneering *Opticks* (1704), though Claver was more interested in the two treatises on curvilinear figures, 'Nuton's [Newton's] Trigonometry', as he called it, that were included in this first edition.
- Works on Philosophy and Religion: Sir Kenelm Digby's *Two Treatises of Bodies and Man's Soul* (1669 edn), arguing that the soul must be immaterial and immortal; Dr William Cave's two books on the history and lives of the Apostles; Henry Maurice's books in defence of episcopacy; and the non-juror, Charles Leslie's *A Short and Easie Method with the Deists* (1st edn, 1698), attacking the view that, from close observation of the natural world, it was more reasonable to believe in a Supreme Being who was the creator of the universe than it was to have faith in a Christian God.
- A travel book: the translation of the Danish merchant and diplomat Evert Ysbrant Ides's very popular *Three Years Travels from Moscow over-land to China* (1706).
- Works of literature: two volumes of Cicero's writings; John Dryden's *Fables Ancient and Modern* (1st edn 1700); and a four-volume collection of *Poems on Affairs of State* (1697–1707), the last volume of which included two pieces that were later censored for having cast aspersions on the queen and her relationship with the duchess of Marlborough.

For Betty's education, Claver bought a book on French grammar and the French *Dictionary* (1st edn, 1699) by Abel Boyer, a Tory journalist and Huguenot refugee. More surprising was his purchase of a study of human sexuality; a translation of Dr Nicolas Venette's *The Mysteries of Conjugal Love Reveal'd* (2nd edn, 1707). Although Venette, dean of the Royal College of Physicians at La Rochelle, drew upon the views of ancient and modern writers in an academic manner, his commentaries were quite salacious. The Preface advised 'A Woman may be instructed by this Book, how to rule her amorous Inclinations, and manage the Reputation of her Daughters', but this just served as a cover for the earthy tales within. Most of the text consisted of short chapters containing teasing answers to straightforward questions: 'At what Age a young Man, and a young Woman, ought to Marry?' (25 and 20, respectively); 'Which is the most amorous, the Man or the Woman?' (undoubtedly, the woman); 'What hour of the Day one ought to kiss one's Wife?' ('All hours are proper'); 'After what manner married People ought to caress?' (preferably, in legal ways); 'Whether there is an Art in getting Boys or Girls?' (Yes; a boy especially 'when the cold North Wind blows at full Moon').[15] Whatever Claver and Molly may have made of *The Mysteries,* it did not matter. By the spring, Molly was expecting her second child.

20

'DRINK IF YOU PLEASE'

The arrival of the spring of 1709 was hugely welcome. In the previous autumn Claver had lost his brother-in-law, Betty's uncle Edmund Dawe, at the age of thirty-eight.[1] And since December, a Great Frost had settled over the whole of Europe freezing the land and rivers more severely than at any time in the previous five hundred years. By the beginning of the traditional new year on 25th March, there were signs that Molly was pregnant again, and Claver was thinking about keeping a diary to record his thoughts and feelings about key moments of each day. On Sunday 17th April he noted that he had been 'at ye Palace with the Bishop sick in Bed with a Cold'. Then, reflecting on the preceding months he wrote, 'This Winter just past was the most cold and snowy that ever was rememberd by any one. The greatest snow (when I went to Pill [Pylle]) was Jan: 24'. That was the night of a full moon. But the worst was yet to come. The unprecedented weather did so much damage across Europe and at home, as frost and floods destroyed animals and crops, it was not long before food supplies became scarce and famines followed.

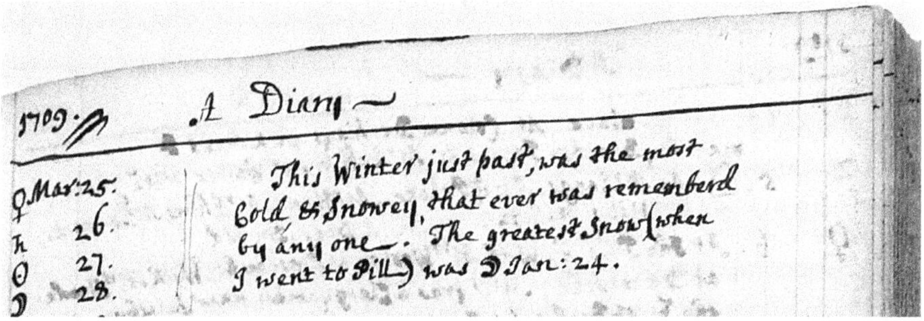

FIGURE 12 The start of Claver Morris's diary, 1709
The diary begins on New Year's Day, 25th March, but there are no further entries until 14th April when Claver records he 'supp'd & Danc'd late' that night

DOI: 10.4324/9781003333654-22

By the end of the summer, over 13,000 'Poor Palatine' German refugees had arrived in England exhausted by war and famine, and in France over half a million people had starved to death. In the previous December the Allies had claimed another famously expensive victory after successfully besieging Lille for four months at the cost of sixteen thousand of their own men. Although Britain was surviving in the war and faring much better from the famine, across the recently united kingdoms (since the Act of Union had abolished the Scottish parliament in 1707) there was still far more hunger and hardship in 1709 than in most other years. In May, several hundred colliers armed with cudgels marched four miles from Kingswood into Bristol, where they were joined by other labourers protesting against the high price of wheat and its shipment to the troops in Flanders. After securing a promise that corn would now be sold at no more than six shillings and eight pence per bushel (twice its usual price), most of the colliers dispersed. But some stormed the council house, broke its windows and fought with the local militia before making their escape.[2]

At Claver's house in the East Liberty there was very little prospect of anyone running short of food. Molly, who enjoyed taking trips to Bath, also liked to cook, and Claver himself recorded ruefully in May that he now weighed over 214 pounds (97 kilograms), having put on over sixteen pounds in about a year. The household bills had also grown from £28 a year, twenty years ago, to well over £80, plus £20 for Molly.[3] The household was a little larger now as there were always two or three live-in maids as well as a man-servant to feed and clothe, though they had their own quarters in a hall behind the house. Whereas Grace and Claver had lived very comfortably together at the chantry house, Claver, Molly and Betty were a family that had guests for dinner and supper almost every day. Anyone looking for good company, with music, singing, dancing and a little gambling to accompany a plentiful supply of fine food and drink, would not leave disappointed. With a daily stream of guests to entertain, the household bills were bound to soar.

According to the cook-maid, Anne Carpender, Claver's man, John Curtis, was a little too fond of the strong October beer they brewed, and when John offered his resignation over this, Claver told him that 'he should do as he thought best'. Since Claver also took this opportunity 'to tell him some of his Faults', John Curtis did not stay for long.[4] But he was soon replaced by William Clark from Evercreech, who agreed to a salary of £4 a year. That was a pound more than the cook-maid earned, but a pound less than Curtis had been paid. Since Will Clark accompanied Claver almost everywhere, riding with him to visit friends and patients, and always running errands, it was important that he was capable and trustworthy. This also applied to Anne the cook-maid. In July 1709, when a tenant sent a present of a roasting pig, and the bishop sent a haunch of venison from the buck that had been raised within the palace grounds, Claver would not have kept a cook who could not turn such gifts into delicious meals for him and guests. He expected to enjoy dining on venison pasties and potted venison for several days.

When he first arrived in Wells with Grace, Claver had an income of £90 a year from the rent of their houses in Crane Court, and less than £50 a year from his fees for 'Advice and Prescriptions'. But, due largely to the value of his marriages to Elizabeth and Molly, and to the strength of the medical business he had built, he was now far more financially secure. In addition to his lands in north Somerset, at Ebdon and Felton across the Mendips, which he leased for £80 and £30 each year, he had acquired an estate at Sand Park in Wedmore, which he leased to John and James Tucker for £52 a year. He also enjoyed an income from his land and properties at West Bradley and Pilton, which together brought in another £100. There were also several smaller sources of income, such as the £11 in interest which he gained from his loan of £220 to the trustees of John Morse's estate at Lympsham, six miles from Axbridge,[5] and a similar amount each year from the rearing of oxen on his fields at Dulcote where he bought more land which he let for another £26 a year.[6]

The ownership of land and buildings was the safest form of investment and one of the oldest measures of social status, but it was not cost-free. This was due especially to the annual Land Tax which was now at a record four shillings in the pound. It was collected by unpaid local commissioners like Claver (meeting in the local taverns) according to a fixed amount for each town or parish. There were also other national and local taxes which needed to be paid, such as the Window Tax, based on the number of windows in a house, the Church Rate and the Poor Rate, as well as the expenses of maintaining and improving buildings and the regular costs of hedging, fencing and ditching the land to safeguard animals and crops. To maintain his landed income of about £300 a year, Claver would pay about £60 in 'Expensa', including a pound in land tax on his new house. Land was not his only source of income, however. In 1709, he earned £139 from his fees as a physician; a sum that would rise to nearly £260 over the next few years. With a total income of well over £400 a year, the Morris family could enjoy many of the luxuries of life.

For Claver, this meant the finest clothes and all the trappings of a gentleman's estate, though by 1709 he had not replaced his coach-horses, Duke and Buck; Duke was prone to eye infections and Buck, the better horse, had died after being gored by a stray bull. It also meant having time to read new books and to conduct experiments in his laboratory where he could make medicines at his furnaces and create all kind of implements, such as his 'philosophical globe lantern', his silver toothbrush, a milk-warmer, a conical-shaped glass flask, and an 'Instrument to rule Musick-Paper', all according to his own designs. And it meant that he could fully enjoy the company of friends.

One day every month Claver attended a 'mutual entertainment', fuelled by copious amounts of food and drink, at the house of a member of 'the moon feast club'. The alignment of these meetings with full moons, to aid the journeys home, was not important as most members, and probably their horses, usually preferred to stay the night. Membership of the club was defined to include the members' wives, though few showed any interest in attending. Claver, however, was a regular host along with Maurice Berkeley and Thomas Horner. John Whitehand, the vicar at Shepton Mallet, also hosted sessions and sold Claver old copies of John Webster's treatise against witchcraft, *The Displaying of Supposed Witchcraft* (1677), and works by the Commonwealth's great atheistic philosopher Thomas Hobbes, who had been born in Wiltshire. Spiritual guidance from Whitehand was not needed here, for the interests of the club were unashamedly sublunary. Several of the members were musicians and most were Claver's patients, and when they met each month the aim of their 'mutual entertainment' was simply to eat, drink and be merry.[7]

Above all, having time and money made it possible for Claver not only to collect musical instruments and practise the violin, harpsichord, double bass, flute and oboe, but also to devote his energies toward the development of another, far more important club, his very own 'Musick Clubb'. This was something that he had started with the help of choral vicars in the 1690s, but it was now exceptional by any standards, drawing players and audiences from far and wide.[8]

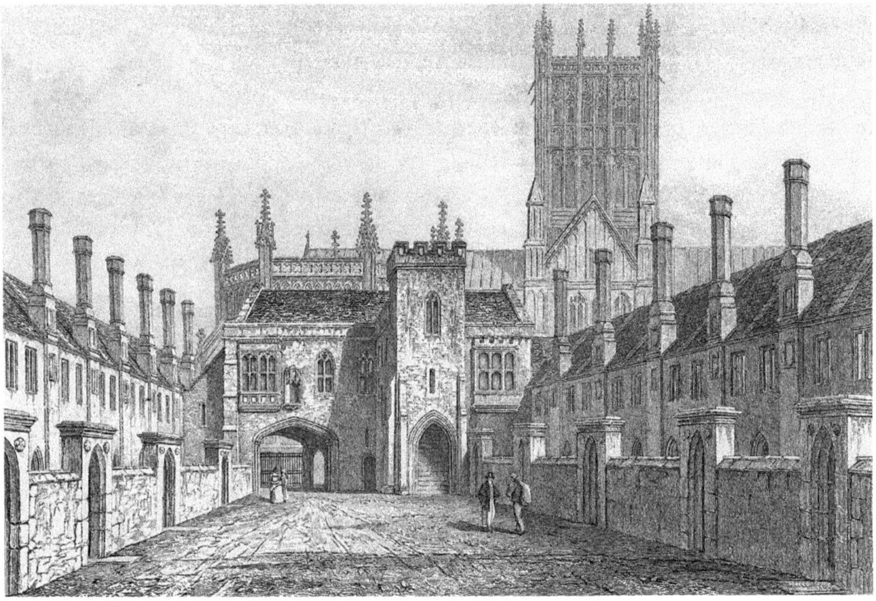

FIGURE 13 The Vicars' Close
Looking south, the staircase leads to the Vicars' Hall and to the passageway over the Chain Gate

Under Claver's direction, the club met every Tuesday evening in the medieval Vicars' Hall on the first floor of the gatehouse at the bottom of the Close. The Hall led into the cathedral, across the enclosed footbridge of the Chain Gate and down the stone stairs to the Chapter House. It included an organ, and was large enough for the 'Clubbers' to add a wooden gallery. Being served by its own fireplace, kitchen, bakehouse and brewery, the Hall had been designed originally to provide a meeting and dining room to support the communal living of over forty single men, the early vicars choral who had been in Catholic holy orders.[9] Yet it could accommodate well over a hundred guests on special occasions, such as the concerts held on the 22nd November every year in honour of St Cecilia, the patron saint of music and musicians. Claver was so passionate about his club he seldom missed a weekly meeting, let alone the celebration of St Cecilia's Day, and he often rode long distances in bad weather to ensure that he arrived in time to play his part.

Although the club was dominated by Claver and his male companions, it was not a male preserve. Women came to sing and play, to dance and listen not only to old folk and Renaissance tunes, but to whatever modern music Claver and fellow members could acquire from booksellers such as Edward Lewis at London, Henry Hammond at Bath, John Miller of Sherborne, and other suppliers in Salisbury, Exeter or wherever the latest music could be found. Claver himself bought bundles of anthems, sonatas, concertos and other music by dozens of composers, including Tomaso Albinoni, William Croft, Arcangelo Corelli, George Frederic Handel, Henry Purcell, Alessandro Scarlatti, Agostino Steffani, Giovani Tibaldi, Giuseppe Valentini and Antonio Vivaldi, and often paid to have more copies made.

This was not only a club where amateur and professional musicians sang and played, but also a place where anyone who enjoyed music was welcome to listen or join in, especially as the sixpenny fee for guests was usually overlooked. It was also an important public space, quite unlike the church, the marketplace or inn. At the club it was possible for men and women of various social ranks to mix and make new friends within a relatively relaxed, but respectable environment. And for men like Claver, it was a place where, for at least a few hours every week, the joys of hearing and playing music could transcend their everyday concerns.

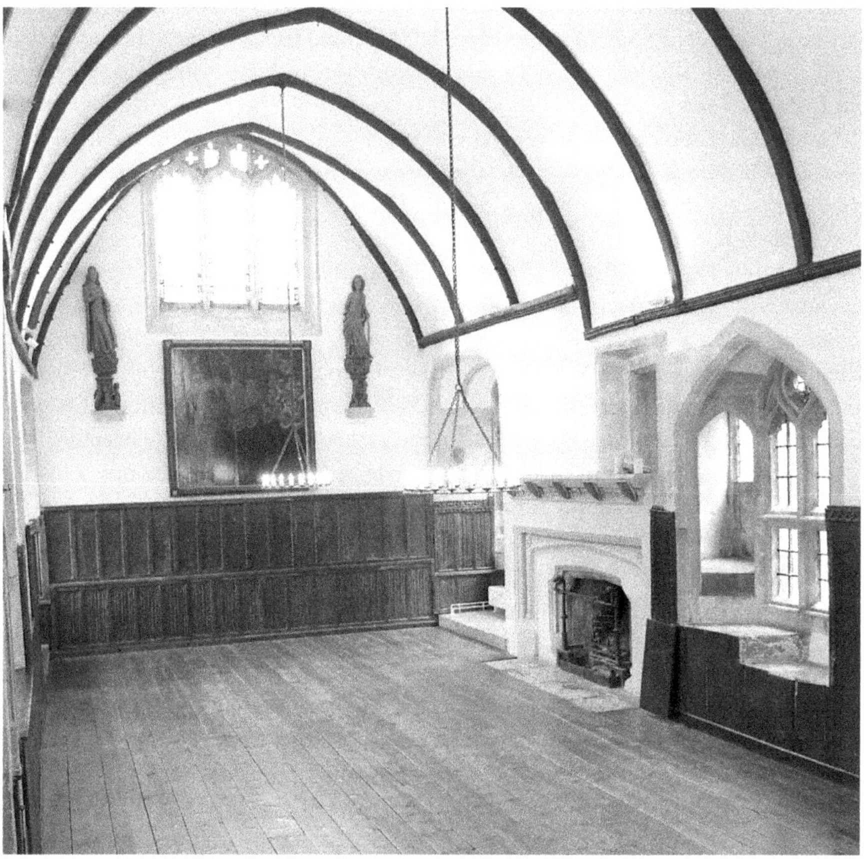

FIGURE 14 The Vicars' Hall
Designed as a communal dining-room above the gateway to the Close, this is where the music club met on Tuesday evenings and held concerts

In the summer of 1709 Betty Morris was either away at school or staying with Sir Dewey Bulkeley's family at Fordingbridge near Salisbury. Molly was planning a trip home to Devon, and as she was five months pregnant, her father sent his coach and horses to fetch her and her maid from Wells. At Sadborow, there was time for a family reunion as Molly's married sister Anne had come from the Isle of Wight with her husband John Leigh and their fourteen-year-old daughter. Molly's father, and her unmarried sister Elizabeth, still lived in the manor at Sadborow, and the four children of her deceased brother lived close by, though the eldest, William, was now supposed to be studying at Oxford.

While Molly was away, Claver continued in his rounds, visiting patients such as the Mattocks families of Wells and East Harptree on the Mendips, and Elizabeth Strode at Downside where during one evening she was 'taken with an Hysterical Passion, & an intolerable Paine in her Head'. She soon recovered, but it was not an evening that Claver could easily forget. After dinner and games of cribbage, some of the guests had the temerity to ask him if he thought that God had punished Bishop Kidder for the injury that he had done to Claver, even working a miracle on the night of the terrible storm in 1703 to bring about his death. Claver had no difficulty in 'setting them right' about his feelings, but he could barely disguise his anger that his dispute with Kidder was still a topic of discussion and speculation six years after the bishop's shocking death.[10]

A few days later, on 11th July, he hired a coach-and-six to take him and his friend George Wiltshire (a choral vicar who gave Betty singing lessons) to Somerton, where they stopped at the Red Lion for a couple of hours before going on to Sadborow.[11] After a day's rest at the Bragges, they went a further thirty-five miles west to Exeter to visit Molly's uncle, Edward Drewe, a canon of the cathedral and the archdeacon of Cornwall who had visited Molly and Claver at Wells earlier in the year. The archdeacon was a member of the old gentry family of Drewes from the Grange at Broadhembury, an estate near Honiton that he would inherit from his brother in the Spring. After a few days' lodging at the Half Moon and dining with the Drewes, Claver and Wiltshire returned to Wells via Sadborow, where Molly had been staying.

At home in the Liberty, Claver was met by another of his relations, George Farewell, the husband of his former sister-in-law Anne Dawe. Farewell's family owned the manors at Holbrook and Horsington near Wincanton, and after years of study at Oxford and Cambridge, at the age of thirty-three, he had just been appointed rector of South Cadbury, a few miles from his family home. At the end of May he had also been made a prebend of the cathedral, and to celebrate the appointment Claver hosted a dinner for him with over twenty guests who all stayed till the early hours, including most of the senior clergy of the diocese.[12] Since Claver loved to entertain well into the night, George was always welcome. Having been treated to a crown's worth of claret, he came home with Claver who had hired a coach to collect Molly and her maid on Thursday 21st July. When Claver and his family returned to Wells from Sadborow, they brought with them Molly's sister Anne Leigh, her fourteen-year-old daughter and their maid who travelled behind in Major Bragge's best coach.

To celebrate the return of Molly with her guests, they all sat in the garden in the evening where, with the help of several of the choral vicars, Claver organised a concert. And the next day, after writing to Betty and drawing up prescriptions, at five o'clock, he took his niece, his maids and a few other guests on a two-mile walk over Milton Hill to visit the famous caves at Wookey Hole. They had no guide, just candles to help them through the subterranean caverns, but they were clearly not deterred by local legends about the old witch who was believed to be living there. On Sunday they dined on venison and went to church, and on Monday evening Claver organised a ball for the entertainment of his niece. Before the week was out, his 'sister Leigh' and niece had been taken to another ball, to an evening at the music club, to see the rare books in the cathedral library, to the springs and moat of the bishop's palace, and on a tour across the bishop's deer park to see the paper-making mills at Dulcote. When they left in a stagecoach for Bath on Saturday evening, 30th July, Claver gave his niece a book on the kings of England and a copy of Abel Boyer's edition of the works of the Jewish historian Flavius Josephus. He then went to bathe, as several medics were now recommending, in the cool of a spring-water pond, 'Nabb's Hole'.

Two days later, on Monday 1st August, he went to watch the hay-making at Dulcote and West Pennard, and on Tuesday morning he had to 'lay a-bed out of order in a cold', though he still made it to the music meeting in the evening. The next day he recorded that he was 'so sick of a Fever with a Violent Pain in my Head, Stomach & Limbs', he could not get out of bed. In the afternoon he took a purgative made with salt of tartar (potassium carbonate) 'which work'd upward 7 times & downward near as often'. Believing that 'twas all over in 2 hours or less', he took two more electuaries (medicines sweetened with honey) and went to bed.

On Wednesday he could not resist joining his friends for the moon-feast meeting at Maurice Berkeley's home at Pylle. He spent the day in the garden's summer-house, eating a little tench, taking hartshorn jelly (made from the decoction of burnt deer-antlers, used to treat diarrhoea), sipping beer and drinking half a glass of punch, but when he left for home, he was feeling worse again. After a day of sitting in his 'sweating chair', on Saturday 6th August, the surgeon Christopher Lucas was called and took sixteen ounces (0.45 litres) of blood from his right arm. Then, for the next two weeks he was so ill he could not even write to Betty, let alone keep his diary.

During these anxious days, Lucas, Cupper and several of the choral vicars took turns as bedside 'watchers'. Claver noted later that 'all doubted my recovery' from what 'appeared to be the Spotted Fever'. A week later, however, after he had been to church and his friend George Wiltshire had sung to him 'An Anthem of Thanksgiving for Recovery for a Dangerous Sickness' composed by a former organist of the cathedral, John Jackson, he was ready to take a trip to see the Leighs at Bath. As he was still recovering, he made pills of Aethiops Mercurialis-Mineralis (black sulphide mercury), a treatment for scrofula, hereditary syphilis and other skin complaints.[13]

Claver only stayed a couple of days in Bath, just long enough to say goodbye to the Leighs before they set off for home on the Isle of Wight. He also had time for dinner with John and Abigail Prowse, whose one-year-old son, Tommy, he had been treating at the bishop's palace ever since Abigail had become pregnant and had suffered from a miscarriage in the summer. There were other friends and patients who needed his attention too, particularly the family of Sir Henry and Lady Sarah Gould at Sharpham Park on the Somerset moors, where their son's wife, Honora, was ill with a tertian ague (malaria). Sir Henry's daughter, Sarah, was also in need of help. Having married the soldier and profligate gambler Colonel Edmund Fielding (much against her parents' wishes), she was now living at Sharpham with her two babies, Henry and Catherine Fielding, born in 1707 and 1708, and with a third child on the way.

At their house in the Liberty, Molly was also waiting to give birth, but mostly without Claver to keep her company since he rarely spent a whole day at home. In September, he made several trips to Axbridge (where he had many patients and was invited to dinner by the mayor and corporation), to Downside, Mells and Shapwick. But it was often music rather than medicine that kept him on the move. He took a trip to Bath with George Wiltshire, from where they went on to stay with John Harrington at his manor in Kelston, a few miles away. Here they could enjoy playing music not only with a family of highly talented musicians, but at a place where there were often concerts with famous guest performers.[14] Claver himself was well known for his music club and knowledge of musical instruments. In September he brought the professional lutenist Thomas Deane to play in Wells, and at Shepton Mallet he was invited to give his opinion on the installation of a new organ in the church. He also took Christopher Lucas and James Nicholls, a choral vicar who taught Betty the violin, on a four-day trip to Salisbury where they all dined with Betty at the Angel, attended concerts and watched her dance at school.

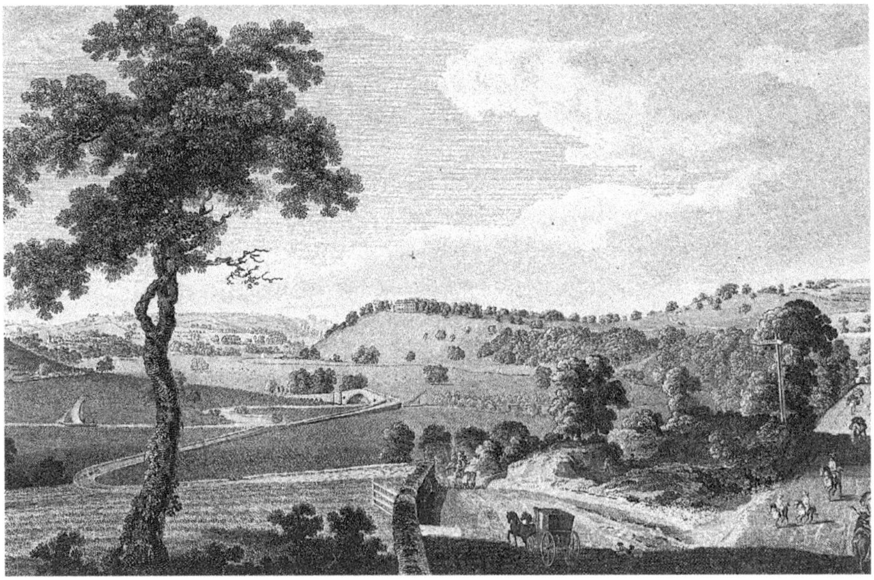

FIGURE 15 The road from Bath to Kelston
After the Harringtons sold their Elizabethan mansion next to the church in 1759, it was demolished and a new one (shown here) was built on the top of the hill above the village

Claver's music club was now well known for the growing number of its guests, and for music that was reckoned to be 'the best they ever heard'. Even so, the conversation of some guests occasionally stretched Claver's patience to the limit. One guest, an army captain, asked Claver 'how a spirit could throw a bed-staff'. This question related to the well-documented story of how a family in Wiltshire had been haunted for years by the demon of a vagrant drummer-boy, William Drury, after his drum had been confiscated by a magistrate in 1661. Supported by living witnesses, the story had been extensively recounted (together with a similar one, from Shepton Mallet) in a book by Joseph Glanvill, the rector of Bath Abbey. Its veracity was widely accepted, especially as Drury had been imprisoned and Glanvill had argued that the demon's throwing of the bed-staff at a clergyman was proof of the existence of witches, ghosts and spirits.

Claver had no patience with such stories, which could so easily turn into tragedies, particularly with the connivance of the clergy. It was less than thirty years since the execution at Exeter of three poor elderly women for 'bewitching several persons, destroying ships at sea, and cattle by land'. It was said that they had consorted with the devil to cause their neighbours at Bideford great pain and suffering. Moreover, the church had played a vital role in ensuring their conviction for witchcraft.[15] So, in response to questions about the drummer-boy, Claver could barely hide his anger. But he managed to be diplomatic, noting that it 'gave me an occasion to prove beyond his [the army captain's] denying, & I hope satisfaction, that the World was not eternal, & that there were future rewards & Punishments after Death'.[16]

Having lost two wives and three daughters (two as babies), Claver needed to take comfort from beliefs in divine justice and salvation. And he took nothing for granted as he still found time most mornings, or occasionally in the evening, to attend services in the cathedral. After matins on 17th October 1709 – a day that he would otherwise remember for having had a horse and oxen requisitioned for the war effort – Molly went into a labour which lasted for two days. Her helper, Mary Rogers (the wife of George, the choral vicar who Claver paid for copying-out Corelli's compositions), was a somewhat surprising choice as midwife, for she had previously been reprimanded by the dean and chapter for having borne a daughter out of marriage, though she claimed to have been secretly married at the time. But Mary was Molly's choice, and 'the midwife and women with her' decided that as Molly was 'without considerable Pains', 'twas not thought fit to do anything' but wait.[17]

Claver noted but accepted the decision of the women, and on Thursday 20th October he recorded that 'at 20 or 22 Minutes after 6 in the morning exactly my Wife was verily happily deliver'd of a son. I had many Congratulations on that occasion.' In the evening, several friends arrived and they were 'very merry, but temperately so', though they played the card game 'Drink If You Please'.

21

HIGH CRIMES & MISDEMEANOURS

After writing letters to Betty at Salisbury and to his mother at Lydlinch to tell them the good news, Claver sent invitations for his son's christening to be held by candlelight during evening service on Thursday 27th October 1709. It was the responsibility of godparents to ensure that 'the child may be virtuously brought up to lead a godly and Christian life', but their social standing was no less important. Molly's father, Major Bragge, and Maurice Berkeley, the twenty-eight-year-old unmarried son and heir of Colonel Edward, were asked to be the godfathers. Abigail Hooper, the bishop's wife, and Molly's sister, Anne Leigh, the godmothers. As Molly's father at Sadborow was almost seventy, and her sister was living on the Isle of Wight, they were unable to attend, so John Prowse, the bishop's son-in-law, and Anne Farewell (née Dawe), the wife of George, the rector of South Cadbury, stood in for them. It was no surprise that the baby was named William, after his grandfathers, or that after the service there was 'a great Company of Men and Women' at Claver's house. Although some left at four o'clock the next morning 'very well pleased with their entertainment', the house was still so full of well-wishers that Maurice Berkeley and Claver had to share a bed.

It was seventeen days after giving birth that Molly first left her bed to walk a little in her chamber, another week before she left her room to dine, and not until 17th November, when she was covered in a veil and carried in a sedan chair to the cathedral, that she completed the traditional 'churching' ceremony. This was a quiet occasion as the only woman to accompany her was her midwife Mary Rogers, to whom Claver gave two guineas. In the evening, baby Will was sent to stay with his wet-nurse, Jane Nooth, who had given birth to her first child, a girl, in March 1709. She was married to James, a choral vicar, clerk and library cataloguer (for which he earned an extra £2 a year). Although Jane was paid by Claver at the rate of four shillings a week, first and foremost she was Molly's friend, and on days when Will was sick, Molly went to stay with her in Vicars' Close.[1]

DOI: 10.4324/9781003333654-23

As the 22nd November was St Cecilia's Day, with the help of four members of the Harrington family, Thomas Naish the subdean of Salisbury, and other 'Lovers of Musick', Claver prepared a concert, including Purcell's *Hail! Bright Cecilia*, which he reckoned was a great success. But he was greatly irritated by the fact that while sixty-two male guests had each paid half-a-crown for entrance to the Hall, only thirty-three of the women had paid the fee, as many had been smuggled in.

Ironically, concern about the ease with which women could be smuggled in and out of the Close dated back to Medieval times. It had been hoped that by building the Close, the vicars would be kept away from women, 'wholly separated from the tumults of the people, the pomp of the world, and the occasion of evil', so they would be more 'at leisure to serve God'. As the Close only had one entrance, opposite the cathedral, and its gates (one for pedestrians and one for carts) could be locked at night, it was believed that the vicars would be less likely to succumb to temptations of the flesh. But the plan was easily thwarted, as women simply waited in St Andrew Street, just outside the gates. So, the elegant Chain Gate and footbridge over St Andrew Street was built to connect the Close and Vicars' Hall directly with the cathedral's Chapter House. The problem now was that although the two most senior vicars, the Principals, were the only people permitted to have keys to the Close, the gates were often left unlocked, and even a special injunction 'against such as shall be abroad in the Town all the Night' made little difference.[2]

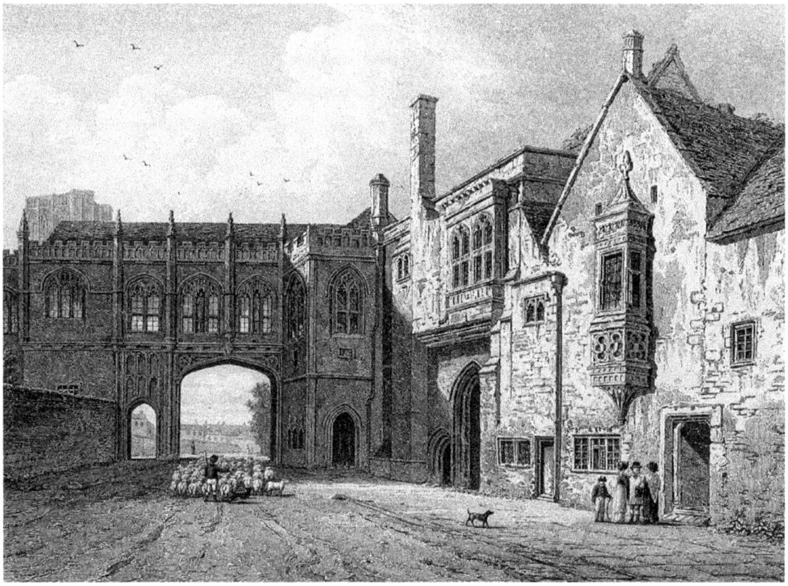

FIGURE 16 The Chain Gate and entrance to Vicars' Close
The sheep are heading west towards the cathedral green

Claver was delighted to see so many women at the meetings and the concerts of the club, not least because he liked to dance. Since the Reformation, the vicars were entitled to have wives living with them in the Close. This greatly reduced fears about some forms of heterosexual misconduct ('incontinence', as it was often called). But the Elizabethan charter for the college, with all its rules about residence, from the prohibition of dogs and horses to the locking of the gates at night, were still in force. Claver knew this very well, for he paid James Nooth to copy out the 'Statute Book of Close Hall' in order to see if there were any way that he could claim a right of access to the Close. It might only save him a minute or two in not having to walk down East Liberty and into St Andrew Street to get to the cathedral, but it would enable him to come and go as he pleased and to smuggle his friends in and out at night. He might also justify his claim on the grounds that, as a physician, he had patients in the Close, and as a musician he ran the club and its concerts in the Hall. There were also precedents: for the convenience of tenants, a few had been granted the use of temporary backdoors that broke though the high walls around the perimeter of the college. But these were desperate arguments with which to break the spirit and the letter of the charter, which is why Claver solicited support.

The plan was to make a passageway from the Back Liberty through to the top end of the Close, coming out by the Vicars' Chapel. This would require the building of a 25-foot wall across the garden of one of the houses that Robert Creighton currently leased and sublet for a profit, and the construction of a door in the wall of the Back Liberty, to which only Claver would have a key. After Creighton had agreed to the idea, Claver sought Hooper's 'connivance' in the plan. After initially agreeing, the bishop then changed his mind. Claver appealed to precedents and to what he saw as the 'plaine Letter & Meaning' of the vicars' Statutes 'which does not forbid any such thing' as a passageway. But Hooper disagreed and angrily replied that 'he was the best Judge' of the Statutes.[3]

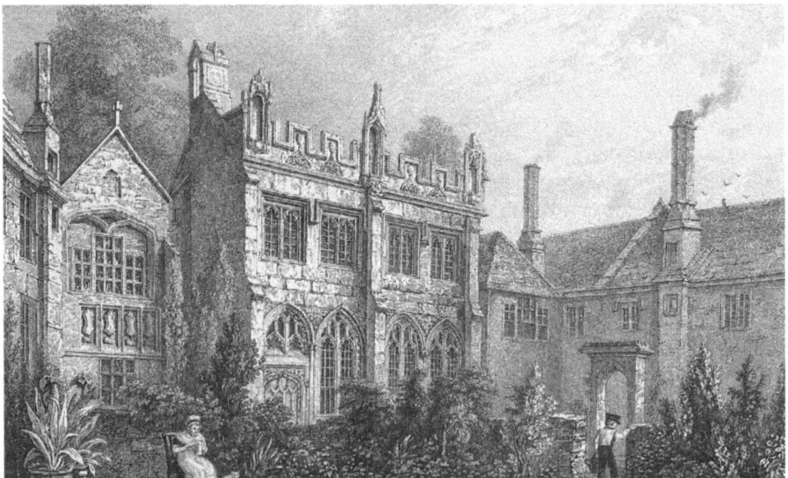

FIGURE 17 The Vicars' Chapel
At the top of the Close, Claver's new passageway into Back Liberty ran between the chapel and the house (to the right) that he sub-let to the schoolmistress, Grace Pierce

Another cause of disagreement with Hooper concerned the theft of books from the cathedral's ancient grammar school. The headmaster, Henry Mills, had been appointed in 1699 at the age of twenty-four, having previously served as the cathedral's librarian. He was a local man who had been educated at the school and at Trinity College, Oxford. In 1702 he had been made a prebend, providing him with a useful income to supplement his salary of £10 a year and the fees that he could collect from the dozen or so boys who boarded at the school. By 1709, he had become one of Claver's and Molly's closest friends. Aside from being a regular drinking companion and member of the music club, Claver supported him by giving money to his schoolboys when they recited texts such as Virgil's *Aeneid*, or held performances of plays such as *Hamlet*, *Julius Caesar*, or *Oedipus Rex*. Mills was also entrusted with the honour of 'churching' Molly just a few months after his own daughter had been accidentally scalded to death by a kettle of boiling water. And the families were so close that although Mills's wife, Mary, often needed prescriptions for her 'ague', Claver never charged for them. So he was naturally inclined to believe his friend when he said that Sam, a son of the archdeacon of Wells, was the person who had been stealing books.

Claver had no quarrel with the archdeacon Samuel Hill, a truculent man of sixty who, somewhat surprisingly, Hooper had made archdeacon in 1705 and a residential canon in 1708, even though, as vicar of Kilmington, he had been a great thorn in the side of Kidder. In fact, Claver still served as physician to Hill's wife and other children, so he probably believed that he was well placed to help Henry Mills by asking Hooper to pass judgement. Though there were witnesses who swore to seeing the seventeen-year-old Sam breaking into the school, Hooper was not inclined to find him guilty. It was then that Creighton, together with five other residential canons and Claver, signed an open letter commending Mills for having 'raised the Reputation of his School far above what former Masters could effect these many Years'. Even so, they could not keep him. Disappointed by Hopper's inaction, Mills left to be headmaster of Whitgift School in Croydon, taking, as was customary, several of the boarders with him, and leaving the cathedral school quite derelict and empty. In some respects, this outcome probably pleased Creighton as he now secured the appointment of his son as the new headmaster, and moved him into the gabled manor-house, next door to Claver.[4] But Claver and Molly had lost a friend, and Sam Hill, the archdeacon's son, was going to cause them even more trouble in the years to come.

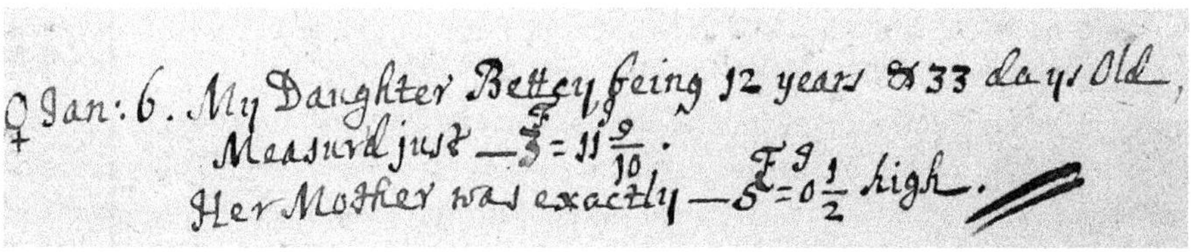

FIGURE 18 Molly and Betty measured, 1710

In January 1710, Claver took his annual reckoning of Molly and Betty's heights, finding, as expected, that his wife still measured 'exactly' half an inch above five foot; a few inches shorter than the average height for women. Betty, at twelve years old, was 'just' one tenth of an inch short of being four foot tall; a figure that must have disappointed her. Since Claver himself, at just over five foot, six and a half inches, was only slightly taller than the average man, he could not have been surprised. But Betty was also quite sensitive and shy, as she had shown the week before at Henry Mills' house when she refused to speak French to the wife of one of Claver's friends. Having corrected her, he noted that 'she fell into Tears, & continued grieving in that way, even after she came home, so long, & so much, that I was doubtful of her hurting her Constitution'. After an apology, she was immediately forgiven and a few weeks later Claver organised a ball for her at which she entertained a dozen of her female friends.[5]

Before the ball, Claver had taken Molly and Betty to see his mother at Lydlinch, staying with George and Anne Farewell at the rectory in South Cadbury on the way. Molly rode very carefully behind Claver's man, John Curtis, and Betty rode behind her father as the roads were 'frozen & very slippery'. Safe at home, on 9th February, Claver was asked by Elias Rebotier, a Huguenot refugee whom the bishop had ordained and recently made his personal chaplain, to sit up one night with him at Dr Cheney's house in Back Liberty. Claver agreed, simply to reassure the Irish family, his patients who were dwelling there, that they were not living in a haunted house. But Rebotier's aim was 'to speak to the Apparition, if any was seen, that had frighted Mrs Irishes Family very much'. So it was no surprise to Claver that by the morning they had 'heard nor saw nothing of ye kind'.[6]

Two days before Christmas, he had also stayed up half the night with Maurice Berkeley and others after playing flute sonatas throughout the day at Major Richard Prater's home in Frome. This late night was due to the appearance of a Catholic, Mr Glin from Mere in Wiltshire, who objected to the Anglican Church's separation from the Church of Rome. Such complaints were meat and drink to Claver, and although 'we did not shut up the Dispute till Half an hour after 2 a clock', he went to bed content as he felt 'it was very visible to the whole company … that I had met with a weak adversary'.[7]

In the new year, he bought more books and music, and a repeater clock for his bedside, made by Christopher Tucker for £7. He bought Betty a small harpsichord (a spinet) for £5, and paid Anthony Walkeley, the organist at Salisbury, two guineas a year to teach her how to play it. He also paid Rachael De Groodt, whose husband he had commissioned to engrave copper portraits of his family, to teach Betty how to paint. As for Will, in mid-March he suffered a serious illness with a high fever for which Claver repeatedly prescribed. Although Will managed to recover, within the next few weeks Claver lost two of his dearest friends. The first, on 26th March, was Judge Henry Gould of Sharpham Park, who died at his chambers in London at the age of sixty-six. Molly and Claver had stayed with the Goulds after their marriage in 1703, and Claver would continue to treat and support his redoubtable widow

Lady Sarah and her children, not least in her fight for custody of her grandchildren, including Henry and Sarah Fielding. The second death was even more shocking.

At the age of thirty-four, John Prowse caught smallpox and died soon after at Westminster on 4th April 1710, while serving as an MP for Somerset. His father-in-law, Bishop Hooper, attending the House of Lords, was with John at the time and managed to persuade him not to settle his whole estate upon his wife Abigail. They agreed she was to be left £1,500 and made the sole executor. The will stated that if she should die before Thomas came of age, six men, including the bishop, Maurice Berkeley, Major Prater and Claver Morris, were to be his guardians.[8] It was a sensible arrangement, not least because, living at the bishop's palace, both Abigail (after a miscarriage in 1709) and her son were frequently in need of medical advice. And Claver's disagreements with the bishop did not seem to matter now, for the friendship between their families deepened. The bishop's wife was godmother to baby Will, and her youngest daughter, the fifteen-year-old Rebecca, was a guest at Betty's ball. Her eldest daughter, Abigail, 'one of the most accomplished women of her time', but now widowed at the age of twenty-six, was so fond of Betty that she made her a silk gown and petticoats.[9]

A few weeks before his death, John Prowse sent Claver a copy of a sixteen-page pamphlet, *The Speech of Henry Sacheverell, D.D. made in Westminster Hall on Tuesday, March 7, 1709/10 [1710],* knowing that this was something he would relish. Ever since the High Church zealot had published his incendiary sermon, *The Perils of False Brethren, both in Church and State,* delivered to the City Fathers at St Paul's Cathedral on 5th November 1709, political and religious tensions had been growing. By 1st December when a second edition of the sermon, with a print-run of 40,000, went on the sale, the whole nation had been inflamed. Sacheverell, a fellow of Magdalen College, Oxford, and chaplain of St Saviours, Southwark, was a vain, ambitious and arrogant young man, well known for the viciousness of his attacks upon Dissenters. For years, his fiery rhetoric had been answered and parodied by dozens of writers, including Daniel Defoe. But he craved attention, and in August 1709 he had delivered a sermon at the assizes in Derby proclaiming that 'our Church and constitution' were being 'shamefully betrayed'. So, in choosing him to preach at St Paul's on 5th November, the Tory Lord Mayor of London knew exactly what to expect, or so he thought.

Instead of focusing on the nation's deliverance from Popery, commemorating the Gunpowder Plot and William of Orange's landing at Torbay, Sacheverell used the pulpit at St Paul's not only to draw attention to the hypocrisy of occasional conformity, but also to challenge the legitimacy of the Glorious Revolution and the folly of granting any form of toleration or 'indulgence' to Dissenters. According to Sacheverell, the sacrament of Holy Communion in the Church of England was now 'rent and divided by factious, and schismatical impostors'. Her pure doctrines 'corrupted and defiled; her primitive worship and discipline profaned and abused; her sacred orders denyed and vilifyed; her priests and professors (like St Paul) calumniated, misrepresented and ridiculed; her altars and sacraments prostituted to hypocrites, Deists, Socinians and atheists'.[10] Weakened by the recent collapse of peace negotiations, another dreadful military 'victory' at Malplaquet, and the arrival 10,000 Calvinist refugees in London, Sacheverell's provocation was too much to bear for the Lord Treasurer Godolphin and Anne's leading ministers. On 15th December the House of Commons voted that Sacheverell should be impeached for 'high crimes and misdemeanours' for which he could be punished with imprisonment for life.

The decision to conduct a 'state trial' in front of all members of the Lords and Commons meant that Christopher Wren had to design an amphitheatre with 2,000 seats and public galleries in Westminster Hall. This was intended to provide a platform for the public to hear the government's justification of the Glorious Revolution, the Act of Toleration and much more. But by the time Sacheverell gave a speech in his own defence, claiming disingenuously that 'when my words were capable of two Senses, the worst and most invidious, tho' at the same time the most strained and unnatural, Construction has always been made of them', everyone in the country had already made up their mind.[11] In the enormous propaganda wars that now raged in the pulpits and the press, it was not difficult for Sacheverell's supporters to portray him as a martyr for the Church. As observed by a furious Sarah, duchess of Marlborough (soon to be dismissed from the royal household after her quarrels with the queen), Sacheverell's followers put 'the air of a saint upon a lewd, drunken, pampered man'.

By the third day of the trial, 1st March 1710, the belief that the Church of England was in mortal danger had grown so great that thousands of church-going Londoners rioted throughout the night to light bonfires in the city and tear down six of its best-known meeting houses. Only the exemplary discipline of the troops used to disperse the mobs kept the number of deaths and injuries in check. Following the case in Wells, Claver went to the coffee house on 4th March 'to see the result of Dr Sacheveril's Trial', and he kept going in anticipation every couple of days until the 21st March when he 'read the ill-news of Dr Sacheverils being found guilty by the Majority of 12 Lords'. In fact, the Lords had found him guilty on 20th March by sixty-nine votes to fifty-two; Bishop Hooper recording his objection, just as his son-in-law John Prowse had voted in December against the Commons' decision to impeach. But, regardless of the verdict, most of the Anglican clergy, and probably most men and women, now regarded Sacheverell as a national hero. When his punishment was merely to be banned from preaching for three years and to have his two most recent sermons burned by the hangman, his victory was complete. During the summer, while Godolphin's ministry collapsed, bells were rung and bonfires lit as thousands of Sacheverell's admirers mobbed him and bought copies of his portrait during his triumphal tour across the country.[12]

In May, Claver bought Betty a small horse and ordered a side-saddle to be made for her, decorated with crimson silks and silver braids. She was now ready to ride all the way to Sadborow to see the Bragges. A few months later, he bought her more presents: a scarlet riding-coat and stockings, satin gowns and aprons, turkey-leather shoes, green-stone earrings, a very fine feather muff, several fans, and a gold watch and chain. In taking as much care over Betty's appearance as he did his own, not to mention her music education, Claver must have hoped that she would be very much her father's daughter, and she was. Her shy refusal to converse in French was quite untypical of her otherwise good and dutiful behaviour. But while Claver's mood was good, the mood in Wells was one of fear and fury, as in most other towns throughout the West. When Thomas Parker, Lord Chief Justice and a leading prosecutor of Sacheverell, arrived for the summer assizes, the city's corporation and many of its gentry chose not to greet him. Hooper showed a little more respect by sending his chaplain Elias Rebotier to excuse his absence, but then he declined to send the judge the customary present of several bottles of fine wine selected from the bishop's cellar.[13] No one would have been surprised.

At the end of April 1710, when a by-election was held to replace John Prowse as an MP, a 'Knight of the Shire', for Somerset, the rich and clever twenty-one-year-old Sir William Wyndham was elected without a contest. He had just acquired £10,000 by marrying Lady Katherine Seymour, the second daughter of Charles Seymour, the 6th duke of Somerset; a Whig magnate who everyone regarded as so preposterously self-important he turned 'pride of rank and birth into a disease'. Such family connections must have helped Sir William, as would the four shillings that Claver spent on election treats, for which Sir William sent a side of venison as thanks. But the fundamental reason for Sir William's success was the fact that he was a High Tory who supported Sacheverell and the plan to negotiate a peace with France.[14]

In 1710, most of the freeholders of Somerset and other counties wanted to make peace with France and to protect the privileges of the established Church. So did most of the voters of great trading and manufacturing centres such as Bristol. Here, about a third of the 25,000 inhabitants were Dissenters who had seen one of their meeting houses torn down during the Sacheverell riots in the spring. Yet, at the general election in October, the strength of High Church feeling was still sufficient for a majority of the city's 3,500 voters to easily overturn the Whig monopoly of power, in favour of two non-resident Tory merchants; the exceptionally wealthy old slave-trader and benefactor Edward Colston, and the warden of the city's Merchant Venturers' Society, Edward Earle. In Wells, the Whiggish William Coward, son of a previous Tory MP from a prominent local family, was turned out of his seat in favour of Claver's young friend Maurice Berkeley. And the second seat was retained (without a contest) by another Edward Colston (nephew and intended heir of the Bristol slave-trader), though he had hardly set foot inside the town.[15] So it was unsurprising that at the general election in October 1710, Sir William Wyndham was re-elected as Knight of the Shire for Somerset, again without a contest, during the Tories' landslide victory.

The size of the Tory majority in the Commons meant that Robert Harley, the moderate Tory leader of Anne's new ministry, had to bring a number of hard-line members of the party into government. So, Sir William Wyndham, being an energetic and talented new MP, was appointed Master of the Buckhounds. This was more than just an honorary post as Anne still liked to hunt in her single-seated chariot, and after Sir William's appointment Claver spent another six shillings and sixpence treating his supporters at Ilchester. A year later, Lady Catherine miscarried after a narrow escape when the Wyndham's £6,000 house in Piccadilly was destroyed by fire, killing two of the maids who tried to jump to safety. But, with the patronage of his friend and mentor Bolingbroke, Sir William prospered. In 1712 he was made Secretary-at-War with the responsibility for disbanding British regiments.[16] Such a rapid rise to power pleased supporters, but what friends like Claver could not have known was just how far Sir William might be prepared to go in opposing the Hanoverian succession at the death of Anne.

22

AMONG THE GENTRY

The fear and hatred sewn across the nation by Sacheverell and his trial did not abate after the new Tory-dominated House of Commons met in November 1710. Before the first session ended in June 1711, new laws were introduced to strengthen the privileges of the established church and landed gentry. An Occasional Conformity Act was passed to prevent anyone in England who was not an Anglican from holding any kind of national or local office. Anyone, such as a town councillor, caught attending a meeting house would be subject to a fine of £40 and permanently barred from government employment. In the hope of reducing the number of Whiggish lawyers, army officers, foreigners and bankers who were being elected as MPs, a Landed Qualifications Act was also passed, restricting membership of the Commons to persons born in England or its dominions who had a landed income of at least £300 per annum if they were standing for a borough, and £600 per annum for a county seat. And a New Churches Act was passed with the aim of reducing the growth of Dissent in London's suburbs by paying for the building of fifty new churches from public funds.

Although the popularity of the ministry's leader, Robert Harley, rose greatly after a French spy stabbed him in the chest in an attempted assassination, he could not resist all the demands of hard-line Tories such as Bolingbroke and Wyndham. He was determined, however, to negotiate a peace with France, and this meant dismissing Marlborough from his post as captain-general. A few weeks later, after the opening of the second session of parliament (December 1711 to June 1712), the Whig Secretary-at-War Robert Walpole was arrested, and Marlborough was severely censured for corruption. Harley's friend, the Anglican clergyman Jonathan Swift, had already prepared the ground for Marlborough's fall and the negotiation of a secret peace with France in a scathing attack upon the war effort, *The Conduct of the Allies, and of the Late Ministry, in Beginning and Carrying on the Present War* (1711).

DOI: 10.4324/9781003333654-24

Claver was pleased to read the tract, which had sold 11,000 copies before the end of January 1712.[1] And in that month the Tories rode the wave of hostility towards refugees, particularly the new influx of 13,000 'Poor Palatines', by repealing the Whigs' 1709 Act for Naturalising Foreign Protestants.

Under the 1709 Act, all immigrants could become naturalised subjects if they were prepared to take the statutory oaths of allegiance to the crown and the holy sacrament of *any* Protestant denomination. It was believed that this would show British solidarity with Protestants throughout the continent; most obviously, the hundreds of thousands of Huguenots who had fled from persecution, slavery, and forcible conversion in France ever since the 1680s when Louis XIV had finally abolished their 'toleration'. But the 1709 Act would also reassure the thousands of Protestants who had fled from the Jacobite War in Ireland after the Glorious Revolution and, more immediately, the thousands of Palatine refugees who were now arriving, devastated by war and famine. It was further hoped that the 1709 Act would provide some recognition of the benefits of immigration as 'a means of advancing the wealth and strength of the nation'. But hard-line Tories believed that 'aliens' would always be a security risk, owing to their allegiance to their native countries. They would 'endanger our ancient polity and government' by holding public offices and voting in elections, and 'by frequent intermarriages' they would 'go a great way to blot out and extinguish the English race'. So it was no surprise that many Tories were eager to put a stop to foreigners being allowed 'to send over the scum of their countries to make ourselves, who already abound in Poor, yet poorer'.[2]

Like the majority of the country, Claver was a firm supporter of the Church of England and wanted to shore up its defences against Dissent, and to outlaw practices such as occasional conformity. But, unlike many other Anglicans he had no difficulty in socialising with Dissenters. Some, such as Elizabeth Strode of Downside, the eldest daughter and heir of the notorious Ned, were among his oldest friends and most valued patients. In the four years since Sacheverell's trial, Elizabeth had congratulated him on the birth of his son, submitted land-tax appeals to him, dined with him, and paid him £70 for his prescriptions and expenses in making over twenty trips to Bath, where she often resided for the season.[3] Elizabeth, her younger sister Mercy, and their relatives who were also Claver's patients, found nothing objectionable in his commitment to the established church. Friendship with members of more radical groups, such as the Quakers, was more difficult, due to what most people regarded as their subversive social attitudes and puritanical way of life. So, like most Anglicans, Claver did not mix socially with them, but he knew several Quaker families, such as the Middles and Simms of Pilton and Bristol, the Fears of Glastonbury, and the Maynards of Street, and he did not hesitate to offer them prescriptions and advice.[4]

Like most of the country, Claver believed that several of the Allies, especially the Dutch, had prolonged the war with France for no good reason (but at great cost to Britain). But he was sympathetic to the plight of foreign refugees. The first great surge came in the years soon after Louis XIV's abolition of any toleration in the Revocation of the Edict of Nantes, issued in the same month as Claver's marriage to Grace in October 1685. At that time, James II and most of his ministers and bishops pondered over their response, not wanting to offend Louis XIV or to support the growth of Protestant dissent at home. But Bishop Ken had used his pulpit to denounce the cruelties of Louis XIV's policies and demanded that the refugees should be recognised as 'brethren, members of Christ whom we should take in and cherish'.

Ken's plea was all the more impressive coming from 'a bishop who had undergone the censure of being inclined to Popery'. But he meant what he said and, just when Grace and Claver arrived to make their home in Wells, in April 1686 he sent a famous letter to all the clergy of his diocese urging them to do everything they could 'to contribute freely and cheerfully to the relief of these distressed [refugee] Christians'. Claver gave five shillings, the dean and chapter donated £40 from the cathedral's funds, and the king gave £1,500. But by far the largest contribution to the fund came from Ken himself; £4,000, almost all his worldly wealth. He had no regrets. By the end of 1686, the fund had raised over £42,000 in support of the poverty-stricken refugees. It was an unprecedented sum that would not be matched either by the £38,000 raised for the Irish Protestant refugees in 1689, or by the £22,000 raised for the Palatines, many of whom were sent on to America or (usually against their will) to Ireland.[5]

Most of the Huguenots who arrived in Somerset, such as the weavers, sailors and traders who settled in Bristol, were from working families, but not all were poor.[6] Men like James Gendrault of Golden Square in London, who was naturalised by royal authority in 1686, were of such standing that they were able to marry into titled families, as he did when he married Jane, a daughter of Maurice Berkeley of Bruton, 3rd viscount Fitzhardinge, who had been one of Claver's patients until his death in 1690. Consequently, James and Jane Gendrault, now living in the Liberty, became Claver's friends and they called for him when each of their three children were born. Within a year of James's death in 1707, Jane re-married, this time to Christopher Keen, a London merchant from a local family. It was not a happy marriage, possibly because Keen was something of a ladies' man, which might explain why, in 1709, Claver overheard the pair arguing fiercely about her not going to bed all night. But Claver was no less fond of Jane, with whom he enjoyed dancing, and although Betty was too shy to converse with her in French, both of Jane's daughters (by James Gendrault) came to Betty's ball.[7]

In the three years following Sacheverell's trial, much of Claver's professional time was devoted to looking after members of the Berkeley and Wyndham families. In addition to frequent visits to Colonel Berkeley's widow, Elizabeth, and her two unmarried children, Elizabeth and young Maurice, the MP for Wells, who all lived at Pylle,[8] there was now another branch of the family at the village of Maiden Bradley in Wiltshire, twenty miles west of Wells. Here, a massive new Palladian mansion, Bradley House, had recently been completed, built by the exceptionally arrogant, dissolute and shrewd old Tory magnate Sir Edward Seymour (a cousin and political rival of Charles Seymour, 'the proud duke' of Somerset) who had died in February 1708.

A few weeks earlier, Sir Edward's only daughter, Anne, had married William Berkeley, the younger brother of Maurice, and Claver was now given responsibility for looking after the whole family: Anne and her baby sons and daughter; her widowed mother, Lady Seymour; her brothers, Francis and Charles; and her half-brother the new Sir Edward (5th baronet) and his wife, Laetitia Popham, a cousin. Looking after this family entailed regular trips to Bradley House, where he would often stay overnight and lose several shillings playing cards. But sometimes he was called much further afield to the Woodlands estate in Dorset where another branch of the Seymour family lived. Travelling in winter was physically demanding, but it was always financially rewarding; for just treating the widowed Lady Seymour in the eighteen months before her death in March 1714, Claver's fees and expenses came to nearly £40.[9]

The Horners were another gentry family that often called upon Claver's services in these years. Their manor at Mells, a village outside Frome, was known to everyone, at least in verse. According to the nursery rhyme, this is what 'Little Jack' John Horner (steward to the abbot of Glastonbury during the Reformation) found when he 'Put in his thumb and pulled out a plum' from the pie that he was expected to deliver. Under the pastry, the abbot had hidden the deeds to properties that appealed to Henry VIII's rapacious appetite for England's monasteries. But, rather than return the documents to their rightful owner, 'Little Jack' simply kept the deeds to the manor of Mells, and made a fortune. Apocryphal or not, by the time 'Little Jack's' descendant, the nineteen-year-old Thomas Horner succeeded to the manor on the death of his father in 1708, the family estate had lost a large slice of its wealth. Even so, by 1709, Thomas was a great dining companion of William Berkeley and other members of the moon-feast club (as well as Claver's music club), and they often stayed at each other's homes when the weather was intemperate, or they had consumed too much beer and wine. No doubt, 'the half a buck' that Thomas Horner sent, and the hare delivered by Maurice Berkeley's huntsman to Claver's house in the summer of 1710 were intended for the monthly feasts.

In 1711, Thomas Horner was appointed high sheriff of Somerset, and two years later he was elected 'without opposition' alongside his fellow Tory, Sir William Wyndham, as a Knight of the Shire for Somerset. Both men were still just twenty-three. On 17th November 1713, Thomas married Susanna Strangways, a month before her father (a former Jacobite MP and very wealthy landowner from Dorset) died. Susanna's widowed mother now moved to Milton Clevedon, between Shepton Mallet and Bruton, where she had recently rebuilt one of the Strangways' manors at a cost of £6,000. So, Susanna was often there with her mother. Later, she would gain the whole of her family's estate, as well as a national reputation for being 'a very salacious Englishwoman'. In 1714, however, in spite of the visits he made, Claver was unable to save her baby son.[10]

With so many wealthy gentry families all calling for Claver's services, his financial dependance upon the senior clergy of the diocese was much reduced. He now also enjoyed a landed income of about £300 a year, and there were still patients in the city who depended upon him for support. One of these was his old friend William Westley. Having lost all five of his young children and, more recently, his wife (who even William Penn thought 'very kinde'), Westley had married Frideswide, the widow of the Rev. Edmund Brickenden, by whom she had two daughters. It was probably a mistake. Within a month of the marriage in April 1710, the new Mrs Westley was ill and would call for Claver at least thirty-six more times over the next four years, at a guinea a visit. And when William came to make his prosaic but charitable will, his thoughts were all for his first wife and his friends.[11]

As Claver's income from his work as a physician rose to £260 a year, he too could easily afford small acts of charity in addition to the free treatments he sometimes offered to the poorest of his patients. He gave half a guinea to Mrs Moss, 'she being Poor & sending Mrs Rogers [the midwife] to beg something of me', and he gave two guineas to Elizabeth Alford, 'being old and indigent, to help support her and keep her from being burthensome to Sturminster' parish. He also paid over two guineas for the nursing, washing, board and lodging of young Martha Alford for three weeks after her father had brought her to him to be cured of smallpox.[12] And although Claver felt he had to dismiss Will's maid 'for the misfortune of having [the] King's Evil [scrofula or tuberculosis of lymph nodes in the neck], & infecting my little son with it', he gave her six months' wages in compensation. He paid one of his labourers, John Parsons, his weekly wages even when he could not work, and when his man, Will Clark, caught smallpox, Claver paid his wages and for medicines and nursing, as well as someone to do Will's work.[13] He gave freely to street musicians, Morris dancers and travellers, such as the juggler who showed Betty tricks, and the dancers at Wells to whom he gave four shillings and sixpence to encourage them in 'these Diversions for the advantage of the Town'. He also gave twenty pence towards a bull-baiting at the Crown.[14]

There were other little acts of charity that Claver undertook outside the city, giving a few shillings to the parish poor or contributing to fund-raising ventures such as for the new organ at John Whitehand's church in Shepton Mallet.[15] But most of his good works were at places where he held land. So at Pilton, where he was beset with difficulties trying to build a fishpond to raise the six brace of carp that the Berkeleys had donated, and to recover the costs of pigeons that a parishioner had shot, he paid over two guineas for twelve dozen cushions 'for ye People to kneel on'.[16] A year later, at Pilton and Wedmore, he spent several pounds on folio editions of Thomas Comber's *A Companion to the Temple and Closet; or a help to public and private devotion* (1684–1702) and a guide to The Common Prayer Book, as well as desks and chains to secure the books.[17]

Having been elected by the parish vestry in West Bradley, Claver took on the responsibility of being an 'Overseer of the Poor'. This meant collecting the poor rate for the parish, distributing funds of about £30 a year to the needy, and keeping a good record of how all the sums were raised and spent. Since Claver was the second-highest taxpayer in the parish, paying over £3 every year, he had a financial interest in this unpaid work, and he enjoyed keeping meticulous accounts. But if he had not served the parish well and fairly, he would soon have been replaced. Instead, his probity ensured he was re-instated every year alongside another Overseer, usually chosen from among the wealthier but still illiterate parishioners; men like his tenant Henry Bull.[18]

Being such a regular visitor and well-known figure among the farmers in these marshy villages, Claver would have understood their way of life as akin to his own experiences growing up in the cattle-grazing lands of Blackmore Vale. He would also have known that disputes were mostly settled locally, often with the help of an arbitrator such as himself, except in cases where there had been a serious offence. So, when the vicar of Pilton reported acts of fornication or adultery to the church authorities there was little that Claver or anyone else could do. Having admitted her 'incontinence' with George Ramsey, in August 1712 Grace Hurly was required to stand in front of the pulpit in a white sheet and with a white wand in her hand at Sunday service, before confessing her 'heinous sin' to the congregation and asking for forgiveness. Although this was a standard penance, it was nevertheless a humiliating experience which George Ramsey was not required to share. Claver did not know either Grace or George, but a few years later, when other acts of fornication came to light at Pilton, he was unable to intervene on behalf of families he knew well. Only occasionally, as when William Hawkins stood before the congregation to say that he had defamed the widow Alice Andrews by calling her a whore, were men shamed in a similar, though less traumatic, way.[19]

23

QUEEN ANNE'S PEACE

During the three years of Tory government and legislation following Sacheverell's trial in 1710, Claver watched carefully over the development of his son and daughter. In January 1711, after sixty-four weeks of wet-nursing, baby Will was finally brought home from Jane Nooth's, though it would not be until September that he was taking his first steps. And although in the following year he caught scrofula from his maid, by July 1713 he had recovered well enough to be sent to Grace Pierce's dame school in Vicars' Close, for elementary education along with his new maid Mary Bedford, at a fee of a shilling each per month. In September 1712, Molly provided her son with a legacy of £300 that she had inherited from a cousin, and when Claver measured Will on his fourth birthday, 20th October 1713, he was just a fraction short of three feet tall.[1]

Betty was thriving too. She was still at school in Salisbury, and in the holidays would ride her pony around Wells and its surrounding villages, though on a trip to Dulcote to watch the reaping of the wheat she got caught in such a storm that a local boy had to bring her home. Occasionally, she accompanied her father on his trips to Bath to see his patients there, sometimes staying at the lodging house of the Three Tuns inn, near the abbey and the thermal baths. They bought green and bohea teas to take home for Molly, at five and seven shillings and sixpence for a quarter pound. In December 1712, Betty, now aged fifteen and exactly four-and-a-half feet tall, was also enjoying acting in 'a Tragedie' in which she had the leading part. In his notes, Claver told himself that she would not develop an abiding love for such a low profession, and that her interest in acting was only 'for diversion'.[2]

Two months earlier, Molly's father, Major Bragge, now seventy-two, had made his will, leaving £2,000, gold coins and his coach and horses to Elizabeth, his unmarried 'dutiful daughter' who lived with him at Sadborow. His main heir was his twenty-two-year-old spendthrift grandson William Bragge, whose younger brother

DOI: 10.4324/9781003333654-25

and sister each inherited £1,000. There was also £500 for his seventeen-year-old granddaughter, Anne Leigh, from the Isle of Wight, and another £500 for his grandson Will at Wells, when he reached the age of twenty-one. And to each of his servants, Major Bragge left five years' worth of wages. But for Betty, being no blood relation, there was nothing.[3]

Although Major Bragge paid Betty no attention (though she attended his funeral in March 1713), she was the apple of her father's eye. She had now left school in Salisbury but was still learning the harpsichord, with lessons (at four guineas a year) from the choral vicar William Broderip, who had just been appointed organist for the cathedral at £20 a year. She would make good use of her musical abilities when she went with Claver to stay with the Harringtons at Kelston, where she gave over six shillings in tips to servants and lost another shilling playing cards. Claver paid for these expenses and for items such as a prayer-book, bound in red turkey-leather, that he purchased from Henry Hammond at Bath for seven shillings, on top of the £5 pocket money he gave to Betty every year. But it was largely the cost of Betty's clothes, shoes, hats and accessories, made for her in Wells and London, that brought the annual tally of 'Clothes & Necessities for my Daughter' to nearly £30. This was much more than Claver, for all his fashion-conscious dressing, ever spent upon himself; and he even paid for one of his tailors to go to Bath 'to see [how] the fashionable make clothes'.[4] Yet no amount of money could keep Betty in good health.

Betty had caught smallpox at nine years old in 1706, when her baby sister had died from the disease. At the time, Claver and Molly feared they would lose Betty too, but she recovered and was now, so they hoped, immune. In April 1713, however, she began suffering from another serious illness, probably phthisis (tuberculosis), or 'consumption' as it was often called. It was a long-held belief, from ancient medicine, that asses could not catch phthisis, and that their milk, being the 'thinnest and less fat' compared with other milks, could 'nourish and cleanse' a patient, when taken 'fresh and hot' each morning. So, Claver secured a good supply of asses' milk and paid Margaret Bedford and Mrs Keen's maid to attend to Betty 'in her most Dangerous Sickness'. He also prepared his own remedies based upon very expensive bottles of white wine, and bought Betty food she loved; chocolate and baskets of strawberries grown at Axbridge. As word of the seriousness of her condition spread, a local huntsman brought her a hare for supper.[5] Whatever the efficacy of her treatments, when Betty was reckoned out of danger after thirteen weeks of suffering, it was time for a double celebration. The queen proclaimed that Tuesday 7th July 1713 would be a Day of Thanksgiving for the peace that Britain and all the Grand Alliance partners (except Austria and Hanover) had signed with France in the Treaty of Utrecht.

For the great majority of people, the peace represented an enormous relief after decades of unrelenting war, so it was no exaggeration when the *London Gazette* reported that the country was filled with 'Bells, Bonfires and Illuminations'. At Wells, the corporation set the tone by treating the public to a hogshead of ale to be drunk in the marketplace. Claver and his friends prepared for Thanksgiving Day by practising one of William Broderip's anthems, 'God is our Hope and Strength', to be performed in the cathedral where William played the organ. Bishop Hooper was not present at the service as he was delivering the Thanksgiving sermon to parliament at St Paul's cathedral. In this, he barely mentioned the defence of the realm or the terrible price of the military 'victories' that had been won. He was looking to the future: 'the Triumph now is for an Intire, Finish'd Victory; over not the Enemy only, over War it self: A Triumph truly Christian.' It was a noble sentiment. In Wells, however, Claver's thoughts were probably much closer to the public mood, giving thanks 'for this very Happy Peace, after a long and Insidious War for the advantage of the Dutch, fomented by the Dissenters, & treacherous Low-Churchmen for the Destruction of the True Church of England'.[6]

Under the terms of peace, Louis XIV renounced any union of the French and Spanish crowns; fully recognised the legitimacy of the Hanoverian succession at the death of Anne; and promised never to acknowledge that 'the Pretender', James II's son, had any rightful claim. But peace did nothing to unite the nation. Fuelled by the propaganda of Daniel Defoe, Jonathan Swift, Richard Steele, Mary Manley and a host of other writers, the Tory party was now deeply split between those, led by Robert Harley, who were largely committed to a Hanoverian succession (or at least to a Protestant one, if James Francis Edward Stuart could be persuaded to convert), and those led by Viscount Bolingbroke who were in secret negotiations with the Pretender and considering rebellion. Claver was in the former camp, but a number of his friends – including Sir William Wyndham and Thomas Horner who, riding on the popularity of peace, were elected MPs for Somerset during the Tory landslide victory in the autumn of 1713 – most definitely were not.

The problem for the Tories was that, on Anne's death, the best they could expect from the House of Hanover was to be swept from power. For everybody knew that Hanover was bitterly opposed to the Treaty of Utrecht and believed that peace with France was largely a ruse to bring in the Pretender. Consequently, when Anne became dangerously ill at Christmas 1713 and a few weeks later the famous author Richard Steele published *The Crisis,* a tract selling 40,000 copies which claimed that the Hanoverian succession was in danger, the sense of national emergency reached fever pitch. The Tory-dominated House of Commons had little choice but to condemn Steele for his 'malicious insinuations' that the government was secretly supporting the Pretender, but this simply confirmed most people's fears that the Hanoverian succession was at risk.[7] Leading members of the ministry, such as Bolingbroke and Wyndham, now tried to unite the Tories by attacking their old enemies, the Dissenters, and introducing a Schism Bill that would stamp out Dissenters' academies and schools. But on the day this law was due to come into force, 1st August 1714, Anne died. Sophia, the eighty-three-year-old Electress of Hanover had died two months earlier, so her son was proclaimed as George I.

For Claver and most people, Anne had been 'a most excellent Queen'; a 'much lamented and most gracious Queen' for whom, to show his respect, he bought *two* sets of mourning suits of very fine black cloth. Anne had not left a will that might attempt to overturn the Act of Settlement (1701) by bequeathing Britain to her half-brother James the Pretender, as the Jacobites had hoped. James, for his part, had made it clear that he would not renounce his Catholicism. For most moderate Tories, unwilling to commit treason, there was therefore no option but to accept the new Hanoverian regime. But that choice was not made any easier by the fact that at the age of fifty-four, George I was hard to like. He was a foreigner who had been cuckolded by his wife, who now lived under house arrest in Saxony. He lacked charisma and good looks, and he was often accompanied by his German mistress. Worse still was the fact that, politically, he was in the pocket of the Whigs.[8] Having dismissed Anne's Tory ministry in favour of the Whigs, by the time George was crowned at Westminster on 20th October 1714, a large part of the populace, particularly in the south and west, had had enough.

At Bristol, hearing a rumour that the Whigs were preparing to burn an effigy of Sacheverell, on the night of the coronation 'a horde of 500 colliers and labourers' gathered to loot Dissenters' homes and meeting houses and spoil all of the corporation's official celebrations. At least one rioter was killed, as well as a Quaker who tried to quell the mob. There were similar disturbances at Bath, Bridgwater, Dorchester, Salisbury, Taunton and other towns.[9] Claver normally went to the Crown where, for four shillings a year he subscribed to *Wye's Letter* and other papers to keep abreast of all the news. Now he picked up a new edition of *A Cat may look on a Queen*, a long satire in which its Whig author mocked Queen Anne's 'pretended virtues' and dark complexion. The writer sneered, 'I'll praise no Colour but what resembles the Night, and as 'tis Queen Anne's Complexion, 'tis a sort of Loyalty now to admire (or perhaps to look on) a Black woman.' The appearance of one more 'Abusive lying Pamphlet', as Claver called it, among the hundreds of others revelling in the Tories' loss of power, was simply a reflection of how deeply divided the country had become.[10]

Considering Claver's growing animosity towards the Whigs, it was fortunate in 1714 that he had no time for Jacobite intrigue. For five weeks in the summer, his family all went to Sadborow to stay with Molly's sister and her nephew William who had just inherited the Bragge estate. And they made another visit in the autumn, after William had sent Claver sixteen gallons of claret smuggled from across the Channel. Claver went to Sadborow and Lyme Regis too, and twice to Lydlinch to see his mother, but he did not linger anywhere. In addition to seeing the patients who came to his house for treatment, and undertaking local visits, he spent much of his time on horseback, often riding five hundred miles a month to attend to patients' needs. In fact, there were few large villages or towns within a day's ride of Wells where Claver did not have patients, and the number of people seeking his 'Advice in Physick' was rising, especially among the gentry.

In 1709, John Coxe from Wiltshire had married Margaret Hippisley at the village of Ston Easton, ten miles north of Wells, and had settled at the manor there. By 1713, Margaret, not yet twenty-one, was having her first child, and Claver was repeatedly called upon to prescribe. After the birth of two girls, she lost her first son, John, in November 1714.[11] A mile away, at the manor of Farrington Gurney, John Mogg, a former sheriff of the county, and his wife Dorothy, owners of land and coal mines in the region, had been among Claver's regular patients for several years. Their son, Richard, had his own family now, and their daughter Dorothy was about to be married to Thomas Churchey of Wincanton, so Claver became their families' doctor too.[12]

Further south, in 1714 he made his first visit to Montacute House, the home of Edward Phelips, who had just been dismissed as Comptroller of the Mint. Edward had been in dispute with his aunt Lady Edith Phelips ever since his uncle, Sir Edward, had died in 1699, leaving him an annuity of just £60 while the main family estates were placed under the authority of his indomitable aunt until her death. The fact that Edward had married his uncle's eldest and most favoured daughter, Ann, in 1702 (and after Ann's death, her sister) led to fresh disputes. But, by the time that Claver arrived at Christmas 1714, at least the family had found a way to live together in the great Elizabethan mansion. So Claver prescribed for Edith, Edward and his children, Ann and Bridget, and he also no doubt discussed the misfortunes of the Tory party since George I's accession. Edward also had his own grounds for complaint. He had been Tory MP for Ilchester since 1708, and won the most votes in the contested election of 1715. But a bailiff rigged the result, so Edward lost his seat until he was elected as a Knight of the Shire for Somerset in 1722.[13]

Thirty miles south of Wells, at East Coker on the Dorset border, William and Joanna Helyar were also regular old-gentry patients. William had inherited Coker Court and other estates in Somerset and Devon, and a sugar plantation in Jamaica with all its 'Stock of Negroes, Copper and other Utensils' from his Royalist father in 1697. Without any sense of incongruity, his father had also left £600 to be raised from the profits of his slave plantation to support the poorest residents of East Coker in the almshouses built by his grandfather. It was not until Christmas Day in 1710 that Claver began treating Joanna and her five children, and he visited them throughout the next few years. It was during his visit on 11th October 1714 that Joanna died.[14]

William paid Claver five guineas for treating Joanna, and Claver returned two weeks later to prescribe for Robert, one of the sons. But Claver was not called upon to administer at Coker Court again, though this was not the end of his relationship with the squire. William Helyar, whose mother had been a Wyndham, had been elected with Sir Edward Wyndham as a moderate Tory MP for Ilchester in the Convention Parliament of 1689–1690, voting in favour of William of Orange's accession to the throne. But although he had also been a sheriff of Somerset, he did not stand again for parliament until 1715. It was probably the twenty-six-year-old Sir William Wyndham, who persuaded William Helyar to stand in 1715 after a new parliament had been summoned in January by George I. The riots at the coronation had shown the depth of hostility towards the king and his Whig ministers, and there were unbending Tories such as Viscount Bolingbroke, Sir William Wyndham and James Butler, the 2nd duke of Ormond, who, having been dismissed from their high offices, were harbouring new ambitions. It was clear, however, that in the electorate as a whole, public opinion had shifted firmly in favour of the Hanoverian regime.

Sir William Wyndham and Thomas Horner were elected (uncontested) as the two Knights of the Shire for Somerset in the Tory landslide of 1713. But, in 1715, when Horner chose to stand with Maurice Berkeley as the candidates for Wells, Wyndham needed a new running mate who would appeal to the electorate of the county. For this, William Helyar fitted the bill perfectly. In theory, all adult males who owned freehold property worth £2 a year in rents were entitled to vote in the county elections. And as the number of freeholders in most counties ran into the thousands, votes cast for Knights of the Shires were generally regarded as the truest expression of 'the sense of the nation' as a whole. In the general election of February 1715, the Whigs took twenty-two of the nation's county seats from the Tories, and lost just one, so it was abundantly clear that the Whigs had secured an unprecedented victory in every sense. But not in Somerset.

Lending his hand to the Tory cause, in November 1714 Claver had already attended two meetings of freeholders in Wells who had promised to support the Wyndham and Helyar ticket.[15] At Somerton on 9th February 1715, he spent seven shillings and six pence in electoral treats, and paid for ten horses to carry freeholders to and from the poll at Ilchester. In the event, his contribution might have helped, but the contest was not close. William Helyar polled 2,789 and Sir William 2,664 votes; way more than their Whig contestants. On 4th February, Thomas Horner and Maurice Berkeley had been elected as MPs for Wells, with 44 and 43 votes respectively, twice as many as their rivals.[16] Thus, all four of Claver's friends were now able to use parliament to oppose the government and, as he must have suspected, at least two of them were prepared to do much more.

The decisive Whig victory in the general election of February 1715 did not allay Tory fears that the Whigs would allow the Church of England to be undermined to appease the interests of foreigners and Dissenters. In London and throughout the country during the spring and summer of 1715 there were scores of popular riots and disturbances attacking Dissenters' meeting houses, and relaying Jacobite chants. At Bristol, Bath, Marlborough, Frome and Norton St Philip on 10th June (the Pretender's birthday), James Francis Edward Stuart was proclaimed King James III.[17] In response to such treasonable acts, the government did what it believed was necessary to secure the state: Robert Harley (committed to the Tower); Bolingbroke (fled to France to become the Pretender's Secretary of State); and the duke of Ormond (a former Captain-General who also fled to France) were all impeached. The Riot Act was passed, making it punishable by death (with the authorities indemnified for any use of lethal force) for anyone in a group of twelve or more people not to disperse within an hour of a public reading of the Act. And the Habeas Corpus Act of 1679 was suspended, making it far easier to keep people imprisoned without good evidence for their arrest.

Heartened by the popular riots, the poet, playwright and Jacobite George Granville, Lord Lansdown (former Treasurer of the Household) and Sir William Wyndham took the lead in planning a rebellion in the West. It was to be centred on Bath, where 100 gentlemen would gather to bear arms, expecting to be led by the duke of Ormond when he set sail from France. Although on 6th September the earl of Mar raised an army in Scotland under the Pretender's standard, by the end of the month the plans for a rebellion in the West had run adrift. The prospect of French support was scuppered by the death of Louis XIV, and the government's discovery of the conspiracy led to warrants for the arrest of three Jacobite peers and six MPs. Lord Lansdown was soon arrested for high treason and imprisoned in the Tower, and after a dramatic escape from his home at Orchard Wyndham, Sir William handed himself in at the beginning of October. He had hoped that his father-in-law, the duke of Somerset, would be able to procure a pardon, but he was disappointed and found himself confined to the Tower until June 1716.[18] By then, the rebellion in Scotland had been defeated, dozens of Jacobites had been executed and hundreds transported to the colonies. Moreover, the Whigs had strengthened their hold on the government by passing the Septennial Act which extended the maximum life of the present and future parliaments to seven years.

24

FAMILY & FRIENDS

The good citizens of Wells – or at least the freemen of the city who were granted a vote in the re-election of Thomas Horner as MP in June 1716 – clearly liked his politics. For although his victory in 1715 was overturned in the House of Commons by the Whigs, and he was very lucky to escape arrest for his support of the Western uprising, in 1716 he was re-elected with a great majority, securing 221 votes against a Whig candidate from Dorset who polled just ninety-five.[1] As a trusted physician who travelled regularly between the houses of the landed gentry in the region, no-one was better placed than Claver to carry confidential messages and papers to and from conspirators such as Horner and the Wyndhams. But if he did lend assistance, as his framing of a print of the duke of Ormond (impeached for high treason) might suggest, he wisely left no paper trace and kept any secret missions to himself.

What would certainly have attracted suspicion was the arrival of Mary Evans and her maid at Claver's house in January 1716. Mary, whom Claver had known since she was a child, was the daughter and heir of John and Anne Evans, who had rented the old chantry house to Grace and Claver when they had come to Wells in 1686. Having lost both of her parents, Mary, now in her thirties, was one of richest ladies in the city, with land and properties around Wells, and an estate in Cornwall, worth over £225 a year. She was also unmarried and, like her parents, Roman Catholic. As well as the old chantry house in the Back Liberty and a house in Chamberlain Street, Mary owned manors and farms in the nearby villages of Burcott, Godney, and Dulcote.[2] So she was never short of a place to stay. Being a rich, single Catholic woman, however, at a time when all Catholics, especially after the Jacobite Rebellion, were regarded with suspicion and often treated to abuse, she would not find it easy living on her own. At Claver and Molly's home, she could live very comfortably and safely, and share all the respect and good company that the Morris family enjoyed.

DOI: 10.4324/9781003333654-26

It was probably Molly who invited Mary to come and live in her for, after accepting twenty moidores (worth about £27) in a silver purse from Mary for the first eleven months of her board and lodging, Claver immediately passed three of the gold coins to his wife.[3] Whatever suspicions Mary's presence might have aroused in Wells, they were not anything with which Molly could not cope. With Claver so often absent, Molly must have welcomed Mary's companionship and genteel company in the house for she took Mary on visits to see friends, and to stay with her sister and nephew at Sadborow.

Betty also enjoyed Mrs Evans' company. Now eighteen, she accompanied her on trips to enjoy the sights and company of Bath, where Mrs Evans' mother had been buried in 1706. On these trips Betty could dress in the latest fashions, showing off her embroidered silk gowns, fans and headdresses, gold studs and a diamond and topaz ring. She was now old enough to take trips on her own. As well as visits to see relations at Sadborow, South Cadbury and Lydlinch, she stayed with the Harringtons at Kelston and the Berkeley family at Pylle. She took the stagecoach to Exeter to stay with the Drewes of Broadhembury, and rode to Bath, where she stayed with the rector of the abbey, archdeacon William Hunt and Elizabeth his wife. Betty also stayed at the grand new mansion of Bradley House, where Sir Edward Seymour, the 5th baronet, lived with his wife, eight daughters and four sons.

On top of her £5 a year in pocket money, Claver lent Betty extra money to support her trips – though he noted that he did not expect to be repaid. He also supported Betty's love of theatre, treating her to see a French juggler, rope dancers and 'a play acted by a Deaf Man, a Paralytick Woman, & a Girl taught by these two', at the Crown. And he took Betty and her friends to see Jones's Company of Players (where, unsurprisingly considering Betty's love of fruit, they also feasted on some pears); Nicholas Rowe's *The Tragedy of Jane Shore* (1714); one of Tom Durfey's trilogy of plays with music by Purcell, *The Comical History of Don Quixote* (1694); and Thomas Otway's *The Orphan, or the Unhappy Marriage* (1680).[4]

Will was six years old in 1716, and although he was still attending the dame school in Vicars' Close, he was now also having reading and Latin lessons from Thomas Gravill, a choral vicar who lived with his wife and three young children in the Close. Will was being prepared for admission as a day-boy at the cathedral's grammar school (dressed in a scarlet coat and breeches), where Robert Creighton, the precentor's son, was the headmaster. Another choral vicar, James Nicholls, who lived with his family in Chamberlain Street, was teaching Will how to dance, charging Claver two guineas a year plus a little more for music and candles. Yet, being Claver's son was never going to be easy in terms of matching his father's boundless energy and determination to succeed. So when William Bragge, who preferred parties to studies, sent his man to deliver 'a spaniel puppy dog' to his cousin Will, he might well have hoped this little gift would bring young Will amusement and diversion.[5]

Will was not the only boy who was a member of the Morris household in 1716, as Claver had taken on a new apprentice, Jack Watts, probably as a favour to his father, William, who was Claver's tailor. William was instructed to make his son a livery suit, for which he was paid £8 and, as part of the indenture, Jack would now be bound to work for and 'live obediently' with Claver for the next ten years. Such agreements were a common way of training children for particular trades and professions, and Claver might hope to educate young Jack to be an apothecary or surgeon. But, if Jack were to be a full member of the Morris household, as well as working hard he would need to be able to make a contribution to its music. So Claver immediately paid £4 for Jack to have an intensive course of lessons on the violin, or until the teacher had 'perfected' him.[6]

Although by 1716, there were eleven members of the Morris household – Claver, Molly, Betty and Will; Mary Evans and her maid; Will Clark and Jack Watts, Claver's man and boy; and the three maids, Elizabeth Stone, Sarah Bampfield and young Molley Mitchell, who lived in the servants' quarters in the back garden – there was always room for guests. Friends, relations and players at the music club often came to stay for a day or two, and sometimes longer as when the London musician John Shojan was given bed and board for eight months, during which time Claver paid him 'to perfect' Betty on the violin.[7] She had been taught to sing and dance, and was still having lessons on the harpsichord, and she liked to recite and act. So, when it came to the 'entertainments' held the house at least once or twice a week, Betty could always lend a hand.

Across the road, Claver had not given up on plans to build a passageway between the Back Liberty and the Vicars' Close, despite the vicars' Statutes and the ruling of the bishop. So, in 1715, he purchased the leases for two of the vicars' houses at the top end of the Close for £35 from the subdean Henry Layng, and by 1716 had fixed a set of stairs, doors and locks to give him private access. He was pleased with the arrangement, and it meant that he could now rent one of the houses to Grace Pierce, the mistress of Will's school. But this exercise of what he believed to be his legal right would store up problems for the future. He also exercised his landowner's right to take action at the quarter sessions in January 1717 against a poacher 'for beating out a hare & hunting it with greyhounds' on his manor at Perridge in Pilton. But his most persistent problem at Perridge was that the fishpond he had spent years building, inspecting, filling and repairing, and that he reckoned ought to hold 113,501 gallons, was still leaking.[8]

The dean and chapter had their problems too, for the government was ready to demonstrate that it would not tolerate any sign of Jacobite resistance in the West. In August 1716, a month before the Wells assize, it sent a troop of soldiers to the city as a show of force. It was over thirty years since Monmouth's rebels had 'robbed and defaced' the cathedral and Judge Jeffreys had presided over a 'bloody assize' in the marketplace, but memories of these events had not faded from the public mind. So, when soldiers were allowed during Sunday services to 'enter the cathedral church in a military manner and make it a place of arms and exercise', contrary to the laws of the realm and 'to the great offence and disturbance of the congregation', it was not only the dean and chapter that were appalled. Yet, all they could do was to write to the commanding officer, asking him 'to give such order that the like practice may for the future be forborn'. At the age of seventy-six, bishop Hooper, a moderate Tory and supporter of the Hanoverian succession, had largely disengaged from politics, so he chose not to intervene.[9]

While the government regarded the clergy and gentry of Wells and the West with great suspicion, it was Catholics who were generally held responsible for the Jacobite rebellion. To punish and diminish them, they were now required to register their names and properties at the quarter sessions, and were fined and threatened with the confiscation of their estates. Bath and Wells had always had a small but notable number of Catholic residents, like Mary Evans and her parents, and they were required to pay double the annual land-tax rate. But not all Catholics were rich. In 1715, Mary registered her 'Papist estates' as being worth £225 a year, and her relatives, John and Thomas Evans, listed theirs. But her friend and relation Mary Muttlebury, who had recently inherited Wookey manor, two miles from Wells, managed to avoid declaring any of her family's wealth, probably by making regular visits to the parish church. In Sadler Street, the Market Place and High Street, where there had been eight Catholics among the 158 Land Tax payers in 1709, most were listed again in 1715.[10]

Aside from Mary Evans, the Pearce family – including Joseph (leaseholder of the Swan in Sadler Street), Elias (a baker), Thomas, and James (believed to be a priest) – were probably the most prominent local Catholics. But there were two mercers, James and Jonas Browne (who held property in Dorset); and a widow, Margaret Woolmer of Burcott (where Mary Evans owned the manor), who also registered estates. A bodice-maker and a chandler were among those who managed to keep their names out of the books. So did the family of Jonas Bourne, a woollen draper in the High Street, whose son, Thomas, was one of Claver's tailors. He and all the others were well known to Claver. Mary Muttlebury and Margaret Woolmer came to dinner at his house, and ten years earlier on the basis of his friendship with the Muttleburys he had lent them £360 to extend the mortgage on their lease of Wookey manor.[11] There were also Catholic families further afield that Claver knew and prescribed for, such as the Beaumonts of Ston Easton and Francis Carne of Bath (Steward of the Catholic James, Lord Waldegrave at Chewton Mendip). And Claver was still visiting Mary Greene and Charles Willoughby, the Catholic aunt and the cousin of his first wife Grace, at the villages of Knoyle and Donhead in Wiltshire; villages in which there were Catholics, living next to an even larger congregation at Wardour, the great estate of the Catholic Henry, Lord Arundel.[12]

For all his objections to Catholicism, Claver counted on Catholics as his friends, and that meant he would try to support and protect them from unjust treatment; for the 1715 Rebellion had not been led by Catholics but High Churchmen like Sir William Wyndham. After the discovery of another Jacobite conspiracy in 1722, led in Devon by another of his young friends, Sir Coplestone Warwick Bampfylde, Claver served as a collector of a new tax on 'Papists and other Persons' who refused to take three oaths of loyalty. The claim that all Catholics were 'Notoriously concerned in Contriving, Stirring up, and Supporting the said Rebellions, Insurrections and Conspiracies, by which it most manifestly appears, that they take themselves to be obliged, by the Principles they profess, to be Enemies of his Majesty and the present happy Establishment', was quite untrue. But Somerset was required to raise £915 (of a national sum of £100,000) from those who refused to take the oaths. Claver chose a gentleman attorney with whom he had worked as a Land Tax officer, Richard Comes (sheriff of the county in 1722), to help him collect the tax, but it was a fractious business. In the process, he tried to secure reductions in the contributions made by Mary Evans and his tailor Thomas Bourne, but without success.[13]

Although by 1717 the Tory party was hopelessly split between the majority who accepted the accession of King George and the minority who would not, the party was united in its opposition to government by the Whigs. In Wells this meant that to make it harder for the Whig majority in the Commons to overturn the city's election of Tory MPs (as it had done by ousting Thomas Horner and Maurice Berkeley in May 1716), the mayor and corporation were happy to increase the number of freemen entitled to a vote. The process began in January 1717 when seventy-two citizens, led by the Town Clerk, John Gutch, petitioned to be freemen. Yet, although Horner had been restored to his place with a huge majority in the by-election in June 1716, the new freemen of the city could not prevent the Whig majority in the Commons from ousting him again, in April 1717, in favour of John Dodd, the twenty-four-year-old Whig candidate from Dorset. So, after Robert Taylor the grocer was made mayor in September, a new round of Tory admissions to membership of the city's guilds took place.

In 1705, the corporation had rejected Claver's application to join a guild, though at the same time it had admitted several of his friends, including William Berkeley and John Prowse. Twelve years later, Claver was among the twenty-three men who were now admitted as freemen of the Mercers' Company, and others joined as members of the Inn-holders' and Hammerers' guilds. The list of twenty-three was quite extraordinary. It began with two Jacobites, Sir William Wyndham and Sir Coplestone Bampfylde. Third and fourth were Thomas Prowse (the nine-year-old son of John, the former MP for Somerset, and grandson of the bishop) and William Bragge of Sadborow. The next three on the list were William Malet (barrister of the Middle Temple, living in East Liberty), John Horner (a relative of Thomas Horner, the ousted MP), and Davidge Gould (another barrister of the Middle Temple, the son and heir of Sir Henry of Sharpham Park). Claver was eighth on the list, followed by John Burland, a young gentleman from Stogursey, ten miles west of Bridgwater. All were well known to Claver, though not all were from the gentry. When, among a group of sixteen of them, Claver took the oaths of loyalty and signed his name to become a burgess of the city on 26th November 1717, three of the group were unable to sign, so they just drew a cross to make their mark.[14]

Although it cost him £8 in drinks and fees, and a donation towards the upkeep of the city's almshouses,[15] after years of exclusion, it must have given Claver tremendous satisfaction that in 1717 he had finally received the civic recognition that he felt that he deserved, especially as this came at the end of a hard year. In the spring he had lost two of his best friends. At the age of thirty-six, Will's godfather, Maurice Berkeley of Pylle, MP for Wells, a music lover and popular member of the moon-feast club, had died after months of illness during which Claver had been his doctor. Being single, he left most of his estate to his younger brother William, but all his books went to Wadham College, Oxford, and all his clothes plus £100 to his servant, William Wood.[16]

The second death was less expected but equally distressing. George Farewell, rector of South Cadbury, had been married to Anne Dawe, the sister of Elizabeth, Claver's second wife. When George died in April 1717, he left a wife and two young sons, George and Thomas. It seemed that his will – leaving his estates in trust to Anne for her life and then to George, with £500 bequeathed to Thomas – was quite straightforward. But it was disputed in court by William Dawe, the self-styled 'next friend' of the four-year-old Thomas, against his nine-year-old brother, mother, and the two executors, Nathaniel Farewell (George's brother) and Claver Morris. By the autumn, Anne was sufficiently distressed for Claver to reserve one of his houses in Vicars' Close as a place for her and the sons to live.[17] And he would keep a close eye on the future of them all, not only out of his unswerving loyalty towards his former friend, but also because he cared for Anne and was determined to support her sons.

PART THREE

1718–1727

25

THE LETTER

1718 was a year that no-one in the Morris household was ever likely to forget, though at first there were no great changes to report. Almost every day, Claver continued to visit patients and to offer advice and prescriptions at his house. His reputation was now so well established that on top of this regular work he was also called upon in all kind of emergencies, for there were no hospitals to treat the sick.

In mid-January, an inexperienced young midwife, Gertrude Hanne, suddenly arrived on horse, fearing for the life of her patient, the wife of John Cannon, a poor clerk from Shepton Mallet. During a long labour, in accordance with superstition, Mrs Cannon had drunk a glass of her husband's urine to hasten the delivery of her baby, and this had seemed to work. But a few days later, she became so ill, the midwife was advised by local women 'in this critical juncture' to consult 'a[n] eminent physician in Wells, one Dr. Claver Morris' to save the mother's life. From what he could discern from Gertrude's account of Mrs Cannon's condition, Claver clearly feared the worst, and said as much. But he drew up a prescription to be made up and administered immediately by Reynold Oak, the apothecary he knew at Shepton. Much to everyone's relief, the treatment soon 'had its intended effect', for which John Cannon cheerfully recorded in his diary that he 'praised God and the doctor'.[1]

Such emergencies were not uncommon and they did not disturb the regular pattern of daily life in the Morris household in 1718. Will Clark was now working independently, but still helping out occasionally. Thus, George Champion was brought into service and kitted out in the Morris and Bragge livery. Mary Gould had replaced Sarah Bampfield as one of Molly's maids, and Mary Evans and her maid were now fully settled in as residents. Molly, now fifty-one, was worried about the health of Elizabeth her sister, still living at Sadborow with her nephew William Bragge. Will Morris was growing tall at eight years old, learning French

DOI: 10.4324/9781003333654-28

and Latin at the cathedral grammar school, and had received a legacy of £50. Betty was just twenty, still taking lessons on the harpsichord and violin, but enjoying travelling, either on behalf of her parents or on visits of her own. Claver too was well and often travelling, not only locally but across the county. Even in the cold of January and February he went to stay and play music with the Harringtons at Kelston (twice), the Horners at Mells (three times), and made trips to Lydlinch, Sadborow, Axbridge, Somerton, North Cadbury, Farrington Gurney, Pylle and Chewton Mendip.

The household expenses were rising, even though the cost of alcohol had fallen as gallons of smuggled 'French Claret' and 'White Lisbon Wine' were now being delivered by William Bragge's coachmen, both for local consumption and for re-distribution. Claver was still purchasing books on medicine, mathematics, history and religion; usually losing a few shillings playing cards and backgammon at the places where he stayed (though he won ten shillings on a horserace at Maesbury Castle on the Mendips); and paying for new music and expenses for the meetings of his club. This was thriving and its reputation was strong enough to attract the attention of the former prime minister, Robert Harley, earl of Oxford, who had been released from the Tower of London in the summer of 1717, with all charges against him dropped. He was still banned from Court, but on Tuesday evening, 8th July 1718 he arrived at Vicars' Hall to enjoy the music with his wife, Lady Sarah, and his old friend, the poet and diplomat Matthew Prior, who had also been kept in custody and impeached.

Claver rarely missed any meetings of the club, and these occasions, together with his household's gathering on Sunday evenings, were probably the only times each week when anyone could be fairly sure where he would be. Even at six o'clock on any morning when he was at matins, he could be called away with little notice to attend a patient's needs. But Tuesday and Sunday evenings were almost invariably reserved. On Tuesdays he would play and sing, and sometimes dance, often late into the night among his friends. On Sundays he would read to his household from one of several books designed to promote a clear understanding of what it meant to lead a Christian life. His texts were taken from a series of moral guides first published anonymously at the time of the Restoration: *The Whole Duty of Man* (1658), *The Gentleman's Calling* (1660), *The Causes of the Decay of Christian Piety* (1667), and *The Ladies Calling* (1673). Since then, these books had become immensely popular among Anglicans, and their author, the Royalist divine, Richard Allestree, had been rewarded with the post of Regius Professor of Divinity at Oxford University in 1663. Claver took each text in turn, reading and commenting on selected passages every week until it was completed.

Each book had its merits, but it was from *The Whole Duty of Man Laid Down in a Plain Way for the Use of the Meanest Reader* that he read the most. This was because it consisted of seventeen chapters, one to be read every Sunday, on topics such as love, humility and obedience; each chapter giving 'a short and plain direction' to good Christians on how 'to behave themselves so in this world, [so] that they may be happy for ever in the next'.[2] As every member of the household, whether literate or not, learned what Allestree (and Claver) thought about their duty to God, to their neighbours and themselves, a shared understanding of good conduct developed. This served the household well, for there were rarely any signs of bad behaviour that Claver thought worthy of recall. But things could change, especially when high standards were not upheld elsewhere.

Across the road, the conduct of the choral vicars was a regular topic of discussion among the dean and chapter, and on 1st July 1718 the dean warned the vicars that their negligence in the performance of their duties was notorious and would not be tolerated. It made no difference. On the following day William Hill, the eldest son of Samuel, the former archdeacon of Wells who had been such a bitter opponent of Bishop Kidder, failed to turn up to read prayers at a service led by Dr Edmund Archer, the archdeacon of Taunton. And ten days later, another choral vicar, Farewell Perry, who had only just been appointed, was suspended for refusing to apologise for the 'neglect of his duties and want of respect in not bowing to the dean in church'. So all the vicars were summoned to the Chapter House, where they listened to the dean's enumeration of their duties and his stricture that 'their whole behaviour' should be 'exemplary, sober and religious, so as not to dishonour this church or discredit religion, in the service of which they are so immediately concerned'.[3]

In their defence, the vicars might well have claimed that they were only following the self-serving, often venal and hypocritical example of so many of their superiors; though few would dare to say as much. But when young Farewell Perry, a new friend of Claver who had only been ordained in 1717, could not bring himself to seek a pardon from the dean, it was Claver who could not hold his tongue. During a visit from Dr Archer and his wife, Claver raised the subject by saying that he 'regretted that the Solemn Worship of God should be abated, & ungracefully performed because the Dean thought himself not humbly enough Bowed to & reverenced'. Archer replied: 'tis no great matter whether He is worshiped or not, if it must be done by such a fellow as Perry who does not pay Respect to his Superiors'. Claver had no time for bad behaviour, or for Dr Matthew Brailsford, the sixty-year-old unmarried dean and prebend of Lincoln cathedral who, in thirty years as dean, would leave almost no trace of any work accomplished at Wells, let alone any legacy of note.[4] But Archer's response was shocking, especially as it was before a witness.

Sitting at the parlour table listening to Archer on 20th July was the surgeon Christopher Lucas, who had become one of Claver's closest friends. Ever since he had looked after Claver during his serious illness in 1709, Claver had taken him on visits to treat patients, and he had also sent him to administer to Molly's father at Sadborow before Major Bragge's death in 1713. Usually, Lucas's treatments would entail a simple venesection, letting out about a pint of blood. But he also conducted more complex operations as when he cut off the tendon of a boy's tibialis posterior muscle, exposing the nerves and vessels in order to get to the 'foul bones' of the leg. Lucas had a twin sister, being one of the last two children of a working family from the Quantock Hills, forty miles from Wells. Thus, he had done well to become Claver's most trusted surgeon, and although he could still only afford to live in lodgings in the High Street with his wife, they were often invited to dine with Claver's family in the Liberty.[5] Even so, over the hot summer days of 1718 neither Lucas nor any of Claver's other friends had any sense of something furtive going on.

Part of the reason for Claver's lack of insight was due to his frequent absences from home, often attending to the needs of patients. After Betty had spent ten days at Horsington with her recently widowed aunt Anne Farewell, Claver took Betty on a trip to Lydlinch to see her grandmother in July, stopping off at Francis (Frank) and Dorothy Newman's manor at North Cadbury to inspect Dorothy's ganglion. In September, he also took Betty and her friend, Sarah Edwards, on one of his trips to Bath, where Molly's sister, Anne Leigh from the Isle of Wight, had been staying for the season. He did not find time to accompany Molly on her trips to Sadborow, though Mary Evans did. Rather, he stayed away for days looking after families such as the Horners at Mells, and the Pitts at Bath and Cricket Malherbie, near Chard. He also made trips to Kelston, where he was always welcome to play Vivaldi's concertos and Handel's anthems and symphonies with the Harringtons and some of the best musicians in the country. And he spent days in his laboratory and on visits to the local joiner and blacksmith, Tom Parfitt, to oversee a range of innovations and adjustments that Tom was making to improve his harpsichord, though without very much success.

With so much confidence in his own observations and opinions, it was unsurprising that Claver had an argument with his draper William Salmon, a former mayor of Wells, on 26th August 1718 at his shop in the High Street. This was about Isaac Newton's claim in *Opticks* (1704) that white light is a mixture of coloured rays. Claver soon corrected Salmon by demonstrating 'the insufficiency and fallaciousness of Dr Newton's Notion & Hypothesis of Colours'; and, no doubt, he had instruments in his own laboratory to prove the point.[6] After work in his laboratory, on the following day he went to Bath to treat Anne Leigh and old William Pitt of Kensington, eating at the new dining room of the Three Tuns inn.[7] And on Friday 29th August he returned to Wells with Samuel Pitt, William's son, just in time to witness the preternatural darkness caused by a total eclipse of the moon.

The significance of these days would only emerge later, and only after further days of Claver's absence during November. After daily trips to the Mendips to prescribe for Mrs Moss and her new-born daughter, and getting lost in the fog three times on his journeys home, Claver's final service was as a pall-bearer at her funeral on 19th November. So, it was a relief that he could now focus on preparations for the St Cecilia's Day concert by his music club on the 22nd. For the concert he was delighted to have William Douglas, the celebrated 'Black-moor [black-skinned] Trumpeter', reckoned by Claver to be 'one of the best in England on that instrument', performing 'two Sonatas very finely' and dining and staying for two days with him at his home.[8] On the 24th he took delivery of £700 in cash from Mr Samuel Child in payment for the sale of his estate at Felton; money that was probably passed to Molly to help her shore up her family's finances at Sadborow.[9] And the next day he travelled to Sir John Trevelyan's great estate at Nettlecombe Court on the edge of Exmoor. Here he found that Lady Susanna, under the care of the distinguished physician Dr William Musgrave FRS, was 'quite worn out, but not just dead'. So he stayed for several days for a fee of twelve guineas, treating her 'Atrophy & Hectick-Fever' with a vitriol (diluted sulphuric acid) which caused her to vomit four times before it 'did her some good'.[10]

When Sir John Trevelyan, MP for Minehead, arrived from London on the 29th, Claver left Nettlecombe to ride twenty miles to Hestercombe House near Taunton to administer to one of the largest landowners in Somerset, Sir Francis Warre, a former MP for the town who had been imprisoned in 1715 on account of his part in Sir William Wyndham's plans for a rebellion. Claver's diagnosis was that Sir Francis had been seized with 'a Dropsie to the Brain' (cerebral oedema), so he told Lady Warre that his chances of recovery were 'as improbable as to throw 6 upon 6 Dies'. Had Margaret, their only surviving daughter, been present, they might have tried some of the local remedies and recipes that she had begun collecting. But she had left Hestercombe in October after marrying John Bampfylde, MP for Exeter and brother of the Jacobite MP for Devon, Sir Coplestone Bampfylde, and there was no time to spare. At midnight on the next day, Sir Francis died.[11]

When Claver arrived home after riding thirty miles across Sedgemoor in the wind and rain on Monday 1st December, it was nearly dark. But he would not rest until he had opened the mail that had been delivered while he was away. Sitting in his study in the candlelight wearing his horn-rimmed reading glasses he broke the seals of all his letters, expecting to learn how patients were progressing and where he might be travelling next. The week before, he had given Betty leave to visit Dorothy Newman at North Cadbury Court, on the road to Sherborne and Lydlinch. Betty knew the Newmans well, as they were friends of her aunt Anne Farewell, who lived nearby and with whom she also often stayed. As Betty was not at home in Wells, when Claver saw a letter from the Newmans, he must have expected to hear that she was still with them or had gone to see her aunt. But Frank Newman's news was shocking: 'Mr Burland came to his House Wednesday in the Evening, & told him he was married to her [Betty] Aug. 28 last, which she also own'd.'

In his diary Claver recalled that Frank 'express'd a very great Concernment knowing the great Aversion I had to this Match which I had always express'd & taken all the Pains I possibly could to prevent'.[12] But if Frank found it hard to write the letter, Claver found it unbearable to read. Not only had Betty totally disobeyed him, disregarding everything she had been taught about her duty to her family and faith; she had also exposed herself and her family to ridicule and gossip as stories of her clandestine marriage spread. It seemed that in this the most important decision she would ever make, she had simply ruined her whole life. As for John Burland, to show such wanton disregard for a lady's honour and reputation was unforgivable, and certainly despicable in someone who claimed to be a gentleman, descended from an ancient family.

As the only son of John and Margaret Burland, Betty's husband had inherited the manor of Steyning at Stogursey, a village near the Quantocks, on the death of his father in 1713. He was then seventeen, and his mother had died ten years before.

He had not, therefore, enjoyed the opportunity often afforded to first sons to go to university before taking over the family estates and, in John's case, these were already heavily encumbered with legal disputes and debts. Claver would remember meeting him before Christmas in 1712, when he was still sixteen, as he came to his house in the Liberty seeking medical attention, and was charged ten shillings for the consultation. This was probably when John first met Betty too, when she was aged just fifteen.[13]

Two years later, John paid for another consultation. More recently, in November 1717, he and Claver had stood together in the marketplace to be elected freemen of the city. As there were gentry families in and around Wells with whom John could stay, Betty now had plenty of opportunities to see him on her travels. In this there was no secret, for as Claver saw the development of their friendship, he made it clear to both of them that there was absolutely no prospect of them marrying with his consent. It was not that Burland had a shameful reputation, but he had not attended university and had very little money. So, this was a most 'disadvantageous' match as far as Claver was concerned. And with plenty of eligible young men for Betty to choose from (not least among the sons of her father's friends), Claver knew that she could have made a far more advantageous match.

As Claver reflected on the travesty, and tried to control his fury that his treasured daughter had defied him and deceived him by keeping her marriage a secret for three months, he could recall that Betty had been sick in bed when he had returned to Wells on the afternoon of Saturday 16th August, and on the night of Thursday 28th August he had lodged at Bath. That was the night when, with extraordinary guile and caution, John and Betty must have sneaked into the cathedral like a couple of foxes in order make their marriage vows. Knowing that the news was out, on the morning of 2nd December, Betty wrote to Molly imploring her to intercede to get a pardon for her and John. And after receiving Molly's reply, she sent another letter the next day, as well as one to Will. But Claver would not be moved. He insisted on knowing who was responsible for marrying his twenty-year-old daughter without parental consent, under cover of darkness, and if there were any way this marriage could be undone. So, on Saturday 6th December, he went to his old friends, first to the precentor Robert Creighton and then to Marshall Brydges, chancellor of the bishop's court, to discuss 'the abominable injury the Sacrist had done me'.

The cathedral's sacrist was Thomas Cooper, and his duties were quite clear. These included: sweeping the Choir and Lady Chapel; tolling the chapter bell at the quarters of each day; winding the great clock; carrying the Bible for the canons; lighting candles in the winter; and, most importantly, locking 'all the church doors at such times as are usual'.[14] So, without his keys and assistance at the service, no marriage could have taken place. Yet, even for a very hefty sum, there were probably few priests who would have dared to conduct a clandestine marriage in the cathedral in the middle of the night, given the wrath they could expect from Dr Morris, let alone from the dean and chapter. But Sam Hill, son of the former archdeacon, was one of them.

Sam's elder brother, William, had just been reprimanded for dereliction of duty as a choral vicar, and Sam himself was already well known to Claver. He was the boy who had stolen books from the school library, and who Bishop Hooper had failed to punish in 1710. And in December 1716, at the age of twenty-three, Sam had been ordained by Hooper at the bishop's palace. He was still single and, like his siblings, had been left little money by his father, though he had inherited his English books; the Greek and Latin ones going to William. So, the cash that John Burland offered Sam for his services on 28th August 1718 would surely have been welcome. Yet, when the dean and chapter met on 10th December to discuss the case, the result was clear. They recognised that Betty was 'a minor under the age of 21', 'given away [by the sacrist] without her parents' consent in the cathedral church', and that Sam was 'not entitled to officiate there and without the leave of the president of the chapter [the dean] or any of the canons'. But the marriage was still binding. So, there would be no tortuous investigation and eventual over-ruling of the ceremony, as there had been in the Richard Cupper case. The dean and chapter simply punished Thomas Cooper with suspension for a year, and Sam Hill was 'forbidden to officiate in the cathedral on any pretext whatever'.[15]

This was probably the outcome that Claver had expected, but he still went to the palace the next day to talk about 'the ingrateful & villainous action of Sam Hill'; a complaint that would be resumed every time the bishop called for relief from his gout during the ensuing weeks and months. All that Claver could do to allay his anger now – since he had no mind to forgive – was to maintain his own duties and responsibilities. He continued his industrious routine: visiting patients and trekking over the Mendips with Christopher Lucas, even when the snow was 'up to the Bellys of our Horses'; managing the music club; working in his laboratory and making up prescriptions; writing to friends and patients; and, following a three-week break after hearing about Betty's marriage, completing the reading of *The Whole Duty of Man* to the remaining members of his household. On Christmas Day, he took Communion, had a dozen guests for dinner and invited another dozen to play music. To assist with the evening's entertainment he paid four cathedral choristers four shillings to sing carols.[16] But no amount of festive cheer could hide the fact that someone was missing.

26

THE SEVERANCE

Whatever Molly thought of Betty's decision to marry John Burland, secretly and against her father's wishes, she knew that neither of them had married for anything less than love. Betty would have heard her father warn her repeatedly that John could not afford to support her and a family, and John would have known very well that Claver would never provide a marriage portion for this match. Fortunately for Betty, Molly's pride was not as damaged by her daughter's behaviour as Claver's was, and she quickly tried to heal the wounds. She could not persuade Claver to see or write to Betty, who was staying with Thomas and Susanna Horner at their manor in Mells, but she could certainly make her feelings known. She replied to Betty's letters and, for a New Year's gift, sent on two suits of clothes that had been made for Betty in London, and for which Claver had paid the bill. She might also have quietly used part of the £700 she had received from the sale of the estate at Felton to help keep Betty financially afloat. Unfortunately, Molly had other worries too. Elizabeth her sister was sick, and she now went to visit her at Sadborow each month. No less concerning was the fact that, on New Year's Day, Will her son was struck with measles.

Everyone feared that Will, at nine years old, was 'very likely to Die in the Measels, though they were come out'. So, on 2nd January 1719, when Will asked to see his sister and John Burland, they were allowed a visit. Claver avoided them, but Betty stayed on to watch over Will throughout the night. Then Claver resumed his nursing, giving Will gentle purges, making fresh cordials and dressing his blisters every day. Thankfully, it was not long before Will recovered, and Betty wrote another letter, this time to her father, but he 'would not answer it'. He was quite determined not to give an inch, and this was reflected in his growing irritability with friends his guests. So, when old Peter Hoskins, lord of the manor at Purse Caundle in Dorset, visited with his wife in January, he was treated to far more than a medical consultation as they 'disputed much about Liberty in the Profession of

DOI: 10.4324/9781003333654-29

Religion'. Claver had to remind his guest of 'the Arguments I used to persuade him to the Belief of a Future State [heaven]'. Yet, as Peter Hoskins was good friends with the Catholic Mary Evans and the Muttleburys, it was unlikely that he needed much persuasion, or a lecture from his host.[1]

The anger that Claver felt about his daughter did not subside, and when, on 17th January 1719, a messenger came from Marshall Brydges to find out if he wished to prosecute Sam Hill in the bishop's court (which might lead to Hill being suspended from preaching for three years) he did well to continue to write neatly as he made a note of the meeting in his diary. To add to his concerns, a little later that afternoon, Mrs Watts arrived to ask if her son, young Jack, could be released from the remaining seven years of his apprenticeship, as he had recently been running away when Claver chastised him for his absences. Claver might have asked himself: if an apprentice-boy could not 'live obediently with me', who could? Yet, he gave his consent to the termination of Jack's indenture, and within a week he had replaced him with another boy, Will Lane.[2]

In February, the very wealthy barrister George Mattocks arrived to try to persuade Claver to pay for the renewal of John Burland's interest in land that he had leased. But Mattocks' efforts were 'in vain'. Claver did agree, however, to send Betty over £30 that had been given to her during her minority. He also sent the old gold coins she had acquired, and the medal that her grandmother Anne Dawe had left her, tucked into a wrought-silver purse. Molly carried these valuables to Betty, with the hope that her father's anger would subside. But this was unlikely to happen soon. When Claver saw that Molly had also taken six pairs of gloves to Betty as a gift, he was less than pleased. He wrote in his accounts, this gift was 'notwithstanding she was Married to Mr Burland (Aug: 28 – 1718) without my Knowledge & utterly against my Consent & most earnest Diswasions & endeavours to prevent it'.[3]

Considering his current disposition, it was probably a relief to everyone that in the first six months of 1719, Claver did not spend a great deal of time at home. During these months, he still managed to get to half the weekly meetings of his music club, enjoying such moments as 'the first trial of Hendels Pastoral [*Acis and Galatea*]', which had only premièred at Cannons (the duke of Chandos's country seat in Middlesex where Handel was the resident composer) in the previous summer.[4] Otherwise, on most days, Claver was either travelling to or from the houses of his patients, or lodging with them.

By far the most demanding of his patients were Samuel and Mary Pitt of the manor-house at Cricket Malherbie near Chard; an eight-hour journey in good weather, through Somerton and Ilminster. Claver had been treating the couple, as well as Samuel's parents, quite regularly at Bath and Cricket in 1718, for fees of over £20. On his third visit to Cricket in 1719, for six days at the end of February, Claver found that Mary was suffering from an ague and having fits, and she was not prepared to let him leave. So, it was difficult for him to see his other patients in the region, most notably the Goulds at Chard who were related to the Pitts. On his intended return to Cricket in mid-March, Claver lodged at the Red Lion in Somerton, before going on to Yarty House at Membury in Devon, where he found that Robert Fry's poor daughter Frances was 'so far exhausted by a Consumption of the Lungs and Hectick Fever', he could not prescribe for her, and she died that night.[5]

On 19th March, he went on to Sadborow where, sitting in the parlour in the evening with the shutters closed, he missed the meteor that suddenly lit the sky with 'Light as bright as that from the Sunshine at Noon day', though he heard the great 'rumbling noise, like that made by a Wagon going on rough way for 2 or 3 minutes'. Most people were 'excessively affrighted, and some fell down', maybe fearing this was a portent; though several scientists soon said that it was not. To check that all was well at home, Claver returned to Wells in the morning, where he found that the meteor had been 'seen and heard exactly in the same manner' as at Sadborow.[6] But he was now late in visiting the Pitts. Setting off at 5 p.m. on Saturday 21st, he rode at night to Cricket, arriving there at 1 a.m.

For three weeks over the Easter period, Claver stayed at Cricket, looking after Mrs Pitt with little company to amuse him and just one visit from his nephew William Bragge from Sadborow, seven miles away. By the time he returned to Wells on 11th April, he had earned thirty guineas for this work, and the only 'Unnecessary Expenses' he incurred were the thirty shillings lost at cards; a modest sum considering he had lost forty-seven on visits earlier in the year. Although he had been away for longer than ever before, there was no welcoming party or musical entertainment on the evening of Saturday 11th April when he returned, and after church on Sunday the only guest for dinner was the surgeon, Lucas.

Claver had promised Samuel Pitt he would go to Standerwick Court at Beckington, three miles from Frome, to provide a full report on the suitability of the manor-house, set in 300 acres, a few miles from the Wiltshire Downs, as 'a convenient purchase', though it had recently been sold for £5,700. After writing his report, he went to Bath with Tom Parfitt to see the architectural features of a new house in Trim Street, and to agree with John Harvey (the mason who had made the memorial to Elizabeth in the church at Ditcheat) for the engraving of a coat of arms on George Farewell's tomb. After seeing William Douglas, the virtuoso trumpeter, Claver rode home, but he returned to Bath on his own a few days later to prescribe for a lady staying at Mrs Thornley's house in Abbey Green. Unusually, knowing that there was no Betty to greet him, he was in no hurry to get home, so he stopped at the Lamb in Paulton where he dined. When he arrived that night in Wells he found that Arthur Chichester from Barnstaple in Devon had come to lodge. The next morning, Arthur's friend and Claver's nephew, William Bragge, also arrived to stay.

In other years, 1st May might have given rise to several days of music and entertainments to mark the fact that Claver was now sixty years of age. But all that he recalled of his birthday in 1719 was the fact that he accompanied William Bragge and Arthur Chichester to see troops from the King's Own Regiment of Horse that were camped outside the city, and that the three of them played cards and went to Lucas's lodgings in the evening. In the following week he took Bragge to see Thomas Horner at Mells and Bishop Hooper at the palace, went to a meeting of the music club, bought oxen at the beast fair in Wells, and also a small tortoise-shell box in which to carry testaceous powder; balls of powdered animal shells compounded with a jelly prepared from vipers' skins, used in the treatment of feverish conditions.[7] So his birthday passed without any sense of occasion or celebration.

As soon as Chichester and Bragge had left, on 11th May Claver set out by himself for Steyning 'to enquire about Mr Burlands Estate'. This was a thirty-mile trip through Glastonbury and across the moors, so he spent the night at Cannington, north of Bridgwater, before conducting his enquiries and returning home. Five months had now passed since he had learnt of Betty's marriage, and throughout that time he had refused to see or write to her, let alone conduct any correspondence with her husband. His fury had not begun to subside. Since his three weeks' living with the Pitts, when he had not kept his diary, even his writing had become quite scruffy, and he had certainly not found as much sympathy for his shunning of Betty, either at home or among his friends, as he might have hoped. Lucas had been his closest companion in these months, and he had no remedy for Claver's anguish, other than the occasional letting of a pint of blood from his right arm. So it was good for Claver that, following his trip to Steyning, he began to come to terms with Betty's marriage; or, rather, he started to tackle the root of his own objections to it. Nevertheless, he kept this quiet throughout the exceptionally hot summer, during which time he was engaged with plenty of more-visible activities.

The most immediate concern for Claver's family was the chronic illness of Molly's sister, Elizabeth Bragge, which led to several emergency trips to prescribe for her, and to Molly and Will staying at Sadborow for several weeks. Claver also had urgent calls from other patients; especially from Mrs Margaret Coxe (née Hippisley) at Ston Easton. Her husband had died in 1717, leaving her with young children and an exceptionally obese father, Preston, who often needed medical attention. In particular, her young son John Hippisley-Coxe was often in dire need of help. This meant that Claver had to ride ten miles over the Mendips trusting the sure-footedness of his mare in the moonlight, and on other days to ride through 'the most Violent Storms of Rain & Haile, with Thunder and Lightening'. When it rained like this, the lakes of Sedgemoor flooded, so Claver was forced to walk his young mare through them, as she didn't like crossing rivers and had to be coaxed to swim across the Avon when she refused to board the ferry boat to Kelston.

Other matters in which Claver was engaged were less pressing. He wanted to raise the annual rent of his 110-acre farm at Ebdon, near Weston-super-Mare, from £80 to £90 a year. Naturally, the current leaseholder, Joseph Cook, was not pleased when he heard that another farmer, William Chappel, had eventually offered to pay the full amount. But Claver was delighted to seal the deal, at least until he learned that another farmer would have been willing to pay an additional £5. All of Claver's estates needed attention: whether in overseeing the hedging, ditching and thatching at West Bradley; beating down the ant hills at Sand Park; killing the moles at Dulcote; or just paying the local taxes. But it was in attending to the properties acquired through his marriage to Betty's mother that Claver needed to take most care. He was well aware that in the parishes of Pilton, Pylle and West Pennard, the local gentry families were all related and regarded Betty as one of their own.

At Pilton, Claver gave £10 to supplement the income of the vicarage, and bought 115 hornbeam plants to make 'a hedge for shading and defending the fish-pond' there, though it was still leaking. Nearby at East Pennard, the lord of the manor Gerard Martin had recently married, and as well as being Claver's patients, the Martins were good friends. So, as the Burlands were staying with Gerard and Mary Martin, there were times when Claver had to avoid his daughter while visiting the village. And when he was called upon to prescribe for Anne, the only daughter of Sir Edward Seymour and the wife of William Berkeley, just a mile away at Pylle, he had to avoid the Burlands who were on a visit there as well. On one occasion, as soon as the Burlands left, Anne Berkeley made it clear to Claver that she thought it was high time that he should accept Betty's company again. There were other friends who said the same, but their words seemed to fall on deaf ears.[8]

In fairness to Claver, he was now doing what he believed was most important for his daughter's future; working out how best to settle her husband's debts. So, after his visits to Steyning and other places, he sent for Mattocks to draw up a full account of Burland's estates and to make copies of any deeds and leases. The overall picture was quite clear. From all of his estates, valued at £4,980 in May 1719, John ought to have had an income of about £586 a year; £269 from the lands he owned and £317 from lands he leased. That was a very respectable sum indeed. The problem was that the main estates were mortgaged for £1,400, and another £2,000 was owing due to his father's decision to leave each of his five daughters a marriage portion of £400. Servicing these debts at the usual interest rate of 5 per cent would cost £170 a year. Overall, John might therefore manage to raise his income to about £400 a year.[9] His financial plight was by no means as hopeless as Claver feared – though the disgraceful behaviour that John had shown by marrying Betty without parental consent was quite another matter. In perusing the accounts, one estate, in particular, attracted Claver's attention. This was Spaxton farm near Bridgwater, on which there had been a settlement in 1683. Lord James Waldegrave, whose family had been lords of the manor at Chewton Mendip since Tudor times, also had an interest in the farm. So, in mid-June, on a trip to Kelston, Claver stopped at Bath to speak to Waldegrave's steward about the prospect of purchasing all shares in the farm.[10] Before he could learn the outcome of this meeting, he was called to Sadborow again.

On his first trip to Sadborow in July, he let blood from Molly's sister, Elizabeth, but there was nothing else that he could do to help. She had been sick for over a year and, facing death at the age of forty-eight, had just made her will. On his second trip during 'very hot days', Claver had time for a long walk with Molly's nephew William Bragge, and for a swim in the great fishpond at the manor. And when Elizabeth died on 17th July, as Molly and her nephew were the executors and major beneficiaries of the will, Claver took notes on its legacies before returning home to Wells.

Three days later, he rode back to Sadborow with his friend, the builder Charles Taylor, while Molly went ahead in her nephew's coach. And after Elizabeth was buried in a lead coffin on Wednesday 22nd July, most of her small legacies to relations and godchildren were handed out before Molly and Claver left. At the end of August, Claver set out for Sadborow again, this time to finalise the acquisition of a share of Ashcombe farm in Wayford, which Molly had inherited from her sister, with the provision that £5 of its annual income would be used to endow two parish schools for the education of poor children. But he also found time to enjoy dining with Francis Gwyn at Forde Abbey, and John, 1st earl Poulett, at Hinton St George. And on 27th August he went with a small party of relations on a day out to Charmouth from where they took a boat to Lyme Regis and had dinner at the George.[11]

Claver carefully recorded in his diary how these hot summer days gave way to autumnal wind and rain, but there was no decline in the number of patients that came to his house for consultations and prescriptions, and he still visited their homes across the West Country. Fortunately, many patients were old friends who, like William Westley, lived within walking distance. Some of the more distant patients he visited, such as Alicia Gifford, the eighteen-year-old squire's daughter of Charlton Horethorne near Sherborne, whom he had treated since she was a child, also wrote to him quite regularly about their health, and this placed further demands upon his time.[12]

Since William Westley's marriage to the widow Frideswide Brickenden in 1710, Frideswide had been a constant patient, often coughing up 'fresh blood out of her lungs'. But in September 1719, it was William who died quite quickly at the age of eighty-four, with a request that he be buried in the cathedral next to his first wife Sarah and all of their five children. He had made an elaborate will in 1718, setting out legacies to relatives and friends, and a £100 donation for the support of a new charity school in Wells.[13] Bishop Kidder's eldest daughter, Susanna, who had married Sir Richard Everard of Essex in 1706, was among the beneficiaries. To her, William bequeathed Sarah's diamond ring; there was, however, nothing for Susanna's younger sister, Ann.[14] And in a codicil that William added a few weeks before his death, he bequeathed his carnelian ring to Molly, Claver's wife. William's second wife, Frideswide, and her daughters were not even mentioned.

William had been a well-known figure in Wells for over fifty years, but it was the sudden death of one of the city's MPs, in August 1719, that created the most commotion. John Dodd had only been an MP since 1717, when the Whig majority in the House of Commons had accepted his petition against the election of Thomas Horner. That had led the corporation to try to strengthen the local electorate for any future contest by making many more Tories freemen of the city. But nobody expected John Dodd to die at the age of twenty-six, so no-one was prepared for a by-election.

At first, there was talk of William Bragge standing, though he could ill-afford the costs of living in London for a large part of the year. In the event, Claver's friends, the Taylor brothers and Marshall Brydges, soon settled upon Marshall's brother, the barrister William Brydges, a Serjeant at Law, as their candidate. And, in September, to oil the wheels of the campaign, Claver treated the burgesses of the city to a hogshead (over fifty gallons) of strong beer at the Bull's Head, Ben Taylor's tavern in Wet Lane (Broad Street).[15] Even so, when William Brydges asked to become a burgess of the city, there was 'great consternation and strife' over the fact that he had not previously sought the consent of the mayor and corporation. It was eventually agreed that he should be admitted to prevent 'the ill consequences of the present disorder', but this did not augur well for his election as MP.[16]

Throughout October, Claver had little time for electioneering as Molly's widowed sister, Anne Leigh from the Isle of Wight, arrived with her young daughter and son-in-law, Sir John and Lady Chichester of Youlston Park near Barnstaple, to stay and play backgammon. Claver was a trustee of the young couple's marriage settlement, and after the Chichesters had left, Anne Leigh stayed on for another week with her two servants before taking the coach to Bath.[17] Claver had bought an illicit anker (ten gallons) of claret before they had arrived, having missed out on an even bigger delivery that had been seized by the customs officers of Lyme Regis. So, he was well prepared to toast his son's tenth birthday on 20th October. But he was completely unprepared for the little plot that had been hatched under his own roof.

27
LOSS & RECONCILIATION

On the morning of Friday 23rd October 1719, Claver was still feeling the 'shivering & coldness' from which he had been suffering since Will's birthday, three days earlier. It had stopped him from dining, which was always a bad sign, though he had self-prescribed a purge and herbal tea, and had managed to attend a concert the night before, where he had 'played, but was not well'. Even so, while he was dressing on the Friday morning, he was ambushed by seven women. Betty, Molly, Mary Evans and her maid and the three maids of the household burst into his bedroom without warning, calling upon him to listen to his daughter's pleas. He refused. He ordered Betty to go back down the stairs, and shut his door. When Betty, five months' pregnant, opened it 'with aboundance of Begging and Crying' after nearly a year of banishment, Claver finally gave in; or, as he accounted for this sudden change of heart, 'she forced me to beg God Almighty to bless her'.[1]

Molly insisted that Betty stay for dinner, so it must have soon become apparent that although Betty had been forgiven, her husband certainly had not. Claver was still working on a financial plan for Burland, and although he had been informed of this, Claver avoided any meeting with him whatsoever. Claver also had other important business on his mind; in particular, his work as a trustee of the estate of his former friend and patient Gabriel Odingsells, a wealthy London draper who had retired to Wells and left a large portfolio of properties in Somerset and Dorset to be shared equally between Gabriel and Mary, his son and daughter. Claver had known the family for years: Gabriel, a prospective playwright, often came to dinner and attended music meetings; and Mary had recently married Samuel Morley of London, who had caused additional difficulties by borrowing money against the prospect of his wife's inheritance. To settle the debts and dispose of all the properties of the estate would take Claver years and several court cases to resolve.[2] Meanwhile, he also had important business matters of his own.

DOI: 10.4324/9781003333654-30

Ever since he had acquired land with commoners' rights in several parishes near Glastonbury from his marriage to Betty's mother, he had been considering how best to raise their yield. In particular, he had been toying with the idea of enclosure of the common fields for over twenty years, gradually trying to win support for partitioning and privatising the land among the scores of villagers who had various rights to grow crops, graze animals and collect wood across these fields. In this he was bound to find support, but also to meet resistance from those who had no wish to see their ancient rights and ways of life transformed in the name of profit or improvement. It would be a bold venture, for which there was no precedent in Somerset, to try to bring about enclosure of the commons by an Act of Parliament.[3]

There were also legal issues to resolve, not least to determine who exactly had any rightful claim to use or benefit from the common lands. In June 1719, Thomas Creech had claimed, as vicar of Butleigh and the chapelry of Baltonsborough where there was talk of the enclosure, that he had the right to a tithe or church tax on those commoners of West Bradley (including Claver's tenant, Henry Bull) who grazed their animals upon the fields. Claver had no doubt that the claim was just 'a libel', and even the claims of a former vicar of Butleigh to receive tithes from his parishioners had been opposed by the villagers themselves. But Creech's claim still needed to be settled in the bishop's court.

To establish the facts of the matter, statements were taken from the oldest inhabitants of the nearby villages: John Tucker, a former soldier (aged ninety-eight); Richard Coward, a mason, and Ralph Aish, a miller (both seventy-seven); Edward Hill, a wool-comber (seventy-three); and Thomas Pippin, a farmer (sixty-three). They attested that the 520 acres of Baltonsborough's north wood originally belonged to the abbot of Glastonbury and that, more recently, the ground had been owned by the Berkeleys of Bruton. But they insisted they had never heard of their fathers or other commoners from West Bradley paying tithes to the vicar of Baltonsborough for the grazing of sheep or cattle on the land.[4] Interestingly, there was no mention of the fact that the fields and woods were probably best known locally as places of rape and fornication.[5]

Initially, Claver had asked the barrister George Mattocks to help him fight Thomas Creech's claim, but he was not impressed by Mattocks' work, so in December he asked another barrister, William Malet, to draw up an agreement for enclosing the fields of Baltonsborough woods by Act of Parliament.[6] Alongside Claver's holdings, one of the MPs for Wells, William Piers, great-grandson of a former bishop of the diocese, owned lands in West Bradley and adjoining parishes, as did his close relations, the Cowards of Chamberlain Street and East Pennard. So, like Claver, the powerful Piers and Coward families of Wells also had a financial interest in supporting the passing of an Act.[7]

William Piers had only become one of the MPs for Wells in May 1716, along with his brother-in-law William Coward, when, on petition, the House of Commons unseated the two Tory MPs, Thomas Horner and Maurice Berkeley, who had been elected in 1715. At that general election, Piers had only gathered thirteen votes and Coward twenty-two, but as both he and his brother-in-law were Whigs, it was enough to satisfy the Whig majority in the Commons that they should be awarded Horner and Berkeley's seats. Less than a month later, Coward died, and at the by-election in June 1716 Horner was returned with an even greater majority than he had won in 1715. Again, he was unseated on petition, this time in favour of the young Whig candidate, John Dodd.[8] It was Dodd's unexpected death in August 1719 that plunged Wells into yet another by-election. This time, Claver had a very particular interest in finding someone who would join with Piers in supporting an Act for enclosure of the commons.

Although he still found time to attend to patients, organise a concert for St Cecilia's Day, and set up a marble monument to his former friend George Farewell, throughout November and December much of Claver's time was spent in canvassing for the election of William Brydges.[9] Working closely with the four Taylor brothers,[10] he attended meetings of the city's freemen, spoke and wrote to them individually, treated them to drinks at the city's inns, visited their homes, and helped to fix their leases. He even lent money to repay debts owed to the 'Yeoman and Grazier' Charles Tudway, for the hire of horses.[11] And on election day, Monday 14th December, he went with his nephew William Bragge to church and then to the assize hall in the marketplace to observe the poll.

The franchise had recently been extended by the corporation to over 300 freemen, most of whom would need time to travel from their homes across the county to cast their vote. So, Claver sat with his nephew throughout the day observing the proceedings. Unfortunately, by seven o'clock Jacob Worrall the mayor, an old apothecary-surgeon, was too tired to continue as returning officer, and he adjourned the polling until the morning. Throughout the evening and most of the night, while Claver and his friends were busy drinking at the city's inns, votes were being cast in favour of Thomas Edwards, the rival candidate whose wife had inherited a fortune from her uncle, the Bristol merchant slave-trader and philanthropist Edward Colston. So in the morning it was no surprise that Thomas Edwards was declared the winner by thirty-five votes, though this was one of the closest results in living memory.[12]

The result was a big disappointment to Claver, who paid for a transcript of the poll, no doubt with future elections in mind. Even so, Christmas was a happy time, with over a dozen guests for lunch on Christmas Day, plenty of music and his relationship with Betty fully restored. Among his guests was Betty's cousin, Nancy Dawe, the eleven-year-old daughter of Betty's uncle, Charles Dawe of Charlton Horethorne, near Sherborne. Charles, a widower, had died in 1717, leaving five children who needed to be cared for. So, in November 1719, Nancy had come to live with her aunt Molly, where she would be good company for Will, who was a year younger. Claver also enjoyed her company, especially as she liked to dine and play at cards, and he and Molly were probably hoping and expecting that Nancy would become a permanent member of the household, as this would be a good place for her stay. Yet, on Saturday 16 January, when he returned from a trip to Pilton, Claver rushed to Cupper's shop in the marketplace where Nancy had been 'seized with a most violent Head-Ach', and had her carried home in Molly's sedan chair.

When Claver sat down to write his diary on Sunday evening, his handwriting was as neat and sober as it had ever been: 'Miss Nancey Dawe having continued all the night (with very Short, & at last with no Intermissions) in the most violent & universal Convulsions (her left Leg and Arm being towards the Morning motionless but by being continued with the Convulsed Body) died about 7'. He recorded that Betty and Christopher Lucas had come to help, that he had written to Nancy's aunt Anne Farewell to find out what to do about the funeral, and that he had been to church and had read to his household from *The Causes of the Decay of Christian Piety*. This was what he had to do. It helped him to control his grief, for Nancy was 'the most obliging, Flexible, Good-Natured, Ingenious & Civil Pretty Girl of little more than 11 years old that ever I knew'.

It was fourteen years since Claver and Molly had buried their two-year-old daughter, Mary, in the Lady Chapel, when Betty was just nine. And it was next to the floor-slab marking Mary's grave that Claver now arranged for Nancy to be laid to rest. Following his instructions, the funeral was held on Wednesday 20th January. The biggest bell of the cathedral was rung at 1 p.m. for three quarters of an hour, and then tolled until 3 p.m. when the mourners arrived at the west front of the cathedral to be greeted by the singing of the choir. Nancy's corpse was carried by the man-servants of Morris, Bragge and Burland and escorted by six of Nancy's girl friends in white scarves, and white hoods and gloves. Betty, heavily pregnant, was the chief mourner, followed by six maids; the two who had cared for Nancy during her convulsions at Cupper's shop, and the four (including Betty's maid) who had watched over her at Claver's house throughout the night.

Apart from Claver's family and his friend, the choral vicar and rector of Dulverton William Hill, who took the service, there were only a handful of other mourners: Goody Harvey, who laid the body out; Mrs Browne the hatter's wife, who had supplied the gloves and scarves; and Richard Cupper and Mr Tick, who served the wine. After the funeral service had been sung in the Lady Chapel, where 'everything was performed very decently, & as became the Interment of so Religious, Ingenious & Sweet Tempered a Girl', the great bell was tolled again as the mourners made their way through the 'Mizling-rainy weather' to Claver's house.[13] Five days later, Claver went to the cathedral's sacrist Thomas Cooper, the man who had done him the 'abominable injury' of facilitating Betty's secret marriage in 1718, and paid the fees for Nancy's funeral and grave. There was no more to do but mourn. Yet in the afternoon, Hill Dawe, Nancy's cousin and main heir of the Dawe family's estates, arrived to solicit Claver's help.

As Nancy's aunt Anne Farewell had been too sick to travel, Betty was the only blood relative to attend the funeral. The Dawes, including Nancy's guardian and her siblings, were therefore most conspicuous by their absence. The purpose of Hill Dawe's visit was to ask for Claver's assistance in removing Nancy's uncle, Thomas Dawe, as trustee for Charles Dawe's other children. Although Claver agreed that Thomas Dawe, through neglect and meanness had 'begun to utterly ruine' the children, he declined the offer to be their official guardian. Out of respect to Betty and the memory of her mother, he wanted to maintain a decent relationship with the Dawes. And two years later he would welcome Nancy's sister, Elizabeth (who had just turned twelve and been left abandoned at Mrs Priaux's dancing school at Sherborne ever since her father's death), to stay in Wells during the summer and over Christmas and the New Year.[14] But he clearly felt no other obligation or inclination to befriend the Dawes.

The next day, 26th January 1720, Claver had even more family business to attend to, as Sir John Chichester arrived with a request that he sign a petition to the House of Lords to introduce a Bill that would allow him to sell several of his properties in Devon and on the Isle of Wight to pay off debts. Claver was a trustee of Sir John's marriage settlement with Anne Leigh, Molly's niece, who had given her consent. So he was happy to support the family's petition, and in April 'An Act for Sale of Part of the Estate' was passed.[15] Having attended to these family matters, Claver caught a cold that left him with a fever and bad cough for several weeks. He was much too weak to leave the house, though Betty visited every day, Lucas let blood and Cupper administered vomits that produced 'a great deal of vitreous clammy Phlegm'. He ate a little broth, some turnips and some peas, but he did not touch the half a bushel of oysters that one of his patients, Mr Symes of Bridgwater, had sent. It was only on Thursday 18th February that his spirits began to lift when he heard the news that Betty had been safely delivered of a son.

The christening of Morris Burland was held in the cathedral at 3 p.m. on the 3rd March 1720, with William Bragge as godfather. But there were no great celebrations afterwards at Claver's house, even though he was now quite well again. This was because he was still unwilling to hold any meeting with John Burland. Yet, he was rather pleased with his recovery, recording 'I got up, and after my Breeches only were slipped on (but not fasten'd at the knees) I put on everything excepting my shoose, & compleatly dressed my self in 2 Minutes, by my Wife's Watch which I desired her to observe'.[16] He was also well enough to travel through the snow to Kelston to play music at the Harringtons. On the way, he stopped at Bath to hold another meeting with Lord Waldegrave's steward about Burland's stake in Spaxton farm. After reckoning that Waldegrave's share of the farm was worth £140 a year, Claver offered £840 for a new and longer lease. He still could not bring himself to talk to Burland, but nothing would stop him preparing for the future of his daughter and his grandson.

28

THE COMMON LANDS

Although Claver was disappointed by the defeat of William Brydges at the Wells election, he was still confident that the city's other MP, William Piers, being a Whig, would be able to take his plans for enclosure of the common fields of Baltonsborough, through the parliamentary process. By January, with the help of William Malet, he had drafted the petition to bring in a Bill, and had managed to persuade forty-three 'proprietors' from the surrounding villages who claimed rights to the commons to sign up to the venture. And on 17th February 1720, 'the Petition of *Claver Morris* M. D. and *William Peirs [Piers]* Esquire, on Behalf of themselves and other respective Owners of the Common' was granted in the House of Lords.[1]

The Petition claimed that the partition of 520 acres of common pasture would 'very much tend to the Public good as well as the mutual advantage of all Persons concerned therein', and that in public meetings the proposed commissioners (gentlemen like William Berkeley, Gerard Martin and Marshall Brydges) would 'not give any undue preference in allotment of shares or making allotments' to particular claimants. Two days later, 'An Act for enclosing the Common commonly called *Baltonsbury Common*, in the Parishes of *Baltonsbury* and *Bradly*, in the County of *Somerset*' was introduced. It gave any three of the commissioners the power to settle all disputes and to build new roads where needed. After enclosure, all of the new proprietors would acquire the right to ditch, fence, gate and exchange their land as they saw fit.[2] In his letters from Westminster, Piers reported that during the Lords' debate there were a couple of objections by disaffected Whigs, but there was no division, and after a few amendments the Bill was passed on 12th March. The House of Commons took even less interest in the whole proposal (though it clearly abolished ancient rights), reporting to the Lords on 6th April that it had approved the Bill without amendment. So, on 7th April 1720 the Bill received the king's assent.

DOI: 10.4324/9781003333654-31

Not everyone was pleased. In Wells, during the preparation of the Bill, William Malet had been expelled from his position as a burgess of the city after he had taken offence at the words of a former mayor, Matthew Baron, and challenged him to a duel. Malet's neglect of business due to his extensive absences in London, also tried the patience of the dean and chapter as he failed to meet his duties as their legal officer, for which he was subsequently sacked.[3] And from the village of East Pennard, where Claver's friend Henry Gapper had been vicar, the opposition to enclosure led to a deputation of objectors making their way to parliament.[4] Even so, after due notice had been given, on Monday 4th July the six commissioners chosen to execute the Act all met at West Bradley's inn to begin their work. There at the inn, which Claver owned, he treated them to a rib of beef and cold ox-tongues.

Although he took great interest in the whole business of enclosure, never missing a meeting of the commissioners, throughout the spring and summer Claver had a number of other matters to attend to. He was a commissioner himself, for the collection of the Land Tax, and he had a major dispute to settle with Joseph Cook, his former tenant, over the return of Ebdon farm. He also had to conduct a tricky negotiation with the dean and chapter over the renewal of a lease for his home in the Liberty where he was building a Classically-appointed new 'necessary house' in the back garden and refurbishing his laboratory in the basement. In addition, he had a legacy to resolve regarding William Bragge's payment of £430, and Molly's inheritance of the 180 acres of meadows and pastures of Ashcombe farm, according to her sister's will.[5] There were also other family matters that required attention. He needed to host a visit from Sir John Chichester and family who had come from Bath after Lady Chichester had suffered a miscarriage. And he needed to sort out his son-in law's estate, particularly with regard to Spaxton farm.

After being shunned for eighteen months, it must have come as something of a shock to John Burland when he was suddenly summoned to Claver's house on Whitsunday, 5th June 1720 to discuss his stake in Spaxton farm. Now that the ice was broken, it would not take long for their relationship to heal. A few weeks later, John and Betty were invited to dine for the first time with Claver and Molly. This was good for the delicate baby Morris too, as Claver often needed to prescribe for him at Betty's lodgings, at Mr Browne's, 'the haberdasher of hats', and his wife in Sadler Street.[6] The only unfortunate outcome of Claver's reconciliation with John and Betty was that he encouraged them to invest £200 in South Sea stock in the hope that this would soon yield £2,000. Shares in the company (based on a scheme designed to help pay for the national debt of £50 million) had already risen from £128 in January to over £1,000 in June. And in the frenzy of excitement that led hundreds of investors to believe that fortunes were beckoning, in September Claver himself paid £700 for £100 of stock. By then, the shares were already beginning to fall, and investors were facing ruin.[7]

Although Claver had lost his desire to make the long journey to visit London, he enjoyed trips to see his friends in Bristol and Bath, where he also saw the High Church zealot Sacheverell. The summer was exceptionally wet; on a trip to Bridgwater he spotted a pig drowning in the river Parrett, and on the way home he helped save a little boy from drowning too. In May, it rained 'so long & violently' that the shops in Wells were flooded and the Swan in Sadler Street lost beer worth £40. And on one of his trips to prescribe for Mr and Mrs Seymour and their sons, Conway and William, at Regilbury Court in the Chew Valley, he was 'met with such a storm of Rain' as he crossed the Mendips, he could not return to Wells that day.

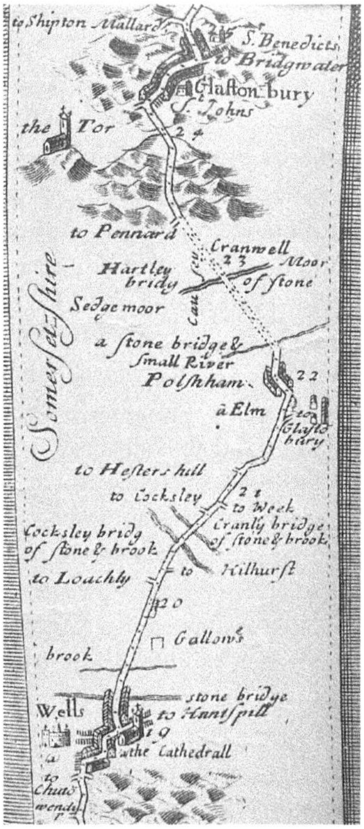

FIGURE 19 The road from Wells to Glastonbury
The road runs for seven miles across the moors, past the city's gallows and Glastonbury Tor

Claver was used to riding in rough weather, and over the next few years he would need to make numerous trips to Glastonbury to support enclosure of the common moors. But at the age of sixty-one he was not travelling as far or staying away from home as much as he had done in previous years. Long journeys to the manors of the gentry were lucrative but tiring, and in 1719 he had made over £310 from the 530 prescriptions he had provided for his wealthy patients. In 1720 his annual income as a physician would fall by £70, and the largest single fee he received was of four guineas for a visit to Bristol to prescribe for a daughter of Mr Andrews, a longstanding patient, formerly of Wells. Almost a third of all his charges now were for five shillings or less, which reflected many of his patients' financial means and his concentration on making a success of his venture into the enclosure of the commons. While the commoners would be grateful for Claver's medical advice at any time, most of them could not afford his usual fees. They probably also appreciated the wider care he took, as local landowner and benefactor, in trying to uphold standards and keep the parish poor-rate low. It was to uphold standards that he went with his tenant Henry Bull to get a warrant for the apprehension of Henry Coxe, a rich farmer from Mark near Wedmore who, according to an unmarried mother in West Bradley, was the father of her baby girl.[8]

At West Bradley inn, the commissioners began their work by visiting the commons, appointing a local man, William Higgins, to provide an exact survey of the land, and hearing the views of anyone who now came forward to claim a share of the terrain. After their second meeting at the inn, Claver was so confident that all was going well, he paid Henry Coxe £45 for his small estate in West Bradley, which included a right of commons that Claver could now add to his collection.[9] At the third meeting of the commissioners, one of them got too drunk to be of use, but by the time of their fifth meeting, over a 'good handsome dinner' at the Swan in Pilton on 7th September, great progress had been made. They had almost completed the partition of the land, and the allocation of allotments to the new proprietors was 'generally according to their good-liking'. So, this was a good time for Claver to present the costs to-date.

Based upon his meticulous accounts, his estimate was that, allowing for three more commissioners' meetings at a cost of £2 each, the total cost of enclosure would come to over £315. This sum included £187 for William Piers' expenses in procuring the Act of Parliament; £60 for making a new stone causeway across the land; £20 to William Higgins for measuring, mapping and dividing up the commons; £16 for producing a fair copy of the execution of the Act and deeds; and several other legal and administrative costs. The commissioners had approved 133 claims or rights to use the common land, and with each rightful claim now due an equal share of the land, the arithmetic was simple: the cost for each new allotment was £2, seven shillings and sixpence. On Claver's advice, it was agreed that each proprietor should bring fifty shillings per allotment for collection at the next commissioners' meeting.[10]

No one quarrelled with the figures, though not everyone was prompt in paying for their share. But after all the work so far, it was quite clear that, at least in economic terms, the venture was going to be a triumph. The 133 commoners' rights were owned by eighty-eight proprietors, the great majority of whom were due one share of the enclosed land. Claver was the biggest shareholder; from his marriage to Elizabeth Jeanes and later purchases at West Bradley he had accumulated fourteen rights to the Baltonsborough commons, which meant that he now held fourteen shares. William Piers had 10 shares from his properties in Baltonsborough, West Bradley and West Pennard, but no one else had more than four. Some of the shareholdings were divided to take account of family inheritances that had been split, as in the case of four infant sisters. Nine proprietors were widows, and five other shareholders were single women. Allowing for the loss of land due to the need for a new causeway and farm tracks, the owner of each share would become the freeholder of a good three acres which, even for pasturage, would usually cost more than fifty shillings just to rent each year.[11]

Claver was delighted with his single plot of forty-two acres which he now named 'Morris Hayes' and soon ditched and planted it with ten varieties of apple trees and two of pears. But not everything was going well. He needed to renew the lease on his house in the Liberty, but was aggrieved to learn that the dean and chapter were unwilling to grant any allowance for the wall he had constructed when he had quietly stolen a slither of his neighbour's garden when his new house had been built over twenty years ago. So, he went to the Chapter House to protest, but the canons would not discuss the matter in his presence. When he received a message later in the day that they would not change their mind, he replied immediately, saying that he knew the dean Matthew Brailsford and the archdeacon Edmund Archer were 'the whole Chapter, at least vertually', and he 'wished they would have acted Honestly this once'. But they would not budge. These 'knavish Rascals' had angered him before, over their treatment of young Farewell Perry who had been suspended for refusing to apologise for not bowing to the dean. A few days later, they angered him again when he observed 'the Foolishness of the Dean' in reprimanding the cathedral's bellringer for not seeking permission to toll the 6 o'clock matins bell at 6.15 a.m. so that, after sunrise, the congregation could see to read the psalms.[12]

Claver knew that the days when he was close to the dean and chapter through his friendship with the precentor Robert Creighton were over. The Creightons were still good friends. They had signalled this by the gift of a magnificent album of over two hundred botanical drawings and watercolours, based upon a fifteenth-century Italian 'herbal', a reference book for medics.[13] But Claver's loss of influence still hurt. Creighton was in his eighties now, as was Bishop Hooper, and neither had the appetite for a fight. At the same time, Claver knew that his own complaints were trivial when compared with the troubles of several of his friends.

In September 1720, one of his oldest friends, Lady Sarah Gould (née Davidge) and her son, the barrister Davidge Gould, called for help in dealing with the distress caused by the death of Davidge's thirty-year-old sister in 1718. Sarah had married Colonel Edmund Fielding without parental consent, and had left six children. The eldest, Henry Fielding, born in April 1707, had been enrolled at Eton, but all the children were in need of care and protection from their father's negligence and gambling. As well as protecting their inheritance, Lady Sarah, now in her seventies, was determined to gain full custody of her grandchildren. This would involve a hearing in the Court of Chancery, where the support of the family doctor could prove pivotal. Claver was pleased, of course, to lend his signature to the cause which, after a great deal of wrangling, Lady Sarah finally won.[14]

Earlier in the summer, an outbreak of smallpox caught Claver by surprise, and he feared that his chambermaid Anne Fisher, 'who never had that Disease', had inadvertently been exposed to it. Catherine Hebdon, a new patient, had caught the worst 'crude confluent' form and, after Claver had prescribed a dozen times, her father was so pleased she had survived that he sent five guineas to express his gratitude. But, when Claver was called upon to treat another woman 'dangerously ill of the Small-Pox', he 'refused to have anything to do with her'. Joan Franklin was the wife of the choral vicar Francis, recently appointed vicar of Chelvey who often preached sermons in the cathedral, most notably on music and on the eating of various meats in Lent; sermons that Claver found so 'very silly' and 'foolish' they sorely tried his patience. Despite the dean and chapter's warnings, Francis Franklin had also foolishly conducted a marriage in the Lady Chapel, without permission. Yet Claver did not disclose his reasons for refusing to treat 'that vicious Woman' Joan. A few weeks before her illness she had lost a baby boy, and a few months later she would lose another two of her young children, probably to smallpox. But she survived, and although Claver did not treat her, he continued to treat and tolerate her husband.[15]

As the disease persisted, Claver's patients avoided trips to Wells, but it appeared in other places too. At Ditcheat, John Wade, a farmer, had first contracted the disease in 1707, when it had blinded him for twelve days and left him badly scarred. Now, after catching it for a second time, it killed him, but only after he had 'infected very many of the Parish who came to visit him in his Sickness not believing he had this Disease again which had so severely affected him so long ago'.[16] Closer to home, Claver also saw the grief of his daughter and her husband when they lost their baby Morris on 6th October 1720. During Morris's seven months of life he had been a sickly child, and Claver regularly prescribed medicines to aid him. But while his death came as no surprise, it probably helped to bring the family together. At the supper party for Will's eleventh birthday two weeks later, Betty and John were the guests of honour.

The threat of smallpox did not deter the commissioners for enclosure from holding meetings throughout the autumn, and they might have concluded their business well before Christmas. At their eighth meeting, however, on 2nd November at the Swan in Pilton, Edmund Bower from Somerton, whose wife was one of Claver's patients, raised objections. He had recently purchased eleven of the new allotments awarded to the commoners, and paid the fees for these. But now he claimed that some of the holdings were on better ground than others, that they were badly measured, and that his own allotments were not joined together. He also said that Claver's share was an acre greater than it should have been. Since all the land had been measured, divided and allocated largely before Bower's purchases, in Claver's view Bower behaved 'with great Insolence to the Commissioners, & little sense'. But, being an attorney, he threatened everyone with lawsuits.[17]

At their ninth meeting, on 1st December over a dish of snipes at the Christopher in Wells, the commissioners were greeted with more complaints about the size of some allotments, due, as Claver thought, to boundary markers having been deliberately moved and the inability of most people to do the tricky maths. So, two weeks later, when they met again, half a dozen of the new proprietors reported that they had hired a man to take new measurements, and that he had affirmed their allotments were too small. 'After much Altercation' the commissioners agreed to get a third measurement of the contested plots before the next meeting. But there were other problems too. Edmund Bower did not attend in person, but he sent his clerk to say that he was still insisting that his allotments were too small and poor, and that he was therefore not prepared, as the commissioners required, to fence them in. For Claver, this was especially annoying as part of his new land shared a border with one of Bower's plots, and he had written to Bower several times to see what could be done. What was also irritating was that his tenant Henry Bull had told him that several beasts had already strayed onto his land, treading down new fences as they went.

Before the commissioners could meet again, Claver and Bower had agreed to fence and ditch their border, but it took a whole night of negotiation at the Christopher to reach agreement. So, on 5th January 1721, when the commissioners met for the eleventh time and learned that the third surveyor had found that Higgins's original measurements were generally quite sound, aside from their signing and securing of new deeds, the commissioners' work was done.[18] This meant that Claver could get on with the management of his Avalon estates. His tenant at West Bradley, Henry Bull, was unhappy to lose the right to Baltonsborough commons, and gave up his lease. So Claver let the estate to the yeoman James Whitehead and his daughter Mary for £52 a year, and the village inn to John Harvey for fifty shillings. At the same time, he bought a twenty-acre tenement from Henry Coxe for £400. At 'Morris Hayes' he spent the best part of a day with six helpers counting the molehills that needed to be destroyed. And after counting 11,400 before nightfall, he reckoned there were still another 500 to mark out.[19]

For all the difficulties of enclosing Baltonsborough commons, Claver was pleased with the result and it was an important step in the economic development of the county. Personally, he had acquired forty-two acres of pasture for just £35, plus his time. With a little more expense he could let the pastures for £20 a year.[20] The small farmers who had paid their fifty shilling fees had the opportunity now to choose how best to work their land, or to sell it at a considerable profit to wealthy farmers; local gentry or men like Claver who could afford to make improvements that would yield even greater profits. So, if this kind of enclosure 'by agreement' set a precedent in Somerset, it might trigger great waves of economic pain and gain, as well as social change. But something would undoubtedly be lost as an ancient and more communal way of life would pass. Like most villagers he encountered, Claver had no romantic notions about communal farming to set against the opportunity he saw to improve the yield and profits of the land. So, in this case, he had no doubts about the value and benefits of the enterprise.

He also recognised that Piers and Malet had played their part. But on a visit to Mells to prescribe for Susanna Horner, when he suggested to her and her husband that Malet might be a good person to stand with William Piers as the MPs for Wells at the next election, the response was scathing. The Horners were not only both 'vehemently' opposed to Malet; they were equally hostile to the idea of Claver supporting Piers. This was unsurprising as it was Thomas Horner who had been unseated as MP for Wells by the petition of the Whig interloper Piers in 1716.

Claver countered with the claim that he knew of no occasion when Piers had 'given his Vote in Parliament once within these 3 Years against the Good of his Country, or Church of England', and left for home. Yet the Horners and most other Tories were not the only ones who would not vote for Piers, who had re-married earlier in the year. On a trip to Somerton, Claver was joined by James Higgins (a relative of William, the surveyor) riding to his house in Street, and he made a point of telling Claver that 'he was much displeased with Mr Peirs [Piers] for Continuing [to keep a] wench he Bread up in Bridewell [prison]'.[21]

29

A CONTESTED ELECTION

There was never a time at Claver's house when life was less than busy. Patients and visitors arrived for consultations and prescriptions, friends and relatives came to dine or stay, and music lovers to play or to be entertained, often drinking and playing games until the early hours. Keeping a simple record of the most important visitors and their purposes, plus his own travels and the vagaries of the weather, was standard fare in Claver's diary entry for each day. And when he had much more to say, it was usually because there was something playing on his mind or just an unexpected episode he wanted to record. So, in January 1721, when he noted that, despite the medicine he had prepared, his cook-maid Mary Gould was 'so ill in [a] Convulsive cough that all concluded she was Dieing', he must have feared the worst. Mary recovered slowly, but a month later there was another scare.

Having refurbished his laboratory, he now spent more time with his microscope and telescope and conducting experiments at his furnace. On Ash Wednesday, while he was mixing sulphur and mercury to make Aethiops Mineralis (black mercuric sulphide, used in the treatment of skin diseases, scrofula and hereditary syphilis), he was 'driven out by the Smoke of Burning'. This did not deter him, but it might have given him the idea of providing demonstrations of chemical reactions for his guests. So, he had 'a blue laboratory vest' made by Watts, and when Elizabeth Berkeley, Susanna Horner, Gerard Martin and John Burland came to visit, he showed them how to produce a great flame by mixing 'strong Spirit of Nitre' (nitric acid) with 'Oyl of Turpentine' (pine oil). A few days later, he was confidently still experimenting with the mixing of nitric acid and various minerals, and using the 1,500 'sparrow bills' (small cast-iron nails) he bought to prepare new medicines.[1]

In March 1721 there was an unfortunate incident when Mary Evans accused the household's maids of paying someone to hang her dog 'which was found and brought to her dead'. The maids all 'vehemently deny'd it' and unless this was an act of anti-Catholicism (an unlikely event in Claver's house), there seemed no obvious

DOI: 10.4324/9781003333654-32

motive unless the dog had been taking chickens or causing a nuisance in the yard. Claver let it pass, especially as he was far more concerned about Molly who, like Mary Gould, had just become 'so ill with a Cough, Spitting & a Fever' she was confined to bed. Two weeks later, she woke in the night with such 'a Convulsive Asthma & Cough' that 'for some time she could hardly Breath'.

One of Claver's remedies for coughs and sneezes, French brandy and lemon juice, might have helped with Molly's recovery, though it did not work with one of his patients, Jacob Worrall, the apothecary-surgeon and former mayor who died in March. Yet Claver was confident that he had saved the life of another resident at this time, the 'very infirme' old clothier Joseph Norton, son of a former mayor, who everyone else believed would be lucky to last two days. And he probably felt the same about Elizabeth Archer, wife of the pompous antiquarian archdeacon of Taunton who had a canon's house in the marketplace and whom Claver regarded as a knave. Elizabeth was Claver's most-visited patient throughout the spring, and she also made a good recovery.[2]

There were plenty of other cheerful moments that Claver noted in his diary. He always liked a wager and had won a bottle of wine from his friend, the choral vicar William Hill, over a disagreement about the dates of William the Conqueror's reign. This win was somewhat against his usual form. He lost £3 to Arthur Chichester who had proved, at Sadborow, that he could throw a hundred stones to land within a yard of each other. And he lost another wager, a guinea to Betty's friend Anne Drewe, when he predicted that 'Ladys of Figure [fashionable women] would leave off wearing Hooped Petticoats' within two years.[3] He noted simple pleasures too: being invited to breakfast and to sip chocolate with Betty and John Burland; overseeing the completion of the portraits of Will and Betty that he had commissioned;[4] and taking delivery of a 'very fine Month-Clock with a Pendulum of 5 feet long' that he had ordered from William Brock of Axbridge for six guineas.[5] He also enjoyed treating Betty to a new riding gown, the best claret on her birthday, and a chintz gown for Christmas.[6] For himself, he purchased a new violin and bow to take to the music club and on his trips to Kelston.[7]

On his sixty-second birthday, when John and Betty came to congratulate him, he wrote to George Smith, a coach-maker at the Dragon & Dolphin in High Holborn. He had decided it was time to enjoy again the luxury of having his own coach and horses. With this in mind, and after charging his pistols for the journey, on Friday 5th May he set out with his son-in-law at 6 a.m. for the forty-five-mile trip to Amesbury, north of Salisbury. Meeting William Berkeley on the way, at the Sign of the Bull in the village of Wylye, they rested for two hours before arriving at the George by 5 p.m. Even before they had all sat down for supper with Sir John Chichester at the inn, Berkeley had found a coach-mare for Claver at a cost of £13. And by 8 a.m. the following morning he had found Claver a second mare for just £12. So, after 'Beef from the Spitt' for breakfast in the famous fair, and Berkeley's purchase of 'two young coach-geldings and a black saddle-horse' for himself, they left to see Stonehenge. Lodging that night at the Ship Inn at Mere, they rose before sunrise the next day and were at home in Wells by 10 a.m.[8]

Claver was delighted with his new mares; one with black feet, the other with white. He had lost his young sorrel horse from a colic in the spring, though it had been 'raked, drenched, clystered & let-blood' several times. This was the horse that disliked boats and water, and had refused to board the ferry-boat to Kelston, over the river Avon, though she was eventually persuaded to swim towards horses on the other side. On other occasions, when riding across the ditches of Sedgemoor, Claver often had to dismount and lead her through the lakes on foot. For someone who spent so much time on horses, Claver was bound to have mixed fortunes with them. Six months earlier, he had needed to replace the pony that he had bought for Will, and in the summer his own new horse was sunk up to its belly while crossing a lake near Street. A fortnight later, on a visit to prescribe for Lady Edith Phelips, his horse fell down 'in a very dirty place', forcing him to stay at the Red Lion at Somerton rather than go to Montacute House in filthy clothes. And there was worse to come. Returning from Somerton in the winter, his mare was so 'frighted at a Young Bear that was lead along', 'she ran down a very Steep and high place into the Hollow Way.' It was only 'by the favourable Providence of Almighty God I was not thrown down'.[9]

At the end of May 1721, Claver was seized with a 'quartan ague' (a type of malaria characterised by severe fevers every three or four days) that gave him 'a very heavy pain' in his limbs and chest. It kept him awake at night and sometimes he was unable to eat anything but a dish of herb pottage in the evening. He took gentle purges, and Cupper took half a litre of blood from his left arm. But for days he felt an 'extreme pain' in his thigh, 'as if the Bone had been grind to pieces'. It did not always stop him from going out, but he had to decline visits to see patients.[10] Just before the onset of this illness, Susan Burland, one of John's sisters, arrived in Wells, and she stayed throughout the summer. Claver and Molly treated her like a member of the family, and she came to dinner several times. But when Claver prescribed for Susan, he probably saw that she had a chronic illness and in September he was an assistant at her funeral. Apart from the friendship that had developed between Claver and his son-in-law, it had been a tricky year. But there was hope of better things to come, for Betty was now expecting another child.

It was important that Betty had a good understanding of her pregnancy, as she could not always rely upon her father's professional opinion in these matters. In February, he had made a bet with Anne Berkeley over whether or not Margaret Malet (the barrister's wife) was pregnant.[11] Margaret was not one of Claver's regular patients and she was good friends with Anne, yet Claver was sufficiently confident in his judgements to wager twenty-five shillings that she was 'not with child'. After returning from London with her husband and young daughter, at the end of August Margaret died, in childbirth. Her funeral was yet another sad occasion, and Claver and John Burland were among the pall-bearers. Wearing mourning scarves, hat-bands, rings and gloves, they met the hearse near Shepton Mallet and followed it to the cathedral for the interment.[12]

Three days later, on 14th September, Claver went with John Burland to the manor at Mells where Susanna Horner (née Strangways) was in the latter stages of her pregnancy. It was a dangerous time as she had previously had several miscarriages and had lost two babies at birth. Claver made another visit in December when he conferred with the physician Dr Wells, and just before Christmas he prescribed again before dining with Susanna and two of her sisters in her chamber.[13] He did not prescribe again, but Susanna gave birth to a healthy daughter, Elizabeth, who became her heir. He never again returned to the manor. A decade later, when Susanna inherited the Strangways' fortune, she was at the centre of a national scandal when, having formed a relationship with Henry Fox MP, she arranged for the secret marriage of Elizabeth, aged thirteen, to Fox's brother, the lover of Lord Hervey.

For Claver, the highlights of 1721 were the trips he took with Nathaniel Farewell (the brother of George, the former rector of South Cadbury), first to Bristol and then to Bath. On the outskirts of Bristol, they went shopping at the White Glass House before drinking at the Nag's Head in Wine Street and sleeping at the White Lion in Broad Street. The next day, they 'bought many things of Mr Tho. Edwards, Ironmonger at the Great-gun in Wine Street', breakfasted on roast beef, drank a pint of wine in Queen Square, and took the ferry to St Mary Redcliffe before returning home in time to attend the weekly meeting of the music club. Three days later, Claver set out for Bath with Nathaniel and his brother-in-law, the choral vicar Farewell Perry, hoping to hear 'the best Player of the Violin in [E]Urope', Francesco Germiniani. They were not disappointed. The Italian virtuoso entertained them 'with his wonderful hand on the violin' and 'with the utmost civility' for two days, at Bath and Kelston.[14]

After the usual festivities and concerts over Christmas, on Friday 19th January 1722, Betty gave birth to a baby girl. She was christened Mary but known as 'Molly', no doubt in honour of the stepmother Betty had known since she was five years old and who had always been a loving parent. On a sunny day in the cathedral at the start of February, Claver and William Bragge (represented by Christopher Lucas) became the godfathers. Unlike Betty's son, Morris, who had had always been a sickly child and who had only lived for seven months, baby Molly seemed quite healthy. It was not until May when she became 'extremely ill' that Claver was called upon for advice and medicine. Two weeks later, however, she had fully recovered and appeared to be doing very well.

In February, Claver also received other news. Since the autumn, he and William Piers had been planning another venture into the tricky business of enclosure, this time of 'the Commons or Tracts of Land called *Common-Moor, Black-Acre* and *South-Moor,* alias *Alder-Moor,* situate, lying, and being in or near the Parish of St John the Baptist in Glastonbury'. The petition to bring in a Bill had been read in the House of Lords in November, sent to the Commons for approval two months later, and agreed without amendment on 14th February. So all that was needed for 'An Act for Inclosing Glastonbury Commons' was the royal assent, and this was granted on 7th March.[15] Three days later, parliament was dissolved. It had been elected in 1715, soon after George I's accession and, although under the Septennial Act (1716) the Whigs had extended its life till 1722, its time had now run out. For years, across the country, Tories had been waiting and preparing for a general election to reverse the great losses they had suffered in 1715. But this time, in Wells, Claver was not going to support them.

His reasoning was simple. Ever since William Piers had become one of the MPs for the city in 1716, after the House of Commons had accepted his petition against the election of Thomas Horner, Claver felt that Piers had always voted for the good of his country and the Church of England. Claver had told the Horners as much in a heated argument in the summer of 1720. Since then, Piers had worked hard and used his influence to secure the passage of the Baltonsborough Enclosure Act, and he was now doing the same for Glastonbury. So, he had become a valuable and trusted friend, even though he was a Whig. The other MP for Wells, Thomas Edwards, had been elected in 1719 with the help of the Colston family and the Bristol Tories, despite the best efforts of Claver and the Taylors to prevent it. And their hopes of unseating Edwards at the general election of 1722 received a tremendous boost when it was reported that Piers had joined with a fellow Whig candidate who could be expected to appeal to voters.[16]

The Hon. George Hamilton, second son of the 6th earl of Abercorn in the Irish House of Lords, was just twenty-two when he married Bridget Coward of Wells in October 1719 and moved into the Coward mansion in Chamberlain Street, probably the largest private residence in Wells. Bridget's father and brother had both been MPs for the city, and Bridget was sole heir to her family's estate. Through Bridget's family connections, George Hamilton could expect to receive considerable support. William Piers was also closely related to the Cowards and, being the great-grandson of a former bishop of Bath and Wells, he too was from a prominent local family. So the Whig partnership of Hamilton and Piers was strong and, as far as Claver was concerned, well proven.

Yet the Tory Thomas Edwards was expecting to be re-elected, and he had found an excellent partner too. Francis Gwyn was not a local man but, having married his cousin Margaret Prideaux in 1690, he had inherited the fortune of her family and its great estate at Forde Abbey, a former monastery in Dorset. At the age of seventy-four, Francis was also a veteran Tory MP, having won fifteen elections in constituencies across the West Country and South Wales since 1673. It was unsurprising, therefore, that before the Wells election in March 1722, Edwards and Gwyn were just as prepared as Piers and Hamilton for a fight. Both sides badgered the mayor Joseph Luff, a tanner by trade, to break the city's by-laws by admitting more of their supporters as freemen and burgesses in order to gain more votes. By 5th March the mayor was quite frightened and exhausted. He reported to the corporation that 'great disorders have of late been committed in the Town', chiefly by new freemen who were 'guilty of Bloodshed, Assaults, Batteries and other breaches of the peace'.

According to Luff, the city was becoming ungovernable: 'great numbers run up and down the streets with Clubbs in their hands, headed by persons of distinction almost every night, huzzahing and crying "Down with the By-Laws"'. The doors of his house in Southover were beaten with clubs and his windows broken, and he was 'afraid of stirring out of his house by night without a guard, for fear of being

Murthered or at least Mayhemed [maimed]'. Even at two o'clock in the afternoon, while the city's Recorder, a Justice of the Peace, was hearing the complaints of people who had been assaulted, Piers and Hamilton interrupted the proceedings to demand that another twenty people were admitted burgesses of the city. So Luff was in no doubt that 'encouraged by two or three persons of distinction … there are such outcries and tumults every night in the streets that the peaceful inhabitants live in continual fear and dread'.[17]

It seems there were high spirits on both sides. Ten days later, when Claver was crossing Sedgemoor, he encountered a 'Wells Rabble on Horse-back [riding out] to meet Mr Gwyn who came to be made a Burgess' of the city. From his home in West Somerset, Sir William Wyndham had posted letters calling for a meeting of the 'Gentlemen of the County' to consider the 'proper persons' to stand as Knights of the Shire for Somerset. In response, Sir John Trevelyan, Sir Coplestone and John Bampfylde, Thomas Horner, Edward Phelips (all Jacobite sympathisers) and many others met at the George in Wells on 16th March. Claver and William Piers attended too, and listened to Sir William and Thomas Horner speak. Then Piers addressed the meeting and offered the assurance that there would be no Whig opposition to the election of two Tories as MPs for Somerset.[18] Even so, the Tory election managers were sufficiently anxious to call upon those present to sign a promise of support, which Claver signed along with several of his friends.[19] As for Wells, however, where the Whigs believed they had a fair chance of success, there would certainly be a contest.

On the day of the Wells election, Friday 23rd March, Claver went with Piers and Hamilton to the assize hall where he cast his two votes. He then watched 'the most unequal Practice of the Mayor' who refused to allow many votes for Piers and Hamilton, accepted a false tally kept by the town clerk, and finally declared Edwards and Gwyn elected, even though Claver believed 'we had a Majority of Voices' on the day. The poll appeared to show an overwhelming victory for the Tories: Edwards and Gwyn winning 235 and 228 votes, respectively; Piers and Hamilton each with 147. And when Claver went to Ilchester on 11th April, Sir William Wyndham and Edward Phelips were chosen as the Tory MPs for Somerset, without a contest. Across the country as a whole, however, the Tories had suffered an even worse defeat than in 1715, and that was before the hearing of petitions in the Commons which could be expected to produce a further reduction in the number of Tory seats. When Piers and Hamilton lodged their complaints about the election they must have reckoned that the prospects of overturning the Wells result were good. So did Claver, who took out a wager with George Mattocks that they would win their case. Over a year later, when half of its members were absent, the House of Commons divided over whether Edwards and Gwyn should be allowed to keep their seats. Somewhat surprisingly, by 142 votes to 123, it was decided that they should.[20]

30

THE GLASTONBURY ENCLOSURE

After being thought of as a lifelong Tory, Claver's decision to support two Whigs in the Wells election of 1722 was bound to have repercussions. Thomas Edwards and Francis Gwyn would never come to see him or invite him to any meeting where they held sway. After the election, Sir John Trevelyan, Sir William Wyndham and Edward Phelips also had no time for him, although he continued to visit Montacute House to look after Lady Phelips and her daughter, Edith. More importantly, he had lost the friendship of the Horners. They did not visit him, accompany him on his trips, or ever invite him to prescribe for them again. These were losses that Claver must have felt, for he had already lost influence and friends among the dean and chapter due to the decline of the aged Robert Creighton and the rise of Dean Brailsford and Archdeacon Archer whom he loathed. But times had changed and he no longer depended upon the patronage of senior clergy or gentry families as he had done when he first arrived in Wells. He had a family, a large house and an income of over £300 a year from his estates as well as over £200 from his work as a physician. Being financially secure, with plenty of old friends as well as two new ones in Piers and Hamilton he was, at the age of sixty-three, still full of energy and ambition.

He might well have thought that after the experience he had gained from overseeing the enclosure of 520 acres of common land at Baltonsborough, the delivery of a second Act of Enclosure would be much easier. This time, he had added his own name to the list of sixteen local 'Esquires' (including Christopher Keen and Davidge Gould) and four other 'Gentlemen' (Marshall Brydges, William Hill, William Salmon, and himself) who could serve as commissioners under the Act, whenever any three or more of them held a public meeting. And their powers were sweeping, for as well as hearing claims and partitioning the land according to its quality, they could build common ditches, drains, roads and gates, and charge all costs to the new proprietors.

DOI: 10.4324/9781003333654-33

The Act stipulated that 'the Commons as they now lie waste and unmanured, are of very little Benefit, Profit or Advantage to the several Owners'. How far the small farmers of Glastonbury agreed with this and believed that enclosure would 'tend very much to the Public Good, as well as to the mutual Advantage of all Persons concerned therein', was a matter of opinion.[1] Nobody would be surprised to learn that, under the pretence of delivering a public benefit, the gentry were prepared to pass new laws (sometimes with dreadful consequences) to protect and promote their own privileges and interests. Yet their willingness to use the rhetoric of public benefit and to subject themselves along with everyone else to the rule of law was no less important.[2] For Claver, delivering enclosure 'by agreement' through an Act of Parliament was a means of ensuring that everyone's rights and interests would be protected, and that everyone would benefit from the privatisation of the common land. But he, like most other people, would expect that the greatest benefits would accrue to those most able to take advantage of the change.

Although the town of Glastonbury had attained a royal charter in 1705, enabling it to govern itself with a mayor and corporation, the parish was still a 'ragged poor place' relative to Wells, with most of its commoners and small farmers still struggling to scratch a living from the soil.[3] There were also many more small farmers who depended upon the 1,250 acres of common land at Glastonbury, than there had been at Baltonsborough. The Glastonbury commoners were also wiser, due to the enclosure that had taken place so recently nearby. So, far from being an easy venture, work on the enclosure of the Glastonbury commons would dominate Claver's life throughout the spring and summer of 1722.

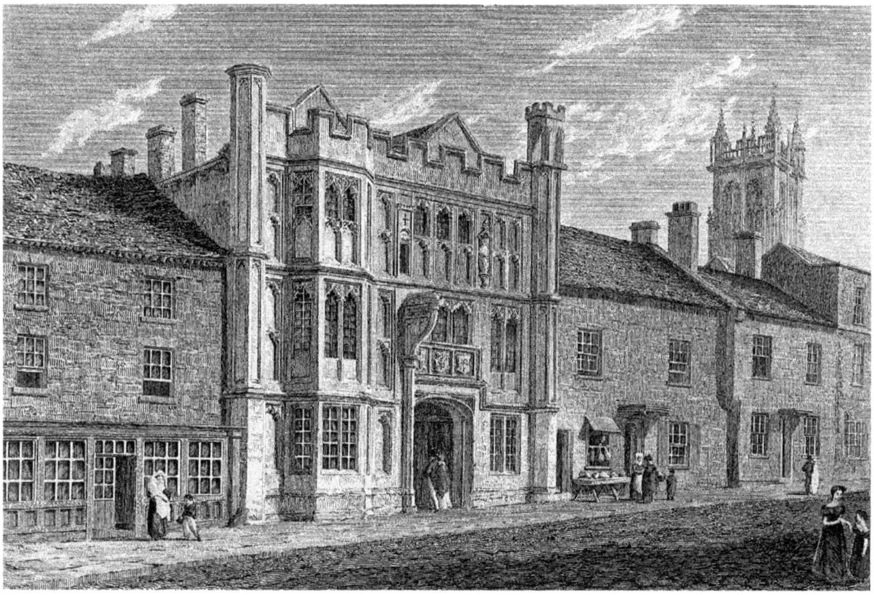

FIGURE 20 The George or Pilgrim's Inn, Glastonbury

At the first meeting of the commissioners at the George or Pilgrim's Inn at Glastonbury on 2nd April the claims for a share of the land were heard. But at the second meeting at the George, Claver was disappointed by the refusal of several of the commissioners to approve the claim of Mrs Leigh of West Bradley, even though he felt her case was strong. Before the third meeting, Abraham Fear, a Quaker, had come to Wells to warn Claver that 'obstinate People' were preparing to drive their animals into the commons, against the commissioners' ruling. And before their fourth meeting, Claver and others went to the moors to meet 'the Chief Inhabitants of Glastonbury', where they valued the land but had 'many altercations' about where to place the drovers' roads. By the time of the fifth meeting at the Bull's Head in Wells on 26th June, a group of commoners had emerged, led by the yeomen William Moxham of Street and James Slade of West Pennard, 'who endeavoured to frustrate the Act' by taking the commissioners to court. They were also refusing to make any contribution towards the costs of enclosure until they had received their shares.[4]

Although William Higgins was employed to measure out the Glastonbury commons, and Claver had a 'perambulator' (odometer) sent from London to provide more readings, it was not easy to determine the relative goodness and value of the various moorlands that were to be enclosed. The job of computing 'how much of each sort [of land] was equivalent to an acre [share]' was left entirely to Claver to work out. So was the process of awarding allotments by drawing tickets from a hat; a process that began on 2nd July at the Bull's Head, but was delayed by Thomas Nicholls, 'a Gentleman of Glastonbury', offering to buy shares in the common moor at 25 shillings per acre, and then changing his mind. It was not until 2:30 a.m. on 3rd July that all allocations were made, and Claver went home to bed. The next day, James Nooth, who had been assisting at the meetings, arrived to say that eight lots had been mistakenly omitted from the draw. Immediately, Claver convened an emergency meeting of the commissioners, proposed a solution, and then went home to make new calculations.

By the time of the seventh meeting, on 6th August at the George, it was reputed that William Moxham, satisfied with his single share of land, was going to withdraw his Chancery suit. But other proprietors now threatened legal action, complaining that their lots were overvalued. And there was another problem. The Enclosure Act had stipulated that 'as there is but a mean and insufficient Maintenance and Provision for the Curate of the said Parish of St John Baptist in Glastonbury', ten acres should be set aside to support his income under the jurisdiction of the bishop of Bath and Wells. This was to be done with the consent of the bishop's three nominees, one of whom was Edmund Archer. So, when James Slade, employed by the bishop to inspect the church's allocation, reported that he was unhappy with the measurement and fencing of the church's land (though it was worth £60 more than he expected), the commissioners knew that this stand-off would not be easy to resolve. There were serious disputes too, over where to place the sluices, ditches and drains that would be needed in the summer months to irrigate everybody's land.

At the eighth meeting, on 29th August in Wells, the commissioners accepted Claver's proposal that each proprietor should make their own ditch, six feet wide and three feet deep, but there were still so many complaints to the commissioners and disputes between the new proprietors themselves that the meeting had to be adjourned. At a reconvened session, Claver suggested that all proprietors should pay expenses according to the number of shares they owned in each moor; a pound for each share held in the Common-Moor and Blackacre, and fifteen shillings for each South-Moor share.[5] But this proposal was overshadowed by news that the bishop's nominees were not ready to sign for the church's land. By 12th September, Claver had meticulously re-measured his own and the church's land and the bishop had agreed to sign, but not in time for Archer to attend the meeting. Then, on 20th September, the bishop's nominees refused to sign on the grounds that they were unhappy with the ditching and fencing of their land. After the commissioners reluctantly agreed to pay for the planting of a hedge, the nominees finally agreed to sign. Unfortunately, by then, Archer could not be found, so more time was spent in dealing with complaints.

The attendance of the curate of St John the Baptist's at a meeting on 26th September might have been expected to help put an end to the procrastinations of the bishop's nominees. Yet he said that while he was happy to have his land well fenced and ditched, he did not want it hedged. Claver explained how this had come to be agreed, but he was too busy listening to other complaints and correcting drafts of the documentation for enclosure that needed to be deposited with a Justice of the Peace, to linger on the curate's case. Even without the curate's complaint, the documentation could not be completed that night, as the proceedings were interrupted by the arrival of an angry shoemaker. He treated the commissioners to such a stream of abuse about his two shares, he was close to being thrown out by George Hamilton when he made his exit. Three days later, the legal documents for dividing the commons between all of the new proprietors were signed, and the main work of the commissioners was done.[6]

There were now over a hundred new proprietors, between them holding over 800 shares in what used to be the commons. Some shares were divided into fourteenths to provide an exact measure of the land to which a particular shareholder was entitled. But most of the new proprietors, like Davidge Gould and James Slade, held a few shares each; each share representing one or two acres of land, depending on its quality. By far the largest landowner was Thomas Nicholls, who held over 100 shares across the moors. Thereafter, there were several other new proprietors with more than a dozen shares, including the Church with fifty-two, Edward Horner with forty-seven, and George Hamilton with thirty-two.[7] Claver was pleased with his nineteen shares, which were all in the best pastures of the Common-Moor. He had purchased a plot of land with a commons right in July for £20, and although the enclosure of all his new holdings had cost him £19, he was soon able to let them for over £24 a year.[8] For all the trouble that the Glastonbury enclosure had given him, it was a sound investment for him and everyone else who had a share. But it was not something that he would want to do again.

At the beginning of the year, he had bargained with Edward Birchmore, a coach-maker in Smithfield, to make him a new 'calesh' for £42, and at the end of May it was ready for collection. Accordingly, George Champion took the two coach-mares to London to bring the carriage home. With its gilt-framed sash windows, and coat-of-arms emblazoned on the brass housings and painted on its panels, it would make a strong impression, though Claver was soon making small 'improvements' to the design that he had commissioned.[9] The calèche arrived just in time to take Will to his new school at Sherborne, an ancient charitable foundation, where they were met by the new headmaster, Benjamin Wilding, MA.

According to one of his pupils, Wilding was a 'strict Grammarian and eminent for grounding his Scholars in a perfect knowledge of the Classicks'. However, 'the Circumstances of his Family (having a scold for wife, but a frugal Economist) and many Children, his Mind was frequently ruffled by domestic Scenes'. And while the headmaster's 'Passions were in Motion, he was often excited to use severe Treatment where Idleness or Dulness appeared' among the students. Wilding had been the vicar of Englishcombe near Bath and master of Bath Grammar School before taking the job at Sherborne in 1720. By 1722, he was already in a lawsuit with the governors over his alleged charging of high fees, in breach of the statutes of the school. He claimed that his fees were unexceptional, and that he had increased the number of boarders from sixteen to eighty. He was also soon embroiled in another controversy when Samuel Dampier, a clothier and Dissenter from Yeovil, led a petition against the compulsory church-going of all students, which effectively excluded local Dissenters' children from entering the day-school, on payment of a shilling. The petitioners won their case; the Court of Chancery ruling that students had a right to attend 'any meeting allowed by law'. Wilding, however, won his case against the governors' efforts to evict him.[10] But rumours of his rough treatment of the pupils persisted.

Staying at the George in Sherborne, Claver did his best to settle Will into his new surroundings: he inspected the lodgings with Wilding's wife, Rachael; ordered a bureau to be made to house Will's clothes; bought a silver spoon as a gift for the headmaster; gave the maids ten shillings; paid £5 for three months of schooling; and spent another ten shillings for Will's lessons on the violin. And before he left for Wells, he went to give five shillings to his niece Elizabeth Dawe, who had been abandoned by her 'villain' of an uncle at a dancing school nearby.[11]

Being left at Sherborne was an upsetting experience for Will who was only twelve years old, and he begged to stay with his father at the George. Leaving Will was difficult for Claver too. Two weeks earlier, during a writing lesson with James Nooth, Will had been told how to hold his pen correctly several times, and when he failed to learn, Claver had run out of patience. He wrote, 'I struck him a Slap on the Hinder part of his Head with the Palm of my Hand'.[12] It made no difference, but in an age when the physical and often brutal punishment of boys was usually considered part of their education, the fact that Claver even recalled the incident was telling. He was desperate to support Will's learning, but as he left the George to return to Wells, he may well have reflected upon Wilding's reputation, as well as his own impatience.

Two months later, on a sunny day in mid-August, Molly and her maid Molley Mitchell took the coach while Claver rode his mare to see how Will had settled in. That night, they all lodged and dined together at the Crown and the next day, at Wilding's house, Molly secured a day's holiday for all the boys. She then took Will to stay for a week with one of the school's governors, Baruch Fox and his family, a mercer who had a shop in Sherborne and an estate three miles away. Baruch was a friend of Molly's nephew, John Bragge, and, along with the Popes, Gillinghams and Newmans of Dorset, he was among Claver and Molly's relations and friends in the county. So Claver had time on his own to visit John Cook's bookshop in the town, where he bought half a dozen old books on theology, and then went to visit his mother at Lydlinch.[13]

Hannah Morris was almost ninety, and though she was in good health, she was keen to sort out her estate by changing the will she had made a few months earlier. She had previously bequeathed £10 to William Goddard, the grandson who had been born in 1685, but as he had no children, she now thought that £5 was quite enough. Similarly, in the spring she had planned to leave a legacy to the maid she shared with Mrs Gillingham, but now she wanted to strike her out, as the maid had not been kind to her. After she had given £30 to Claver to put towards her funeral expenses, he left to ride home on his own to Wells. In October, he returned to Sherborne with Betty and John Burland to see his son again.

In November he rode through the frost and snow to Ashton House, the seat of the Chudleigh family, seven miles south of Exeter, stopping for a night in the Fountain Inn at Taunton on the way. The purpose of this journey was to prescribe for Lady Frances Davie, the young wife of Sir George Chudleigh, who had recently given birth to her fourth child. The only treatment that Claver offered was a vomit, though later, while lodging at the Half Moon in Exeter, he gave her apothecary a prescription and instructions for Lady Davie's future care. It was a successful journey: she soon recovered and paid Claver twelve guineas for his work. Earlier in the year, he had prescribed for other Devon families, the Chichesters and Northmores. In particular, he attended to the 'beautiful' young Florence ('Fuddy') Chichester, a sister of Sir John, who had recently married William Northmore, a former MP for Okehampton. Claver visited Fuddy at the Hotwells spa in Bristol and prescribed for her in Wells when she came with her sisters to spend time with Betty Burland. But her health was not good, and she only lived for another two years.

In mid-December, Claver sent his coach and horses to bring Will home to Wells, along with George and Thomas Farewell, the sons of Anne Farewell (née Dawe), who were also boarders at Sherborne school. George and Thomas's father had been the rector of South Cadbury when he died in 1717, and after a long illness their mother had died in May 1722. To Claver, she had been a woman 'of an unequalled sweetness & beneficence of temper whom every one that knew her most affectionately lamented',[14] and he was highly protective of her sons. Nor had he forgotten another orphan, also one of Betty's cousins. Travelling with the boys in the coach to Wells for the festivities of Christmas was Elizabeth Dawe.

31

'A VERY HOT DRY SUMMER'

After the Christmas prayers and parties, there was still important work to do to complete the Glastonbury enclosure, for when the commissioners met at the George on 3rd January to pay expenses (men like James Nooth, who was owed 20 guineas for attending 18 meetings), it was clear that there was a serious shortfall of over £200 in the accounts. This was because some of the new proprietors (including some of the commissioners) had not paid the rates that had been levied on their shares. It was therefore decided to take the recalcitrants to court. Thomas Nicholls, by far the biggest beneficiary and one of the owners who had not paid his bills, had submitted excessive expenses for the work that he had promised to do; yet he had still not delivered the building of the flood-gates that were vital to protect the land. Claver also had problems with his own property at 'Morris Hayes', part of the Baltonsborough enclosure, where a neighbour had been threatening his tenants, and he would not desist until he had been fined.[1]

In mid-January, after a trip to Kelston where he played Giuseppe Valentini's concertos, it was time to take Will and the other children back to school. At Sherborne, Will was now quartered with the fifteen-year-old George Farewell, but he still preferred to stay with Claver at the Crown. While staying there, Claver took the opportunity to take Will to see his grandmother at Lydlinch, and to visit Edith Phelips at Montacute. He dined with the headmaster and his wife, and a month later, when Wilding came to Wells to ask for 'a Testimonial of his Character' (to help defend himself against the school's governors in court), Claver provided one. He was busy with patients too, though he had recently lost Mary Healy, the wife of Richard, the vicar of St Cuthbert's, who had died childless at the age of thirty-five.[2]

Of particular concern was Anne Starr, sister of one of Claver's former tenants at Worle near Weston-super-Mare, who had recently moved to Wells to lodge above Richard Cupper's shop. Claver had been treating her for years, but her condition was now sufficiently serious for him to ask Lucas to intervene. In February, he

DOI: 10.4324/9781003333654-34

persuaded Lucas 'to push his Probe hard into the Place made for a Seton in Mrs Star's highly swollen knee'. There, 'it luckily broke into the Pelvis where the Abscess had long lain'. And the next day, they 'dilated the orifice of the Impostumation [abscess] in her Knee, and let out a pint of Pus and Ichorous Matter'.[3]

A week later, Claver and Lucas went to Mrs Margaret Coxe's mansion at Ston Easton, where her father Preston Hippisley was in a serious condition. He was fifty-four and reckoned 'exceedingly fat' and unable to travel on account of the leg that he had broken in his youth. To relieve his pain 'Lucas made an Incision into an Abscess which was very large on the left side of his Anus'. After further visits, often struggling through the Mendip fogs, they applied a ligature to Preston's fistula, but it was no cure.[4] They also treated Edward Strode of Pilton without success, for they attended his funeral at the end of March. Just a week later, Claver returned to see Strode's widow, Elizabeth, at the request of William Hill, the choral vicar and rector of Dulverton. His mission was to ask Elizabeth if she would consider a proposal of marriage from his friend. Hill then went himself to see Elizabeth in May, and Claver was asked again to put a good word in on behalf of his young friend; but it was all to no avail.[5]

On his 64th birthday on 1st May, Claver and Lucas went to the marketplace to conduct a post mortem on Anne Starr. She had died the day before, having recently added a codicil to her will. In it, she had left ten shillings to each of Cupper's maids; a suit of clothes to her 'intimate acquaintance' Mary Mattocks (another of Claver's patients); five shillings to one of her brothers; and most of the rest of her estate to her brother Richard Starr. When her hearse left Wells for the burial at Worle on 3rd May, Claver rode behind it for four miles. Only later would he learn that, in the very first item of her will, Anne had left 'Claver Morris, my physician' £20, with the explanation that this was 'for the great care he has taken of me during my long sickness'.[6]

Before the end of the month, William and Anne Berkeley had called upon Claver to prescribe for their two young sons, Edward and Henry, who had been 'seized with the measles' at Sherborne. He must have thought their condition was quite serious as he examined them three times as soon as he arrived on 21st May, and he did not see Will until the evening. He prescribed for 'Neddy and Henry' again on the following morning, and was planning to bring the Farewell boys to Wells with Will, but had to leave them at the school as they had measles too. All four boys recovered and Claver clearly did not blame the school for the outbreak of infections. A fortnight later, he wrote to the headmaster inviting him to visit Mrs Margaret Coxe to discuss the admission of her eight-year-old son and heir, John Hippisley-Coxe, to Sherborne school.

When Benjamin Wilding came to Wells, Claver accompanied him to Ston Easton, and met him again when he took Will back to Sherborne on an 'excessive hot' day in June. After 'a Neck of Veal in Steaks' at the Crown, he returned to Wells 'leaving my Son with his Eyes a little wet'. So, he was pleased to receive a first letter from Will on 2nd August, and immediately wrote one in return. A few days later, in the middle of the heatwave, he was again in Sherborne to prescribe for John,

Mrs Coxe's newly enrolled son. His five-year-old sister Susannah ('Miss Susan') had died in June. Though John recovered quickly, Will was now so sick that Claver felt he needed to stay for several days and sit up with Will all night before he could return to Wells.[7]

The summer months were so hot and dry for farming that Claver took a guinea off his tenants' rents in recognition of the 'excessive dryness and badness of the year'. The months were also hard for working animals. Claver lost his second coach-mare 'Burgess' after an outing with the Burlands in July, though he tried to save her by bloodletting and drenching. He had replaced his other mare in March at Warminster for £14, and in August bought a second one at Devizes for £16. This was just in time to take Molly, the Burlands, George Champion and Molley Mitchell on a 'very hot day' to Sherborne, where they dined with the Wildings and visited relations for several days, though Molly stayed for another week. Claver was now keeping an eye on George for, returning late one evening, he had spotted 'my Man George Champion Hugging and Kissing My Wife's Maid Molley Mitchell'. This would not be troublesome, as long as George went no further without a public declaration of his marital intentions.[8]

Earlier in the summer, the baking weather had been welcome, particularly as it enabled Claver's men to complete the making of a horse-pond and a 'stew pond' (a pool for keeping fish ready to be eaten) next to his cherished and newly-walled main pond on the farm at Pilton. This meant that he had somewhere to keep the fish while their pond was being drained and cleaned. He was so excited at the prospect, he arranged for guests and workers to be treated to a picnic. Hampers containing 'a large Leg of Mutton, & ten pennyworth of Colliflowers & Cabbage, & a Piece of Ruff'd Beef which was Boyld'; 'a large Loaf of Bread, a Cheese, Mustard, Vineger, Salt [and] Butter'; as well as a tablecloth, plates, and knives and forks were prepared and sent. So were refreshments: a barrel of strong October beer, seventy-two pints of bottled October, and twelve pints of 'small' (weak) beer for children.

On the morning of the picnic, Molley Mitchell went to Pilton to dress the mutton, and Claver, Will, and George Champion oversaw the draining of the pond, which took two hours. At 2 p.m. lunch was served to the guests: the builder Charles Taylor and his son; Thomas Swarbrick, the organ-maker; William Hill and others. After sending thirty good-sized carp to absent friends, there were about 190 saved for accommodation in the other ponds. So, by the time that Claver and his guests returned to Wells at 9 p.m., a good day's work had been done. Unfortunately, what nobody could foresee was that the hot dry weather would continue. This meant that there was no water in the well until the end of November, and insufficient water running down the hill to fill the pond until mid-January. By then, the pond had degraded and leaked so badly it would never be filled again.[9]

Claver also had other responsibilities requiring his attention. In addition to his duties as a commissioner for the collection of the Land Tax (now set at two shillings in the pound), and for the maintenance and improvement of the county's watercourses and sewers, in the summer of 1723 he took on the work of collecting a new tax levied upon all Catholic landholders' estates. The tax had been introduced by the Whigs in response to the previous year's discovery of the plot by the bishop of Rochester, Francis Atterbury, to restore the Stuart dynasty. The conspiracy was largely led by disaffected Anglicans and Tories, but it was hoped that by increasing anti-Catholic legislation and taxation (Catholics were already required to pay double the Land-Tax rate), the faith would be suppressed. The tax was onerous, and at least one group of Anglican gentry thought that it would 'certainly be to the Utter Ruin of many' Catholic families in the region.[10] But an even greater danger lay in its sister Act. Alongside the new Papist Tax, designed to raise £100,000, was a new set of oppressive oaths (of allegiance, suppression and abjuration) that men and women had to take before 25th December 1723. And if they refused or failed, under the Oaths Act (1723) their names were to be registered at the quarter sessions. This could lead to the seizure of all their properties by the Forfeited Estates Commission.

From his first meeting on 1st August at the Bull's Head tavern with the other Papist Tax commissioners for Wells (Richard Comes, the county sheriff; and Charles and Matthew Baron, both former mayors), it was clear that Claver would need to take the lead if the annual values of Catholics' estates were to be assessed and charged in time to produce the total sum of over £53 that was required from Wells. So, he worked hard to make progress locally, and he went to Taunton to discuss the problems of collection with the county's commissioners, who were less than helpful.

The Papist Tax was not something that Claver could believe in, and he knew that it was not the Catholic families of Somerset that had conspired with Atterbury to bring in the Pretender. In fact, although he had no scruple in telling Catholics where their beliefs and practices were mistaken, he was far more aggravated by what he regarded as the ignorance and arrogance of some Dissenters. Thus, on 4th August, when Nathaniel Markwick, vicar of the village of East Brent and a prebend of the cathedral, preached a Sunday sermon that smacked of Calvinist doctrines of predestination, it was no surprise that Claver thought it thoroughly 'impertinent & insignificant'. The Papist Tax was also very poorly drafted and administered. But because of his sense of public duty, his position as a respected citizen and his ability to undertake complex calculations, its collection was something that Claver felt well placed to undertake. Naturally, he could also use his position to see what he could do for friends, and he tried to persuade his Catholic neighbours (successfully in the case of William Ball, a resident of Burcott) to take the oaths. He even tried to obtain reductions in the charges faced by friends, such as his lodger Mary Evans and his tailor Thomas Bourne, though in both cases he had no success.[11]

Christopher Lucas was another friend and respected colleague who Claver wanted to support. So, on 22nd August, when Lucas invited him to watch an operation 'to take out a Stone from a Young Fellow by the New Method of cutting throw the Belly', he was keen to see how this was done. The operation was conducted by Samuel Pye, a surgeon from Bristol who described the procedure in an illustrated pamphlet *Some Observations on the Several Methods of Lichotomy* (1724). According to Pye, his patient at Wells was a 'miserably emaciated' nineteen-year-old who had suffered from the affliction since he was a child. On cutting him open, a large stone was found, 'his bladder thick and hard, and strongly contracted to it'. Claver prescribed after the operation, but the boy died a month later, and a post mortem confirmed that 'the neck of the Bladder, where the Stone was lodged [was] very scirrhous and full of deep Ulcers'.[12]

There was no chance of Claver's medicine saving 'the poor Young Fellow', though Pye's 'new method' would eventually become a great success. Meanwhile, Claver still needed to prescribe for men like William Berkeley who were 'tortured by the Stone'. Despite the dangers, Claver also recognised that there were times, as for a patient like Grizelda Irish, when surgery had to be performed as a last resort. She was in her thirties; a woman 'very agreeable in her person, and much more so in her behaviour' according to her family. Claver had been the family doctor since she was a child. So when he 'writ to Mr Gay (surgeon in Hatton Garden) about Cutting off the Cancer from Mrs Grishild Irish's Breast', he must have thought that this was her best chance. In this case, although Robert Gay, an eminent surgeon and former MP for Bath, performed the operation and Claver continued to prescribe, Grizelda died just ten months later.[13]

Claver's diagnosis and advice was more successful when he appeared to save baby 'Biddey', the daughter of George and Bridget Hamilton, who 'everyone despaired of' during her first year of life. The Hamiltons had asked Molly Morris to be Biddey's godmother, and were so grateful for Claver's treatment of their child; they gave him eight guineas as a show of thanks.[14] He also collected over fourteen guineas from Mrs Margaret Coxe at Ston Easton for his care of her and her children, John and Ann. And he collected another fourteen guineas from Margaret's father, though Preston died while Claver was attending to him in December 1723.[15]

Despite these hefty fees and gifts for his work as a physician, Claver's income from his 'Advice and Prescriptions' had fallen to about £200 per year.[16] On the one hand this was due to the fact that he was not travelling as often to the manors of the gentry, and he certainly had fewer patients among the families of the dean and chapter. Far from being within their circle of friendship and preferment, several of the senior clergy now saw Claver as a nuisance and were wilfully obstructive of his work. This was particularly true of his efforts to ensure that everyone in the Liberty paid their fair share of the Land Tax which was, and always had been, levied upon all public offices as well as properties.

Yet, when Claver asked Archdeacon Archer and a couple of his colleagues to pay their taxes, he was met with a series of objections and complaints. In these disputes, Claver was entirely right, but a personal animosity had been smouldering for years, fuelled most recently by Archer's obduracy regarding the fee that Claver paid in ground rent for his house. Archer's austere and haughty manner did not appeal to Claver, nor did his ranting at every kind of non-conformity from the Church of England. Even on a solemn day, such as 30th January, a fast-day commemorating the execution of Charles I in 1649, over which the two men might have shared some common ground, Claver thought that Archer was full of pomposity, having 'preached a silly Sermon very confidently'.[17]

The other reason why Claver's income from prescriptions had fallen was that he was now charging most people less for his prescriptions and advice. He had recently increased his servants' wages by a few shillings every quarter, and had even introduced a new heading 'Money Given, besides of the Dedicated Part' into his Accounts. This was for outgoings that were quite different from the 'Unnecessary Expenses' in which he itemised the small losses incurred from wagers or playing cards and backgammon with his friends. The new category was simply for gratuities and gifts: the sixpences and shillings passed to maids, children and labourers who he happened to encounter on his rounds. Among these items there were also two broader headings under which he recorded his donations. These were for gifts made to 'a poor Family' or to 'a decayed Family'; always two shillings and sixpence for the former, and five shillings for the latter – equivalent to what most labourers would earn in five or six long days of work. Claver could afford these acts of charity and, being of a generous disposition, it pleased him to act in this way. But, as he grew older, it was now important to him to keep a tally of this aspect of his Christian duty.

32

SEEN BY CANDLELIGHT

During the long cold winter, when candles needed to be lit well before supper, Claver seldom went to bed before the clocks struck twelve. Often, especially if there were guests to entertain, he would stay up longer. Sometimes, especially in bad weather, he did not get home till late, as when, after visiting the Seymours at Regilbury, he became so badly lost in the Mendip fog it was not until two o'clock in the morning that he got to bed. Even then, on the frostiest of mornings, he was always an early riser, and for several days each week he was still in the cathedral for matins at six o'clock. When he needed to be up early for a journey, he often only had a few hours of sleep, and on any night he might be woken up by an urgent request to visit a patient at the break of dawn. Occasionally, his nights were interrupted by the stealthy delivery of casks of French brandy, claret and white wine, sent by William Bragge from his ships in the Dorset ports. In spite of his good age, at sixty-three he still had plenty of energy and other interests to pursue.

Trips to Dorset often required an early start, especially in the winter, and while Will was boarding at Sherborne, Claver liked to take him back to school. After each vacation, Will and the Farewell boys would ride in the calèche with Will Clark, accompanied by Claver on his horse. Normally, these were pleasant trips during which they could test the new machine that Claver had 'fixed to my Calesh to Count the Revolutions of the Wheel & consequently the Miles travelled'.[1] They would rest at Ansford Inn on the outskirts of Castle Cary, lodge at the Crown in Sherborne for a night or two, take breakfast with Benjamin Wilding or Baruch Fox, and enjoy a dish of steaks before Claver and his man returned to Wells. It was only ten miles from the school to Lydlinch, so Claver often visited his mother and relations on these trips, as he did with Will in January 1724. But

DOI: 10.4324/9781003333654-35

in early March, he made a different kind of visit to the school. His aim this time was simply to find out 'whether the Report of Mr Wildings excessive Severity to my Son' was true.

He discovered that, since Christmas, Will had often been whipped, though not above three lashes at a time. This was a relief, for Claver had previously objected to Will receiving fourteen lashes in a single thrashing. Wilding professed to love Will, and said that he could make him 'an incomparable Scholar, & the best that ever went from his School'. To prove the point, he called for Will to attend for an oral examination of his ability in Greek and Latin. Will's only fault was evidently that 'he would not take Pains', such as bothering to use a dictionary; a fault that Wilding believed he had almost completely corrected, by 'often whipping him'.

Claver was so impressed by Will's performance in conjugating verbs in Greek, and so committed to supporting his education, he was inclined to agree with Wilding's plan. But when the headmaster revealed that he had just received a letter from Abigail Prowse, Bishop Hooper's daughter, writing to say that Molly Morris was upset by rumours about the whipping of her son, Claver was taken entirely by surprise. Wilding promised that 'he would whip him no more', but Claver feared this strategy might also spoil him. So, they agreed upon 'only moderate Correction which, to a Good-Natured & Flexible though Lazy Boy' like Will, Claver hoped would be effective. It seems that Wilding kept to the agreement, for on this matter Claver did not need to speak to him again. But other boys were not so fortunate. At least one parent removed a son in protest at 'the cruel, barbarous and inhuman' behaviour of the headmaster, which he had verified by 'a strict examination of the flesh'.[2]

Meanwhile, in Wells, a new charity school had been opened for the basic education of twenty poor boys and twenty girls, aged seven to eleven, each to be dressed in a distinctive blue school uniform. The school had been planned with the support of the corporation and the dean and chapter in 1713, when a High Street attorney Philip Hodges offered to build a school house (St Andrew's Lodge) in the Back Liberty, a hundred yards from Claver's home. Claver and sixteen other men from the city's leading families attended the inaugural meeting in 1714 and had since contributed one or two pounds each year to the foundation.[3] There was gossip that some of the workers got drunk on stolen beer during the building of the Lodge, but it was completed by 1720. The first students were admitted under the direction of Thomas Gravill (the choral vicar who had been Will's writing teacher) and Mrs Teek, both of whom were Claver's friends. Part of the mission of the school was to prepare more children for apprenticeships, but when Claver was invited to the school by Hodges in April 1724, he made it clear that he thought this was a bad idea. Perhaps reflecting upon his own disappointing experiences with apprentices, he thought that the enrolment of new ones would not help to address the shortage of good husbandmen and craftspeople in the county. More likely, it would lead the poor children 'to the Army or the Gallows'. Even so, he continued to support the school, and later that year when Hodges became seriously ill he prescribed for him and was a pall-bearer at his funeral.[4]

A few weeks before Claver expressed his opposition to apprenticeships, he had returned to Dorset on hearing of his mother's death. She had been 'confined to her Chamber' for the best part of a year, so it came as no surprise when she died at the age of ninety-two. Claver arranged for a coffin to be engraved, and a hearse to be sent from Blandford Forum to lead a procession the five miles from Hannah's home in Lydlinch to St Nicholas's at Manston; the village where he had grown up and where his brother and sisters had been buried. Before the service on Tuesday 24th March 1724, 'a very large cold Rib of Beef, & of a Gammon of Bacon and Fowles' was served to the parishioners. Later, Hannah was laid to rest under the communion table, next to her husband. Above them, on the chancel wall was Claver's memorial to his first wife Grace and their baby daughter who he had also buried under the altar long ago, and who he had mourned for years.[5]

More cheerfully, at Easter, George Hamilton proposed the formation of a new 'Weekly Society' consisting of a small group of friends who would meet every Saturday at one of their homes to drink and feast. This appealed to Claver, and it seemed especially appropriate after the abstinence he had kept during his Good Friday fast, when he 'neither Eat, nor Drank, nor so much as took any Snuff at all, till past 7 in the Evening'. On Saturday 11th April he hosted the society's first meeting with George Hamilton, John Burland, Christopher Lucas, Richard Comes and Thomas Swarbrick in attendance. Very occasionally, other persons were invited, but the only other regular members of the club were Marshall Brydges and William Hill. Unlike the music club which met on Tuesdays, the meetings of the new 'Weekly Society' were small and required no preparation other than the good services of cooks and maids. But Claver's passion for playing and listening to music had not waned.

Attendance at the music club was boosted by the return of General William Evans' regiment of the 4th Dragoons (Hussars) to Wells, where they had first been posted in the summer of 1723. Not only did army officers and their ladies now come to enjoy the singing and the dancing, but oboists, trumpeters and drummers from the regiment were invited to join in. Two notable Italian musicians also came to Wells to perform, and Claver took them on a grand tour of the cathedral. But he was disappointed that only thirty-two tickets were sold (at two shillings and sixpence each) when the Italians gave a concert.[6] To celebrate his birthday, he went with James Nooth to Kelston, where for two days they contributed to concerts, playing Valentini concertos and Handel's oratorio *Esther* (*c.*1720). And a few weeks later, he took Will and George Farewell on a trip to Bristol where they lodged at

Guilder's Inn. They went on to Bath where they breakfasted at the Harringtons' house in Trim Street, visited the fashionable Orange Grove, and had the famous English trumpeter and flutist, John Baptise Grano, come to entertain them at the new dining-room of the Three Tuns inn.[7]

Claver was determined to get George Farewell a place at Magdalen College, Oxford, and had offered George's guardian and uncle, Nathaniel, £5 a year to help with maintenance. So, he was delighted when Nathaniel finally, if reluctantly, agreed to the proposal. The only disadvantage was that Will would now be without his best friend at boarding school. But Claver and Molly visited regularly, checking that he was not being beaten, and Claver was so pleased to hear that his son was doing well, he sent him a first-rate violin. There was even better news from Betty. On Friday 10th July, after nine hours in labour, at 10.30 in the morning she gave birth to a baby boy. For the proud grandfather, it was auspicious that a new moon had appeared exactly twenty-four hours before. However, Claver was 'extremely tortured with Rheumatick Pains in my Right Shoulder, Arm & from my Head to the lower end of the Shoulder-blade.' The agony persisted for several days, but it did not stop him from seeing Betty and his grandson, or from going, 'though in pain', to his music club.[8]

The baptism of baby John Burland and Betty's 'churching' were moments of celebration during another hot dry summer. As well as his regular visits to see patients and manage his estates, Claver took Molly and Mrs Evans on a trip in the calèche to Ston Easton, where Margaret Coxe treated them to a three-course meal, with seven dishes in each course. And he went on his own, by horseback via Trowbridge, to the village of Poulshot in Wiltshire, where Marshall Brydges had recently been appointed rector. It was only a couple of miles further to Devizes, so they took a tour of the prosperous little town, visiting two very large nursery gardens near the castle and the great malthouse, and stopped at an inn to quench their thirst. When Claver returned to Wells he was 'very much tired', but not inclined to rest. This was because he was so furious to discover that James Whitehead, one of his tenants at West Bradley, had topped over forty maiden oaks without permission, he decided to sue for damages in court. He terminated Whitehead's lease and wrote a new contract very neatly on lined paper, leasing the twelve acres of land to the yeoman William Paddock (who made his mark) for £52 a year.[9] Although he had plenty of similar work managing the rest of his estates, he also had to fulfil his duties as a commissioner for the collection of the Land Tax and the 'Papist Tax', for overseeing of the county's watercourses and sewers, and for completion of the Glastonbury Enclosure Act.

Collecting taxes was never easy, but maintaining the watercourses of the county was no less fraught with difficulty. A particular concern for the commissioners was the flooding of thousands of acres of farmland at Bason Bridge near Burnham-on-Sea, where the bridge was broken and the size of the ditches needed to be doubled.

Samuel Cockerell, lord of the nearby manor of Huntspill, objected to making any contribution, though he boasted that his estate in Somerset alone was worth £10,000, and he threatened the commissioners with no end of legal action until he got his way. Eventually, to protect 4,800 acres of moorland, the commissioners decided that the cost of improvements (£210) should be met by everyone paying a shilling for each acre of land they owned. It was a fair solution, but rather than settle the dispute, it opened up a series of new arguments that ran on for years.[10]

Similarly, although the commons at Glastonbury had been enclosed, there were still problems due to its biggest beneficiary Thomas Nicholls not settling his bills, and a general uncertainty about how the new allotments should be assessed for local rates. Nobody knew for sure to which parish, Glastonbury or Meare, the ancient commons had originally belonged, though Claver insisted that he should not be charged the Glastonbury rates on the land that he had just acquired. For Claver, this was a matter of fair accounting, rather than an attempt to save three shillings. Over the years, he had spent many days walking the commons with the farmers of Glastonbury and listening to their concerns, so he knew there were people who had suffered from enclosure, but who were not entitled to receive relief from the parish rates. In November, he therefore decided that, with the help of the mayor of Glastonbury, he would draw up a list of these 'unrelieved Poor' families, and on 22nd December he took Ben Taylor with him to the Rose and Crown at Glastonbury to distribute £20. Two days later, he wrote a list of 'the Christmas poor' of Wells and gave them 'money as usual'.[11] In the afternoon he went to the cathedral to be a pall-bearer at the funeral of Mrs Keen.

Claver had been friends with Jane Keen (the daughter of Maurice Berkeley) for thirty years. He had been doctor to the children she had borne from her marriage to the Huguenot James Gendrault, and he had supported her following her marriage to Christopher Keen, shortly after her first husband's death. This was not a happy marriage, so it was no surprise to Claver that in the autumn he found the couple quarrelling when he arrived at their house in the marketplace to prescribe for Jane. Though 'very weak', she 'utterly refused' his medicines, saying they would serve no purpose while her husband 'sunk her Strength so often by his ill Usage of her'. During two hours of 'remonstrating and quarrelling' they agreed to part, but could not agree upon the terms. Jane had been paying her husband an allowance of £60 a year, but he wanted £200 to stay away. Under Claver's arbitration, they settled on £150 a year, as soon as an agreement could be signed. This meant that Jane was now willing to take her medicines, and Claver could do his best to look after her. But even after her funeral on Christmas Eve, the rancour did not end.

The main problem was that Jane's son, Charles Gendrault, an army captain and freemason who had come from London to be with his mother during her final illness, believed that his father's will and a signed-but-unsealed statement by his mother, entitled Charles and his sisters to *all* of their mother's jewels and valuables. This view was supported by the attorney William Baron, but Keen and Claver did not concur. After 'Angry Words' between Keen and Gendrault in several meetings at the Mitre, they eventually agreed to share the valuables, though these needed to be retrieved from London where they had been pawned. Christopher Keen was not planning to grieve for long; before the month was out he was in pursuit of another match.[12]

Whatever Keen's shortcomings as a husband, he was certainly of a nervous disposition. Watching Claver make 'Glass of Antimony' in his laboratory one morning – a preparation that required 'a violent Heat' giving rise to 'sulphurous fumes' – Keen was badly frightened when all of the ingredients suddenly exploded and caught fire. For Claver, it was just another unfortunate chemical operation that had led to disappointment; in this case the loss of a substance that could be used to make 'a potent vomit'. But he calmed his friend with a game of backgammon, something they usually only played after supper in the evenings. Claver often lost a few shillings at these games, for although Keen always made mistakes, 'his luck in Throwing was so admirable & even beyond what was usual' he was used to winning.[13]

When Will came home for Easter at the end of March 1725, Claver must have feared the worst. On Good Friday, Will had a headache, but by Easter Sunday it was clear that this was the onset of smallpox. Claver immediately called upon an experienced nurse, Sarah Lovell, to come and look after him, but he knew there was no remedy for this disease. Four days later, on 1st April, the household was in further crisis as Claver noted in his diary 'my Wife being very like to Die, I sate up with her'.

Molly did not have smallpox but a respiratory condition that left her 'labouring her last for Life, & Breathing with the most deplorable difficulty'. Claver made drinks and gargles to ease the pain, and watched over her, as did Betty, Mary Evans and other friends. They knew that Molly did not have long to live. At 2 o'clock on Monday morning, 5th April, Betty arrived in such distress that she ran up the stairs crying out 'Oh! My dear Mother I shall lose my best Friend'. She then collapsed while calling out to Will. Molly, mishearing Betty's cries, thought Will was dead. Though he was still suffering from smallpox, Will had to be dressed so that his mother could see him and, when carefully positioned in the candlelight 'the sight of him seemed to please her', though she was delirious. She said, 'she never saw him look better in her Life'. After kissing his mother, Will was taken back to bed, and Molly died, surrounded by her family and friends. In his diary, Claver drew a small hand pointing to the day's events: 'My Dear Wife who from a Death Sweat grew in her Hands and Arms very cold, left speaking in two or 3 hours, & half an hour after Ten in the Forenoon she Breath[ed] her last'.[14]

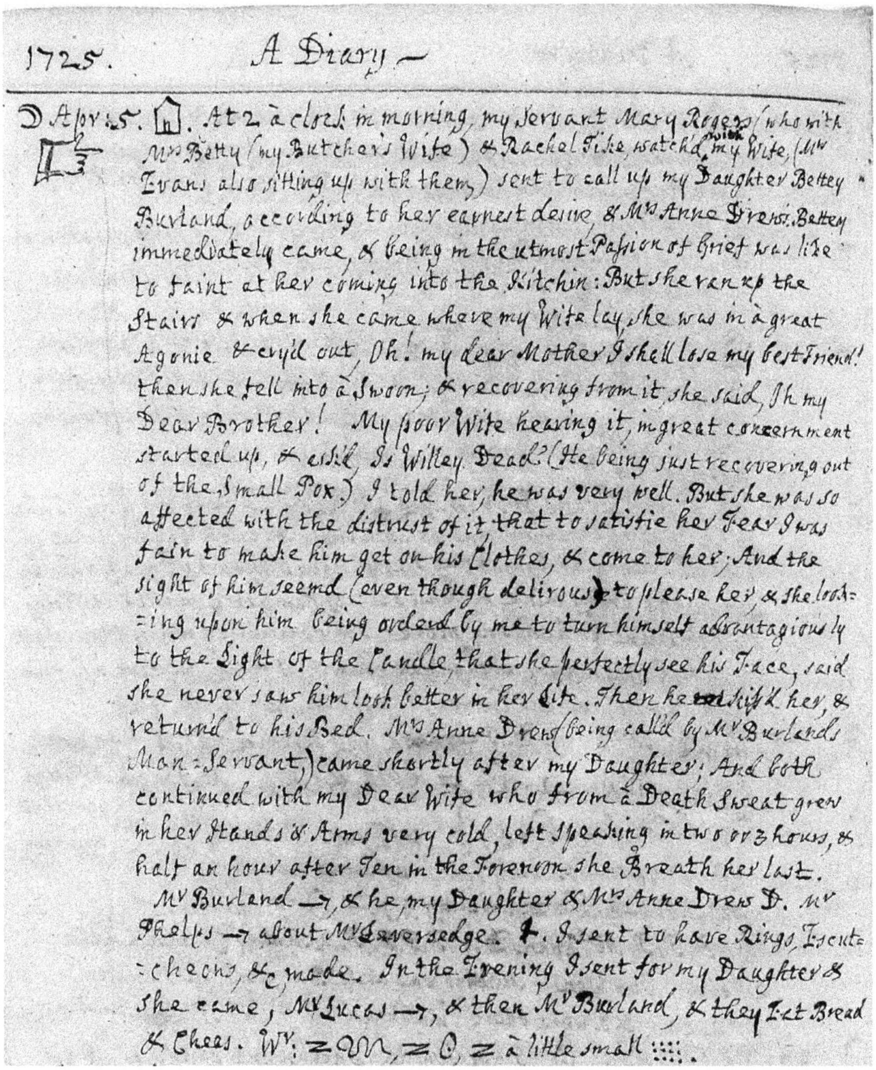

1725. A Diary –

Apr: 5. At 2 a clock in morning, my Servant Mary Rogers (who with Mrs Betty (my Butcher's Wife) & Rachel Fike, watch'd with my Wife, (Mr Evans also sitting up with them,) sent to call up my Daughter Bettey Burland, according to her earnest desire, & Mrs Anne Drew. Bettey immediately came, & being in the utmost Passion of Grief was like to faint at her coming into the Kitchin: But she ran up the Stairs & when she came where my Wife lay, she was in a great Agonie & cry'd out, Oh! my dear Mother I shall lose my best Friend! then she fell into a Swoon; & recovering from it, she said, Oh my Dear Brother! My poor Wife hearing it, in great concernment started up, & ask'd, Is Willey Dead? (He being just recovering out of the Small Pox.) I told her, he was very well. But she was so affected with the distrust of it, that to satisfie her Fear I was fain to make him get on his Clothes, & come to her; And the sight of him seem'd (even though delirous) to please her, & she look=ing upon him being order'd by me to turn himself advantagiously to the Light of the Candle, that she perfectly see his Face, said she never saw him look better in her Life. Then he kiss'd her, & return'd to his Bed. Mrs Anne Drew (being call'd by Mr Burland's Man=Servant,) came shortly after my Daughter; And both continued with my Dear Wife who from a Death Sweat grew in her Hands & Arms very cold, left speaking in two or 3 hours, & half an hour after Ten in the Forenoon she Breath'd her last.

Mr Burland →, & he, my Daughter & Mrs Anne Drew D. Mr Phelps → about Mr Leversedge. I sent to have Rings, Escut=cheons, &c made. In the Evening I sent for my Daughter & she came, Mr Lucas →, & then Mr Burland, & they Eat Bread & Chees. Wr: = M, = O, = a little small ::::.

FIGURE 21 Claver's diary, 5th April 1725

The next day, Molly was laid in a coffin in a very fine burial dress, and arrangements were made for her funeral. Mourning-rings, silk scarves and hat-bands were ordered and over 140 invitations issued. Claver busied himself preparing mulled claret for the guests, and after Marshall Brydges had led the service, they returned to Claver's house. Christopher Keen was among the mourners and 'he went by himself into the Pantry-Chamber, & wept very much'. When most of the guests had left, Claver went and sat with him throughout the night.

33

DINING ALONE

In the days after Molly's funeral, Will's recovery from smallpox was a blessing, and it enabled Claver to focus on settling the family's affairs. He gave 200 sixpenny loaves of bread to the poor of Wells and went through Molly's bedroom cabinet to locate the personal items that she had bequeathed to several friends. These included gifts for Betty; Mrs Evans and her maid; and James Nooth – no doubt for Jane, his wife, who had been Will's nurse. There was also a present for Mary Rogers, the midwife who had delivered Will, though she would soon leave the household, with a few months' extra wages. In settling the accounts, Claver was surprised to find unpaid bills for the butcher, grocer and baker amounting to above £12, for Molly had always said that these were paid. His main concern, however, was for his own health, as he was now so 'very Sick of a continued Tertian Fever', he could not write his diary for ten days, and as soon as he was sufficiently recovered he started to write his will.

Before the will was completed and witnessed by George and Bridget Hamilton and Ben Taylor on 26th May 1725, Claver had missed ten of the weekly meetings of the music club. He was now well enough to attend and to take Will back to school, though it was only by 'Divine Favour' that Will avoided death once again when his horse fell on the way. In the household, there was no further need for Sarah Lovell, who had come to nurse Will in his smallpox. Mary Rogers also left. And Mrs Evans was preparing to leave her lodgings after Molly's death. The household was becoming much smaller and, with no wife or children in residence, much quieter than it had ever been. For someone like Claver, who loved his family and all kinds of company, these changes were hard to bear. After a sunny day, 3rd June, on which he had worked alone in his laboratory and written five prescriptions, he noted bleakly in his diary 'I dined by my self, being the first time I did so above these 20 years'.

The next day he spoke to his maid Hannah Beal about a matter that had been on his mind for some time; 'her too great & foolish Inclination to my Servant Charles

DOI: 10.4324/9781003333654-36

Cook'. Two years earlier, Claver had caught his servant George Champion kissing Molley Mitchell. At that time, Molley was twenty-three and George was twenty-nine, so they were old enough to make their own choices in matters of the heart. But Claver felt protective of Molley whom he had employed since she was sixteen. He need not have worried as the couple were soon married, and although Molley left his service during her first pregnancy, George remained 'my man'. Claver prescribed for Molley when she gave birth to a boy in March 1725, and she would have more children and a very long life with George.[1] But the case of Hannah Beal was quite a different matter.

The root of the problem was that, unlike George Champion, Claver did not fully trust Charles Cook. Despite Claver's warnings, Charles had bolted his chamber one day with Hannah Beal inside, and he had only unfastened the door when William Bragge's coachman had threatened to break it down. Moreover, when, after giving him four months' notice, Claver dismissed his servant with ten shillings, his distrust soon turned to anger as Charles swore and lied. Shortly after, Claver invited Hannah's father to come and dine and talk about the 'Foolish Match' that was being planned. He even employed Hannah's brother in place of Charles, in the hope that this might encourage Hannah to stay and change her mind. But Hannah and Charles were married at St Cuthbert's on 2nd February 1726, though she continued in Claver's service for a few more days until a new maid could be found. Despite his concern and disappointment at the match, Claver parted with Hannah on good terms, and he bought her two silver spoons as a wedding gift.[2]

There was no happy ending to another dispute that came to a head after Molly's death. Claver often prescribed for Mrs Elizabeth Paine before her death in 1726, and was on good terms with most of her family. But he could not tolerate her husband, John. For years, Claver had been in dispute with the old curate over rights of way and the hedging of the boundary between their fields at Dulcote. By 1725 his patience had run out. It seemed that Paine, a 'very disputatious' man, had no interest in reaching an agreement. Even worse, in Claver's view, was the fact that he talked nonsense, claiming 'many Things out of the usual way', such as 'there may be two [kind of] Nothings, & the like'. So, when Paine accused Claver of stealing his soil at Dulcote, Claver retorted by asking him why he would bother to go to church when it was 'certain he would go to the Devil'. After he had told the curate that 'if he Acted like the Devil I could discern no reason why he should not be with him: For he was a very great Rascal, & the most Worthless Fellow in England that had acquired an Estate', there was no chance of any agreement being reached.[3]

Another dispute that had lain dormant also erupted in the summer of 1725, and this one was much more serious. This arose over Claver's claim to have a right of entry from the Back Liberty into the Vicars' Close, through a door and passageway that he had built running between the Vicars' Chapel and the two houses that he leased at the top end of the Close. In 1709, Bishop Hooper had refused to recognise this right of access, but when Claver renewed the leases on his houses in September 1725 and assumed this meant his right to use the passageway had now been granted, he was soon told this was not the case. The vicars choral then asked if they could all have keys to use the passageway themselves, but Claver turned down their request and put a new lock on the door. So, under Hooper's direction, the vicars had no choice but to bar the door and to plead their case in court.

Claver's relationship with the vicars choral had been nurtured over a period of forty years. Aside from a shared love of music, several were among his dearest friends. They often accompanied him on trips to Bath and Kelston (at Claver's expense), took on extra work for him (like the copying of music), and enjoyed the extraordinary hospitality of his home. In return, Claver enjoyed the use of their medieval hall for meetings and concerts of the music club. So, it was no surprise that two of the vicars, James Nooth and James Nicholls, said that they were unwilling to join with their colleagues in a prosecution. Claver told them that they needed to join in, rather than 'incur the Bishop's Displeasure'. But he was not prepared to be lectured by Edward Johnson, one of the vicars' leaders, during a confrontation in the summer of 1726. Johnson watched as Claver's man, Will Clark, sawed off the post that had been erected to block the passageway, telling Claver 'in a very haughty manner' that on behalf of the vicars he would soon set up another one. So Claver responded, 'I would cut it down again, & so would do if they continued to set up a Hundred of them'.

Two weeks later, a warrant for the arrest of Claver and Will Clark for cutting down the vicars' post was delivered to Claver's home, and on 23rd June he was subpoenaed by the Court of Chancery. In their case against Claver's right of access to the Close, the vicars cited their founding statutes and the terms of former leases. But in his 'Answer', Claver challenged everything, including the vicars' interpretation of their statutes which Hooper had upheld in his argument with Claver in 1709.[4] The whole affair was unfortunate and grievous after so many years of friendship. But it was also serious for, whatever the outcome, Claver knew that his long-held permission to use of the Vicars' Hall for meetings of the music club would be withdrawn. He could not expect either the bishop or the dean and chapter, now under Archer's influence, to support his cause. So, in anticipation of the withdrawal of permission, on Tuesday 28th June he sent messages to all members of the club to meet that evening at the Mitre (where Charles Taylor was now the landlord) rather than at the Vicars' Hall.

Among the members at the Mitre were some of Claver's dearest friends: John Burland, Christopher Lucas, Richard Cupper, George Hamilton and Richard Comes. But four of the twelve choral vicars also came. By nine o'clock it was clear that the club could not continue as before, so Claver asked each person how they would like the balance of the club's money (about £10, which he had brought with him) to be spent. Most said that he should be the person to decide, but Claver declined the offer and put the issue to a vote. The result was that everyone agreed the money should be given to 'indigent persons'; five women and two men, living in the city. Among the beneficiaries was Grace Pierce, the old schoolmistress who lived in one of the houses that Claver leased in Vicars' Close, next to the vexatious passageway.

By midnight it was agreed, against the wishes of the vicars, that the club would now meet every Tuesday at the Mitre. Two weeks later, Claver invited the 'club-bers' (including the choral vicars) to his house for supper on a shoulder of mutton, a breast of veal, ox-tongues and a salad. He also served 'a Bowl of Punch, a Bottle of Claret, many Bottles of October Beer, & Ale', after which they played all twelve of Tibaldi's trio sonatas. They had another concert the next day at the Mitre, but everyone must have known that without the support of the choral vicars and the venue of their hall, the extraordinary club that Claver had nurtured for over thirty years, was coming to an end.[5]

Of course, there were other local entertainments to be enjoyed, but nothing quite as much. The various fairs in the marketplace and at Binegar and Priddy on the Mendips often attracted Claver and his friends, and there were always itinerant fiddlers and jugglers performing on the city's streets, and cudgel matches at the Crown. At the Crown there were also performances by travelling theatre groups, such as Power's company from Bristol which put on Congreve's *Love for Love* (1695) to which Claver took Betty and a group of friends in the summer of 1726. He had seen the play before with George Hamilton at the George in Wells, and he also went to see Rowe's *The Tragedy of Jane Shore* a second time. It was with George Hamilton that he went to watch Lewis's company perform Thomas Baker's comedy *Tunbridge-Walks: or the Yeoman of Kent* (1703) at the Crown, but he missed a staging of Thomas Southerne's tragedy *Oroonoko* (1695), giving his ticket to the hatter's wife, Mrs Browne.

Further afield, Claver had often taken trips to Bath both to prescribe for patients and for musical entertainments. But after the death of John Harrington in June 1725, he made no further music trips to Kelston, though he still visited to prescribe and play cards with the family until John's widow, Dorothy, died in the following year. On a three-day visit to Bath in November 1725, he found time to visit the Pump Room and to watch people 'losing their money' gambling at Harrison's Assembly Rooms, but he did not attend a concert. The purpose of this visit was to see two celebrated stonemasons: John Harvey about the design of a memorial for Molly; and Thomas Greenway about the decayed rails and balusters on his house in the Liberty which he wanted to replace with ten new fluted-urns, decorated with flames and foliage.[6] A month later, on Christmas Day, Betty and John Burland and their children, two choristers and a dozen other guests came to his house for dinner and concerts. But with no more music trips to Bath and Kelston, and no hope of an amicable agreement with the vicars choral, Claver's musical world was shrinking.

He still undertook lengthy trips to Sadborow and Sherborne, and occasionally travelled to prescribe for long-standing patients such as the Phelips of Montacute. Sometimes he would stay for several days, as in March 1726 when he was called to prescribe for Edward Phelips' son. On this occasion, Claver worked hard to persuade his co-physician, Dr Williams, that baby Edward should be given a laxative of calomel (mercurous chloride) mixed in a paste with rhubarb and chicory, rather than the drink of 'Milk-water & Lemon-water sweetened with Syrup of Vio[lets]' that Williams had proposed. So he was delighted when 'the Child of 11 months old cast out much Slime by Vomiting twice & Purging thrice', and was soon 'very sensibly amended'.[7] But Claver's enthusiasm for these long trips was on the wane, especially as he still had many other patients close to home.

Inevitably, he was now losing some of the patients that he had been treating for almost forty years. George Long of Downside had died in 1705. He and his wife Mary had been special friends ever since they had lent their coach for Grace's funeral in 1689. Claver was doctor to their children and their grandchildren, but although he made trips to prescribe for Mary, now in her eighties, he could not save her.[8] Set against such losses were calls to treat new patients, such as William Whitchurch and Roger Leversedge, members of two of the oldest and wealthiest families of Frome, where Claver had several patients. Unfortunately, although he rushed to treat Roger on Easter Sunday 1725, Roger's sickness coincided with Molly's final illness, so further advice had to be provided by correspondence.[9] There were new patients too in Wells. Among these were Mrs Elizabeth Palmer, the daughter and heiress of Sir Thomas Wroth, and her sisters-in-law, who all lodged in Wells while Elizabeth's husband, Thomas Palmer, MP for Bridgwater, was at Westminster. Thomas himself had been so 'long afflicted' by a 'calamitous illness' that in his will he called for his coffin to be enclosed in lead after a post mortem (conducted by Christopher Lucas) to find a cause or cure that would save others from this suffering. But his wife and family were also often in need of medical attention.[10]

Though Claver maintained his physician's practice, after Molly's death he spent much more time in his study and laboratory. As one of the trustees of Gabriel Odingsells' estate, he wrestled with responses to new Chancery disputes, the latest being launched by William and Edward Watson, two fishmongers in London.[11] As well as the vicars choral case, there was also a new complaint against him and Nathaniel Farewell, the executors of George Farewell's will.[12] There was also a new case in which he became involved in March 1726, when Mary Pitt arrived to ask if he would be willing to attest in court that her father-in-law, William Pitt (who had died recently at Kensington), was of unsound mind when he made his will. This might have seemed a relatively simple matter, but Claver took time to draft and re-write his report as it was a vexatious business, not least because it involved his friends the Goulds of Sharpham Park.[13]

In the laboratory, Claver made lead plates which he quicksilvered and tied with ribbons to restrict the growth of the ganglion that had developed on Will's hand. He made mithridate; a complex compound that included opium, for use as an antidote to poisons and the plague. Mixed with white wine and water, this was to be taken by Miss Anne Baron and probably several other members of her family.[14] Previously, he had rushed to the assistance of canon Thomas Lessey's wife 'to relieve her from the Ill Effect of the Opium' she had taken by mistake. This was probably one of her husband's medicines, for Claver regularly prescribed for Thomas before his death in March 1726.[15] And in the laboratory, Claver made a paste of macaroons, brandy and arsenic which he mixed with barley-meal to kill the garden rats. The rats soon ate the poison but, inexplicably to Claver, so did half a dozen of his hens.

In January 1726, he would not have been surprised to hear the news that William Bragge had been charged for failure to pay customs duty for the import of wine and brandy on his ships. Casks of wine and brandy had been smuggled up to Wells for years, and just before Christmas, Claver had quietly put another ten gallons of claret 'into the Hole in the Inner Cellar'. But the size of the customs fine, £12,000, was shocking, and could easily lead to the family's ruin; especially as William's extravagances were well known. So were his legal fees which, including the costs of defending him in court, had amounted to the colossal sum of over £450. Most recently, in October 1725, he had arrived for a fortnight's stay at Claver's house with no less than four servants and eight horses. Even on a two-day trip to Bristol accompanied by Betty and John Burland, with Claver and Lucas riding alongside, the young squire needed to take six servants. So, by the age of thirty-six and still a bachelor, he had already spent the family fortune, and when Claver arrived at Sadborow with George Mattocks to see what might be done, he discovered that, in addition to the fine, William had amassed 'vast Debts'.[16]

On the day of his arrival, he noted that the family's chaplain and three maids had been dismissed. William's younger sister, Mary, had confined herself to her chamber and had not seen her brother for two weeks. She did not know where he was and, for this, she blamed her cousin Pattey Drewe, who had also taken to her room. But if Claver and George had access to the family's papers it would not have taken long to work out what was wrong. In 1722, a survey had been conducted of the Bragge properties in Dorset, Somerset and Devon with a view to mortgaging more of the estates. By 1725, Sadborow and the manor of Thorncombe had been mortgaged to Mary, William's sister, and further debts accrued. By 1726, William was barely solvent: his debts amounting to £1,300 less than the total value of his assets, £23,850.[17]

During the summer, William's younger brother and sister lodged with Claver to discuss ways of reducing the family's debts, for William himself was now too sick to travel. On 2nd July he wrote his will, needing just sixty-five words to say that he left £50 to his sister Mary and everything else to his brother John, apart from three guineas each for three sets of bell-ringers who would toll the bell at Thorncombe for three hours before and after his interment.[18] Unfortunately, Claver was now too sick to visit Sadborow, having caught a 'Cold with a Rheumatick Fever, which was by little & little every day encreas'd on me'. It left him with a 'most violent Cough with a discharge at last of thick Pus, Fainty Night-Sweating, & quick decay of my Flesh'. He reckoned this was because he was 'under a Consumption and a growing Phthisis' (tuberculosis). For days he could only eat herb porridge for his dinner, and a dish of chocolate, milk and bread for supper.[19]

Betty came to look after him almost every day, and during his recovery, on 17th August 1726 she gave birth to a baby boy. Claver now had three grandchildren, Mary, John and William, to keep an eye on, and although William Bragge died in October and one of his companions, Gerard Martin, followed in December 1726,[20] there was good news about other friends. After the death of his first wife, Christopher Keen had failed in his pursuit of Mrs Burnald, a lady from Lymington in Dorset. But six months later, in September 1725, he had succeeded in marrying

Rose Aldworth, with a £1,400 marriage settlement, from Westminster.[21] At first, this simply meant that Claver won his wager (a bottle of wine at the Mitre) from John Burland and Christopher Lucas. But as soon as Keen returned to Wells, Claver invited him and his new wife to dinner.

Among Claver's other friends, Lucas's reputation and prosperity were growing, not least due to his friendship with such an eminent physician.[22] After Molly's death, Claver's long-term lodger Mary Evans had moved to her manor-house at Dulcote, but they visited each other and remained good friends.[23] He also visited George and Bridget Hamilton who asked him to be a godfather to their son in May 1726. This was an honour that he would normally have been delighted to accept, but this time he refused, knowing that his own health was declining.[24] In September 1726, another friend, Richard Cupper, became the mayor of Wells. He had survived the scandal of an alleged clandestine marriage and he had taken over his father's business as Claver's main apothecary. But he had also advanced his respectability and influence by buying-up places in the best pews of St Cuthbert's church, where the corporation and the city's leading families took their seats.[25]

Far less pleasing to Claver was Hooper's promotion of Edmund Archer to the archdeaconship of Wells in December 1726. The previous archdeacon, Henry Layng, had been one of Claver's patients and a favourite companion for games of backgammon. Being a son-in-law of the precentor Robert Creighton (now nearly ninety), Henry's death also signalled the demise of Creighton's influence over the dean and chapter. Apart from opposing Claver at every turn, Archer was behind the dismissal of several of Claver's friends from their employment by the cathedral's governing body. Being always highly protective of his friends, the removal of William Malet, James Nooth, Farewell Perry and William Hill from their various posts (ostensibly for neglect of duties) would have angered Claver as much as Archer's attitudes and obstructive behaviour towards himself. He might also have blamed Archer for what he saw as the bishop's inexplicable development of 'an Animosity to me, unless it was for my bestowing two Years Labour with Mr [John] Prowse to prevail with him to Marry his Daughter [Abigail Hooper]'; a very 'advantageous' match for the bishop's family.[26] But, by 1727, this hardly mattered.

Through hard work and determination, Claver had led a rewarding life, making the most of the talents and advantages with which he had been blessed. Not least of these was his extraordinary ability to put friendship as well as family at the centre of his life. He made friends so easily he was very rarely on his own. His home was such a hub of medical, musical and social activity as well as hospitality it was no wonder that, until Molly's death, he never dined or supped alone. Wherever he went, with or without an invitation, from the city's inns to the manors of the gentry, his company was welcome.

In March 1727, he took his son to Oxford to settle him into his new surroundings as an undergraduate. There, on 14th March, at the age of seventeen Will was admitted into Balliol College. Considering the troubles that had beset his education at Sherborne, this was a moment when Claver must have swelled with pride. On Sunday 19th March, after riding a few miles on his homeward journey, he reached the village of Eynsham where he was taken ill and died.[27] It was a swift departure from such a full and energetic life, but Claver was prepared. He had completed his will after Molly's death and his own illness in May 1725, taking great care to ensure that his trustees, William Berkeley, Francis Newman, Gerard Martin and Christopher Lucas, knew how to apportion the estate between his son and daughter.

Betty was to have her step-mother Molly's seven-stone diamond ring and £60, plus all of Claver's lands in West Bradley, West Pennard and the former Baltonsborough Commons. She could pass these to her children, each of whom was given £20. Will was to inherit almost everything else; his father's estates at Pilton, Wedmore, Worle and Ashcombe, his properties in Dulcote, the leases on his two houses in Vicars' Close, and his house and garden in the Liberty, together with the brewhouse, coach-house and stables. Books and laboratory equipment were also left to Will, but all of the other contents of the house were to be shared with Betty. The Burlands were entitled to live in the house rent-free, at least until Will was twenty-one. Each trustee and household servant was to receive £5 (except Will Clark who was to be given £10) and Betty was to distribute another £5 in bread among the poor. Finally, Claver wrote a paragraph about his funeral.

He asked for this to be conducted with 'as little shew and trouble as possible' for 'an affectionate member' of the Church of England. He explained that as the day of one's death was better than the day of one's birth – a birth 'carrying us out into a Tempestuous Ocean', a death 'bringing us (if we have done well) from a Turbulent Voyage into a Haven of happiness' – it was his desire that there should be no sign of grief, even among his family and dearest friends. He only asked for one thing more: 'if it be possible, there might be a Consort of Musick of three Sonatas att least in the Room where my body is placed before it be carried off my house to be interred'.[28] In keeping with the spirit of this wish, when people arrived from far and wide for the funeral on Wednesday 29th March, to help keep grief at bay, for Dr Claver Morris, the musicians would have played all day.

EPILOGUE

A plain and simple floor-slab, inscribed with the words 'Claver Morris, M.D. 1726', was laid over the grave, next to Molly and baby Mary in the Lady Chapel. But it was not long before a tall white marble monument, consisting of a bust of Claver above a Latin epitaph and his coat of arms, was fixed to the wall nearby. It said that Claver 'shone brightly' when 'he restored his patients to health' and that 'he hid his light behind a cloud when his right hand gave to the poor, gifts of which his left hand knew nothing'. As well as Claver's charity, the inscription spoke of his mastery of music, chemistry, mathematics, 'anatomy and the study of herbs'. Above all, it extolled his skill 'in the divine art of medicine', in which, through hard work and experiment, he had 'developed remedies that he had invented for the treatment of grievous diseases'. It told the onlooker, 'If you knew him, passer-by, you knew one who was affable, agreeable and highly courteous'; someone who was 'cautious and wise', but vigorous in all his undertakings.[1] He had lived for sixty-seven years.

DOI: 10.4324/9781003333654-37

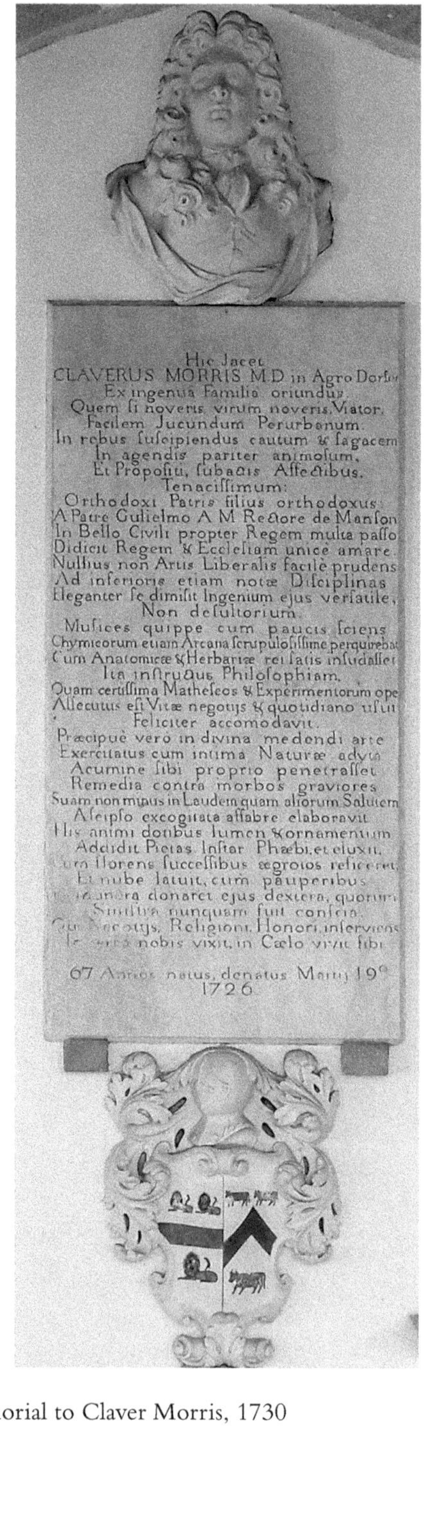

FIGURE 22 The Memorial to Claver Morris, 1730

After the funeral, Betty and John Burland and their children moved into Claver's home in the Liberty, just as he had wished, and a year later Betty gave birth to her second daughter, Margaret. She would have four more children, Claver, William, Robert and Anne; nine in all, over a period of twenty years. Not all lived to adulthood, but most did, including Mary, who married William Hudleston, vicar of St Cuthbert's; Sir John, who married William Berkeley's only daughter and heiress 'Miss Laetitia' and became a baron of the Court of Exchequer; and Claver, who married the daughter of a Gloucestershire squire and became a doctor.[2] In 1738, at the age of twenty-eight Claver's son, Will, died intestate. So, Betty inherited the whole of her father's estate and she continued living in the Liberty with her children and her husband until his death in 1746. After her own death in 1760 at the age of sixty-three, Sir John, her eldest son, inherited the house.[3]

Claver Morris' house (19, The Liberty) is now part of Wells Cathedral School, which has been educating the cathedral's choristers for about a thousand years. Each year, Claver would invite a few choristers to join in his Christmas concerts and sing carols to his guests. The idea that the house he built and suffused with music is now home to young musicians from around the world would have filled him with delight. So would the little gap in the wall across the road. In Claver's time, there was a door (to which he held the only key) in front of the narrow passageway he built between the Vicars' Chapel and the house he rented to Grace Pierce, at the top of Vicars' Close. But now, anyone can walk through the passage from the Liberty into the medieval street where the choral vicars live. At the bottom, the music club no longer meets in the Vicars' Hall but, overlooking the cathedral, the grand houses of the dean and chapter still line St Andrew Street, leading to what used to be the Mitre at the far side of the green.

When Claver was not relaxing or holding meetings at the Mitre (now the Ancient Gatehouse) he was usually reading the papers or drinking at the Crown. The old coaching inn still stands directly opposite the row of shops and houses that were part of Bishop Bekynton's 'New Works' five hundred years ago. The High Cross and Market Hall, where the city's corporation and assize courts used to meet above the traders' stalls, are gone. But most of the landmarks of the market and the city's ancient streets are still in place. So too is the bishop's palace and gardens, around which the moat is now patrolled by swans.

In the cathedral, when a wall between the Lady Chapel and the Choir was taken down, the memorial to Claver was moved from beside his grave to the east side of the grassy churchyard in the middle of the cloisters. Much to the annoyance of the dean and chapter, this was where, in Claver's day, people tried to smuggle in their horses, sheep and cattle for shelter and to graze. But no damage has been done. With so many grand memorials to observe in the cloisters and cathedral, and so much art and beauty all around, in the Lady Chapel a visitor might well pass by a plain floor-slab marked 'Claver Morris, M.D. 1726'. But if they were to pause, they might wonder about his life and world.

CREDITS & PERMISSIONS

I am very grateful to various individuals and organisations for the following images and permissions:

Map of Wells, 1735, from *A Plan of the City of Wells,* drawn by William Symes and engraved by William Toms (1735). Photograph by David Walker, by kind permission of the Wells & Mendip Museum.

Map of Somerset, *c.*1749, engraved by Thomas Kitchen, first published in 1749 and re-issued in *Historical Descriptions of New and Elegant Picturesque Views of the Antiquities of England and Wales* by Henry Boswell (1786). By kind permission of Liam Quin at *fromoldbooks.org*

1. **Marriage to Grace Green,** from Accounts, 1685. Photograph by Craig Stevens.
2. **The Market Place, Wells,** drawn by W. Alexander and S. Prout, and engraved by James Redaway, from *Picturesque Antiquities of English Cities,* by John Britton (1830).
3. **St Cuthbert Street and Church, Wells,** engraved by John Greig from a drawing by Henry Gastineau, from *The Antiquarian Itinerary* by James Storer (1816-18).
4. **The Bishop's Palace, *c.*1733,** drawn and engraved by Samuel & Nathaniel Buck (1733). British Library 004955138. https://www.flickr.com/photos/britishlibrary/50264251428
5. **The West Front of the Cathedral, *c.*1730,** drawn by T. Fourd and engraved by P. Toms, published by J. Smith in London. By permission of the Somerset Archaeological and Natural History Society: SHC, *A/DAS/1/420/28 (item 59).*

6. **Rebels in Wells, 1685,** from the 'Monmouth Rebellion'. Photograph by kind permission of the collection of the Worshipful Company of Makers of Playing Cards.
7. **A Map of Bath, *c*.1706,** from *The History and Antiquities of the County of Somerset* by John Collinson (Bath, 1791). Photograph by Craig Stevens.
8. **A View of Glastonbury,** drawn by Thomas Shew, from *An History of the Abbey of Glaston* by Richard Warner (Bath, 1826). Photograph by Craig Stevens.
9. **Claver Morris's new house, *c*.1700.** Photograph by kind permission of Wells Cathedral School.
10. **Detail from a map of Wells, 1735,** from *A Plan* by William Symes. Photograph by kind permission of the Wells & Mendip Museum.
11. **The astronomical clock,** engraved by James Basire, from *The History and Antiquities of Somersetshire* by William Phelps (1839). Photograph by Craig Stevens.
12. **The start of Claver Morris's diary, 1709.** Photograph by Craig Stevens.
13. **The Vicars' Close,** engraved by George Hollis, from *The History and Antiquities of Somersetshire* by William Phelps (1839). Photograph by Craig Stevens.
14. **The Vicars' Hall.** Photograph by kind permission of the Chapter of Wells Cathedral.
15. **The road from Bath to Kelston,** drawn and engraved by Thomas Bonner, from *The History and Antiquities of the County of Somerset* by John Collinson (Bath, 1791). Photograph by Craig Stevens.
16. **The Chain Gate and entrance to Vicars' Close,** engraved by John Le Keux, from *The History and Antiquities of the Cathedral Church of Wells* by John Britton (1824). Photograph by Craig Stevens.
17. **The Vicars' Chapel,** drawn by William Bartlett and engraved by John Le Keux, from *Picturesque Antiquities of English Cities* by John Britton (1830).
18. **Molly and Betty measured, 1710,** from Expensa. Photograph by Craig Stevens.
19. **The road from Wells to Glastonbury,** detail from John Ogilby's *The Road from Bristol to Weymouth* (1675).
20. **The George or Pilgrim's Inn, Glastonbury,** engraved by George Hollis, from *An History of the Abbey of Glaston* by Richard Warner (Bath, 1826). Photograph by Craig Stevens.
21. **Claver's diary, 5 April 1725.** Photograph by Craig Stevens.
22. **The Memorial to Claver Morris, 1730.** Photograph by David Bevan, by kind permission of the Chapter of Wells Cathedral.
23. **The Claver Morris Manuscript Books.** Photograph by Craig Stevens.

NOTES

All dates are in the 'Old Style' (Julian calendar), except that 1 January is taken as the beginning of the year.

Unless stated otherwise, references to wills in the Notes are cited with their date of signature, rather than their date of probate (as in the Sources), and are from The National Archives.

Throughout the book, words cited from Claver Morris's diary and accounts are given in their original form. The spelling, punctuation and capitalisation of other sources have also been retained, though occasionally some minor changes to typographical conventions (e.g., in the use of italics) have been made.

In the Notes and Sources, place of publication is London, unless stated otherwise.

In the currency of the age, one pound consisted of twenty shillings. There were twelve pennies in a shilling, and four farthings in a penny. The value of a guinea (a gold coin) fluctuated with the price of gold. In 1714, at the beginning of George I's reign, a guinea was worth twenty-one shillings and sixpence, but in 1717 its value was fixed at twenty-one shillings.

Abbreviations

Accounts Claver Morris's book of accounts, 1685–1698.

BRO Bath Record Office.

BHO British History Online.

Canonical Houses Bailey, *The Canonical Houses of Wells* (1982).

Cathedral Monuments *Wells Cathedral: its monumental inscriptions and heraldry,* ed. Jewers (1892).

Cathedral Registers Wells Cathedral Registers of Baptisms, Marriages and Burials, 1660–1982.

CCEd *Clergy of the Church of England Database,* online.

Chapter Book 1666–1683 *Wells Cathedral Chapter Act Book 1666–1683,* ed. Bailey (1973).
Commons Journals *Journals of the House of Commons.*
Collinson *The History and Antiquities of Somerset,* 3 vols, ed. Collinson (1791).
ChAB Chapter Act Book.
CAB Corporation Act Book.
Dean & Chapter *Calendar of the Manuscripts of the Dean and Chapter of Wells (1907–1914).*
DHC Dorset History Centre.
Diary Claver Morris's manuscript diaries for 1709–1710 & 1718–1726.
DNB *Dictionary of National Biography.*
Evelyn *Diary of John Evelyn,* ed. de Beer (1955).
Expensa Claver Morris's books recording his expenses, 1709–1723.
Hardres Accounts Thoresby Hardres's book of accounts, 1674–1685.
Hist. Parl. *The History of Parliament: the House of Commons* (1970–1983).
Life of Ken Plumptre, *The Life of Thomas Ken,* 2 vols (1888–1889).
Kidder *The Life of Richard Kidder. Written by Himself,* ed. Robinson (1924).
Lords Journals *Journals of the House of Lords.*
Luttrell *A Brief Historical Relation of State Affairs,* by Luttrell (1857).
Pharma *Pharmacopoeia Londinensis,* by Salmon (1682).
PR Parish Records.
Recepta Claver Morris's books recording his income, 1709–1723.
SDNQ *Notes & Queries for Somerset and Dorset.*
SHC Somerset Heritage Centre.
TNA The National Archives.
WCA Wells City Archives.
WCL Wells Cathedral Library.
Wells Manor Bailey, *Wells Manor of Canon Grange* (1985).
Wills *Abstracts of Somerset Wills,* ed. Crisp, 6 vols (1887–1890).

Part One, 1659–1697

1. Grace

1. Accounts, October 1685; Lysons, *Environs of London,* II, pp. 45–184; Bryan, *Chelsea,* pp. 4–20; Davies, *Chelsea Old Church,* pp. 190–3; Croot, *A History of the County of Middlesex,* XII, pp. 238–50; Faulkner, *An Historical and Topographical Description of Chelsea,* II, p. 52.
2. Hardres Accounts; Will of Mary Greene, 18 May 1674: *PROB 11/345/95.* Mary Greene probably had relatives of her husband living in the city, though she chose not to name them as executors or trustees. Among the Green(e) families, a John and Grace Greene and their daughter Elizabeth were living in the parish of St Magnus the Martyr, at the head of London Bridge, in 1695: *London Inhabitants,* ed. Glass, p. 127.

3. Hardres Accounts, 1674–1675; Lease of house, 25 February 1675: SHC, *DD/WM/1/52;* Will of John Dennett, probate 1695: *PROB 11/20/726.*
4. Wills of Thoresby Hardres and his father, Thoresby Hardres, 5 June 1691 & 7 March 1685: *PROB 11/405/124* & *PROB 11/386/54.*
5. Abbott, *Life Cycles,* pp. 66–71 & 80–92; Lasocki & Neate, 'Life and Works of Robert Woodcock', pp. 94–5; *London Gazette,* 2316, 30 January 1687.
6. *A Collection of the Yearly Bills of Mortality,* 1685, unpaged; Waller, 'Disease and death', pp. 1–8.
7. Bloom, *Medical Practitioners,* p. 70.
8. *Allegations for Marriage Licences,* ed. Armytage, 19 September 1685, p. 177.
9. *DNB,* 'Adam Littleton'; 'Hearth Tax: Middlesex 1666, Chelsea', in *London Hearth Tax* for 'Adam Littleton' & 'Mr Greene'.
10. *A Sermon at the Funeral*, by Littleton, pp. 24–5; Smith, 'Mary Astell', pp. 44–5.

2. Claver

1. Cressy, *Birth, Marriage and Death,* pp. 97–123.
2. *Acts and Ordinances,* ed. Firth, p. 420.
3. DHC, Lydlinch PR: *PE/LYD; Registers of Lydlinch,* ed. Mayo.
4. In 1686, John Claver was still referring to himself as 'the natural and lawful grandson of William Claver alias Bayly late of Lidlinch': DHC, *MIC/R/258/DA/30.*
5. *Minute Books,* ed. Mayo, pp. 41 & 554.
6. Hutchins, *History of Dorset*, IV, pp. 136–41 & 188–94.
7. *The Desires and Resolutions of the Club-Men,* pp. 1–2.
8. Bayley, *Great Civil War in Dorset,* pp. 259–92.
9. *Minute Books,* ed. Mayo, p. 204*; Dorset Hearth Tax,* ed. Meekings, p. 57.
10. Hutchins, *History of Dorset*, IV, pp. 139–40; Bayley, *Great Civil War in Dorset,* pp. 439–40.
11. Hannah Claver was baptised at Lydlinch on 31 October 1632. All of her children were baptised at Bishop's Caundle: Ruth on 13 October 1651, Hannah on 9 January 1655, William on 7 April 1657, and Claver on 1 May 1659. Lydlinch & Bishop's Caundle PR: DHC, *PE/BCD* & *PE/LYD.*
12. The hearth-tax returns for 1662–1664 list the tax-paying households (and hearths) in each parish: Lydlinch 43 (99), Bishop's Caundle 19 (34), and Manston 17 (52). *Dorset Hearth Tax,* ed. Meekings, pp. 47, 48 & 52.
13. *Survey of Dorsetshire*, ed. Coker, pp. 3–5.
14. An additional reason for moving might have been that the church at Bishop's Caundle was reckoned to stand 'in a very dirty, watery place': Gadd, 'The impact of the landscape', p. 90. Hutchins, *History of Dorset*, IV, pp. 73–7.
15. *Minute Books,* ed. Mayo, pp. 327, 335 & 374–5.
16. Articles of agreement with John Ryves, 29 August 1661: SHC, *DD/WM/1/111.* Squibb, *Dorset Incumbents,* 'Manston'.
17. Mortgage of house at Abbas Combe, 1672: SHC, *DD/WM/1/109.*

18. Accounts, 14 Oct. 1686; Ruth's lease of land at Felton, 2 November 1678: SHC, *DD/WM/1/105* & *114*.
19. Foster (ed.), *Alumni Oxoniensis,* 'William Morris'*;* Manston PR: DHC, *PE/MAN.*
20. Foster (ed.), *Alumni Oxoniensis,* 'Claver Morris'.
21. Ruth was married at Manston on 8 August 1681, and was buried there on 13 November 1683. Of Hannah's children, William was baptised at Manston on 24 July 1685, and his sister Ruth was buried there on 7 February 1689. Manston PR: DHC, *PE/MAN.* The marriage settlements are revealed in *Morris* v. *Shirley* (1687) & *Goddard* (1690): TNA, *C 7/223/36* & *C 8/418/99.*
22. Allen, 'Medical Education', pp. 115–43; Allen, 'Scientific Studies'; Frank, 'Medicine'; Delay, *Germ of an Idea,* pp. 1–15.
23. *Casebooks,* ed. Kassell; Curth, 'Medical Content of English Almanacs', p. 281.
24. Debus, 'Chemistry and the Universities', pp. 173–96; Sloan, *English Medicine,* pp. 70–90.
25. Porter, *Quacks,* pp. 11–30*;* Barry, 'John Houghton', pp. 575–603; Cook, 'Physicians and the New Philosophy' & 'Good Advice and Little Medicine'; Barry, 'Educating Physicians'; Armytage, 'Royal Society and the Apothecaries'; Burnby, *A Study of the English Apothecary;* Loudon, 'Nature of Provincial Medical Practice'; Fanu, 'Lost Half-Century in English Medicine'; Mortimer, 'Diocesan Licensing'; Wear, *Knowledge and Practice.*
26. Dominiguez-Rodriguez, 'Profiting Those that Cannot Understand Latine', pp. 131–52.
27. Haskins, *Ancient Trade Guilds,* pp. 364–8.
28. Subscription books, 1672–1695 & 1685–1730: SHC, *D/D/Bs/42* & *43.* Diocesan Court records, 1671: SHC, *D/D/ca/350.*
29. Will of James Claver, 24 February 1709: *PROB 11/509/309.* James, the son of William Claver (Claver Morris's uncle), was baptised at Bishop's Caundle on 5 April 1655. *Registers of Caundle Bishop,* ed. Mayo.
30. Accounts, 2 November 1686.

3. The Cathedral City

1. Defoe, *A Tour,* I, pp. 266–85*;* Atthill, *Mendip: a New Study*; Croot, *World of the Small Farmer.*
2. Cupper's first wife, Frances, daughter of Francis Sadlier, died in April 1676 and was buried at St Cuthbert's: 'Monumental Inscriptions', ed. Medlycott, p. 50; His second marriage was to Eleanor Carleile on 4 April 1681: Cathedral Registers, p. 66. His shop in the Market Place was leased from the dean and chapter: *Wells Manor,* p. 83.
3. *Wells Manor*, pp. 211–18.
4. *Chapter Book 1666–83,* pp. xxix–xxx.
5. *Illustrated Journeys of Celia Fiennes,* ed. Morris, p. 195**;** Scrase, 'Wells Inns', p. 378. Bristol, the nation's second largest city with a population of about 25,000 had 1,019 beds and 1,377 stables. Bath had 324 beds and 451 stables. Scrase, *Somerset Towns,* pp. 116–22.

6. Wells Receivers' Accounts, September 1685: SHC, *DD/SAS/795/SE/28.*
7. Martha Dowling, Jane Tincklinge, Mary Bartlett, Mary Harler and Jane Bowden. Sessions Book for Wells, 19 January 1677/8: SHC, *DD/SAS/795/SE/29.*
8. Sessions Book for Wells, 1677: SHC, *DD/SAS/795/SE/29.*
9. Sessions Book for Wells, 1 October 1705: SHC, *DD/SAS/795/SE/29.*
10. Dunning, 'The Bishop's Palace' in *Wells Cathedral,* ed. Colchester, pp. 227–47.
11. Casebook of Peter Davis, 1723–1724: SHC, *DD/S/HP/1,* ff. 88–94.
12. Meek, *Wells Liberty and Bishop's Palace,* pp. 6–7; *Wells Manor,* pp. xx–xxiii.
13. WCL, ChAB 1683–1704, 3 October 1685.
14. Dearmer, *Cathedral Church,* pp. 20–44; Malone, *Façade as Spectacle.*

4. The Physician

1. *Wells Manor,* pp. 219–22; Sellers, 'Chantry College', pp. 5–17.
2. See the wills of three William Evans', 20 June 1632, 20 November 1683 & 6 July 1705: *PROB 11/162/104, PROB 11/374/408* & *PROB 11/540/280.* Godney manor deeds: SHC, *DD/BR/mmd/11–12,* & *DD/SAS/C/795/SE/2. Cathedral Monuments,* pp. 3–4. Cathedral Registers, p. 147. *Quarter Session Records,* ed. Harbin, I, pp. 182 & 185–6.
3. *Somerset Protestation Returns*, ed. Howard, pp. 126–33; Scrase, 'Inhabitants of Wells', pp. 17–18; Nott, *Under God's Visitation*, pp. 26 & 64.
4. Westover's diary (1685–1700) and documents: SHC, *DD/X/HKN/1-2*; Hervey, *Wedmore Chronicle,* II, pp. 48–106; Hall, 'Casebook' & 'Pills, Potions'; Neale, 'A Seventeenth-century Doctor'.
5. Accounts, 5 May 1686; Newton, 'Children's Physic', pp. 456–74; Osborn, 'Role of Domestic Knowledge', pp. 249–50.
6. Accounts, 10 June 1686; *Canonical Houses,* pp. 179–80; Winn, *Pouletts,* pp. 63–4; WCA, Serel's book, p. 15.
7. Thomas Piers, son of the archdeacon William Piers and Mary Coward, was baptised on 13 September 1663 and buried on 23 June 1686. Having lost a seven-month-old son in November 1685, and knowing that he was sick and that his wife Mary was pregnant again, he made his will on 3 April 1686: *Wills,* IV, p. 81. He left £100 in trust for his unborn son: SHC, *DD/PINC/9/5.* This son, Thomas, was baptised on 26 August 1686 and lived until 1753. Mary died in 1724 (aged 70). *Cathedral Monuments,* p. 236.
8. *Pharma.*, p. 160; *Pharmacopoeia,* by Culpeper, p. 257.
9. *Pharma.*, 'Of Beasts', pp. 197–221.
10. *Pharma.*, p. 282.
11. *Pharma.*, 'Of Antimony', pp. 319–48; Berrios, 'Madness from the Womb', pp. 223–35.
12. *Pharma.*, p. 42; Le Fanu, 'Lost Half-Century', p. 329.
13. *Pharma.*, p. 122.

5. The Monmouth Rebellion

1. Evelyn, 23 December 1683–1685, February 1684; Andrews, *Famous Frosts,* pp. 17–40.
2. Bush, *Somerset Stories,* p. 75.
3. *Daffy's Original,* by Daffy*;* Ashton, *Social Life,* pp. 5–6; Homan, 'Daffy'; Osborn, 'Role of Domestic Knowledge', pp. 362–4.
4. *Wells Manor,* pp. 65–7; *Canonical Houses,* p. 67; Wills of Thomas & William Westley, 1661 & 1719: *PROB 11/309/275* & *PROB 11/570/323; Chapter Book 1666–1683,* pp. xxii & 55; Nott, *Under God's Visitation,* pp. 30–1 & 96; St Cuthbert PR; *Cathedral Monuments,* pp. 19 & 25–7.
5. *Evelyn,* 15 July 1685; Toulmin, *History of Taunton,* pp. 130–74.
6. WCL, ChAB 1683–1704, 18 June 1685.
7. *Evelyn,* 8 July 1685.
8. *London Gazette,* 2048, 6 July 1685; WCL, ChAB 1683–1704, 1 July & 7 October 1685*; Dean & Chapter,* II, p. 458; Imray, *Wells Old Almshouse,* pp. 68–9.
9. *London Gazette,* 2049, 8 July 1685; Wigfield, *Monmouth Rebellion;* Chandler, *Sedgemoor 1685,* pp. 65–6; Baines, *Monmouth Rebellion,* pp. 5–7; Timmons, 'Executions', pp. 286–91; St Cuthbert PR.
10. Chandler, *Sedgemoor 1685,* pp. 85–6.
11. Evans, *A Chronological Outline,* pp. 235–9; Baines, *Monmouth Rebellion,* pp. 6–8; Muddiman (ed.), *Bloody Assizes,* p. 34; Quarter Session order book, '1685': SHC, *Q/SO/7/456.*
12. Bird was later reprieved after paying for a pardon. Wigfield, *Monmouth Rebels,* p. 173; Baines, *Monmouth Rebellion,* pp. 9–24; Johnson, 'Wells and the Monmouth Rebellion'.
13. Wigfield, *Monmouth Rebellion,* pp. 116–17. George Bisse was buried at Martock in January 1702: Grigson, *Genealogical,* p. 46.
14. Wigfield, *Monmouth Rebels,* pp. viii-ix.
15. *London Gazette,* 2120, 11 March 1686*;* Baines, *Monmouth Rebellion,* pp. 12–13; Wigfield, *Monmouth Rebels,* pp. 29, 32 & 124; Zook, 'Bloody Assizes'.
16. *Report on the Manuscripts,* ed. Bennett, p. 264; *Dean & Chapter,* II, p. 460.
17. See Edward Hobbs, sheriff of Somerset's instructions to the constables of Bath: Collinson, I, p. xlvii; Bush, *Somerset Stories,* pp. 136–41.
18. Wigfield, *Monmouth Rebellion,* p. 88.
19. Bishop's Caundle, Overseers of the poor: DHC, *PE/BCD/OV1/1.*

6. Mother & Child

1. *Canonical Houses,* p. 78; *Chapter Book 1666–1683,* p. xiii.
2. *Chapter Book 1666–1683,* p. xviii; *Canonical Houses,* pp. 162–3; *Wills,* IV, p. 47.
3. As communar he was responsible for managing the chapter's finances, and as master of the fabric he was clerk of the works for the cathedral: *Chapter Book*

1666–1683, pp. iv, viii & xxxvi; *Canonical Houses,* pp. 114 & 152–3; *Cathedral Monuments,* pp. 4–5; Will of Richard Healey, 3 April 1706: *PROB 11/535/318.*

4. Katherine – daughter of William Coward (Recorder of Wells) and husband of William Piers (grandson of the late bishop Piers) – was eighteen when she gave birth to William on 20 May 1686. *Cathedral Monuments,* p. 236; *Chapter Book 1666–1683,* pp. xi–xii; *Canonical Houses,* pp. 126–7.
5. Francis died on 26 January 1688 and was buried five days later: Accounts, 22 & 31 January 1688; Cathedral Registers, 31 January 1688.
6. *DNB,* 'Robert Creighton'; *Chapter Book 1666–1683,* pp. ix–x; Cassan, *Lives of the Bishops,* II, pp. 70–3; Wicks, 'Creighton Family', pp. 335–6.
7. *Cathedral Monuments,* pp. 112–14 & 205–8; *Chapter Book 1666–1683,* pp. xv–xvii; *Wills,* I, p. 76.
8. Robert was baptised on 17 April 1673, Katherine on 15 March 1675, Margaret on 23 February 1677, Frances on 9 July 1679, Frideswide on 12 March 1681: Cathedral Registers, pp. 2–5.
9. Spring, 'Reverend Robert Creighton's Seven Pieces', pp. 32–48; Creighton pieces: WCL, *VC/Music MS.9.*
10. Accounts, March 1689.

7. Visits to New Patients

1. *Evelyn,* 7 January 1689; Accounts, flyleaf dated '26 May 1688'. Claver probably used John Ogilby's road maps to guide his journeys. A decade later, he bought a new set of these maps for £2: Expensa, 3 November 1698.
2. Davies was found guilty and hanged at Salisbury Court, off Fleet Street: *Proceedings of the Old Bailey,* Ordinary's Account, 21 December 1689.
3. *Humble Petition of the Widdows,* anon.
4. Macaulay, *History of England,* II, p. 577.
5. *London Gazette,* 2434 & 2435, 11 & 14 March 1689.
6. *London Gazette,* 2438, 25 March 1689.
7. *London Gazette,* 2433, 7 March 1689.
8. *Obedience Due to the Present King,* by Fullwood, p. 8.
9. *London Gazette,* 2432, 4 March 1689. *Evelyn,* 11 June 1699.
10. Capp, *When Gossips Meet,* pp. 178–81.
11. *London Gazette,* 2433, 7 March 1689.
12. See Ned Ward's characterisation of the Royal College of Physicians, in *London Spy,* ed. Hyland, pp. 99–102.
13. *A True Relation of Two Prodigious Births,* anon., p. 1; *Devonshire Wills,* by Worthy, p. 452. Several of Sir William's relatives were slave owners in Barbados.
14. *A True Relation of A Monstrous Female Child,* anon., p. 1; *Persecution Expos'd,* by Whiting, pp. 32–3; Bondeson, 'Isle Brewers Conjoined Twins', pp. 106–9.
15. *Parish Registers of Street,* ed. Jewers, pp. 66–70; *Wills,* III, p. 109. In March 1703, when Jerrard made his will a few days before his death, he believed that he was dying of a distemper.
16. *Cathedral Monuments,* p. 285; *Wills,* III, p. 122.

17. See the wills of Henry Bull (19 July 1687) and his son (11 August 1694): *PROB 11/410/135* & *PROB 11/428/402*; *Cathedral Monuments,* pp. 46–52; Collinson, III, pp. 426–8; BHO, *History of Somerset,* 8, pp. 160–79; 'Henry Bull', *Hist. Parl., 1660–1690.*
18. Nott, *Under God's Visitation,* pp. 204–5; *Canonical Houses,* p. 57.
19. *Wills,* III, pp. 14–6, & IV, pp. 16–17.
20. *Calendar of Wills,* ed. Fry; Powell, *Ancient Borough of Bridgwater,* p. 288.
21. The will of George's grandson, William Long, 26 January 1736: *PROB 11/699/77; Wills,* II, p. 37; Nott, *Under God's Visitation,* pp. 138–9.
22. *Marriage Allegation Bonds,* ed. Jewers, p. 4; *Wills,* III, p. 103; Leong, *Recipes and Everyday Knowledge,* p. 28.
23. Luttrell, I, p. 612; *Wills,* II, pp. 106–7; Collinson, II, pp. 234–5; 'Thomas Wyndham', *Hist. Parl., 1660–1690*; Green, *March of William of Orange,* p. 35; Fuller-Eliot-Drake, *Family and Heirs of Sir Francis Drake,* II, pp. 62–8; Wyndham, *A Family History,* 'Genealogy I'.
24. Collinson, I, pp. 215–18; *Wills,* VI, pp. 101–2; BHO, *History of Somerset,* 7, pp. 18–42; 'Edward Berkeley', *Hist. Parl., 1660–1690.*

8. Dr Morris

1. *Registers of Bruton,* ed. Hayward, p. 140; 'Maurice Berkeley', *Hist. Parl., 1690–1715.*
2. Cathedral Registers, p. 149: SHC, *DD/WCL/69; Cathedral Monuments,* pp. 124–7; *Wills,* II, pp. 17–18.
3. The monument survives at Manston. Hutchins, *History of Dorset,* IV, pp. 75–6; *Inventory of the Historical Monuments [...] Dorset,* III, p. 144.
4. *Morris* v. *Shirley* (1687): TNA, *C 7/223/36.*
5. *Morris* v. *Goddard* (1690): TNA, *C 8/418/99.* Claver received legal costs of 30 shillings from Goddard in June 1693, and £10 of interest on 'ye 60L he owes me' in January 1697. It appears that Edward Goddard re-married in 1698 and remained on good terms with John Pope. Bishop's transcripts of Stalbridge PR, and Pope's will (1695): Wiltshire and Swindon Heritage Centre, *P5/1696/30.*
6. 'Edward Wyndham', *Hist. Parl. 1660–1690.*
7. 'Hopton Wyndham', *Parl. Hist. 1690–1715*; *DNB,* 'Thomas Thynne, 1st Viscount Weymouth'.
8. Stevenson, *Two Centuries of Life in Down,* pp. 100–6. Eleanor was baptised on 14 February 1650: *Registers of Bruton,* I, ed. Hayward.
9. Accounts, 6 July 1691; Allen, 'Medical Education', p. 121. A certificate for the doctorate, dated 8 July 1692, is folded into Book 1 of the Claver Morris MSS.
10. Accounts, 17 July 1691.

9. Two Bishops

1. *Evelyn,* 7 May 1691.
2. *Life of Ken,* I, p. 226.

3. *Directions for Prayer,* by Ken, p. 5.
4. *A Short Account of the Life,* by Hawkins, pp. 8–9.
5. *Life of Ken,* II, pp. 56–9; *DNB,* 'Thomas Ken'.
6. *Dean & Chapter,* II, pp. 469–70.
7. *Kidder,* pp. 61–4; *Life of Ken,* II, p. 51.
8. Reynolds, *Wells Cathedral,* pp. 241–78; *Kidder,* p. 83.
9. Dearmer, *Cathedral Church,* pp. 134–41.
10. *Chapter Book 1666–1683,* pp. xxiii–xxx.
11. *Dean & Chapter,* II, pp. 458–9, 464 & 467; *A Short Account of the Life,* by Hawkins, p. 13.
12. *Kidder,* p. 64; Accounts, May 1692.
13. Medical Recipe MS book: SHC, *DD/WO/56/10/3; Ladies Cabinet,* by Ruthven, pp. 61 & 108; *Pharmacopoeia,* by Culpeper (1653 edn), pp. 10, 19, 31 & 163; Mortimer, *Time Traveller's Guide,* p. 311.

10. Wicked Practices

1. 'Articles of Visitation', in *Prose Works of Ken,* ed. Round, pp. 485–94; *Life of Ken,* I, pp. 248–50.
2. *Charge of Richard,* by Kidder, pp. 9, 19 & 23.
3. *Charge of Richard,* by Kidder, p. 29.
4. *Kidder,* p. 65.
5. *Kidder,* pp. 65–7.
6. Reynolds, *Wells Cathedral,* pp. clxx–clxxix; WCL, ChAB 1683–1704, 1 July & 27 August 1692, ff. 205 & 211; *Kidder,* pp. 67–72.
7. *Kidder,* pp. 67–8.
8. *Life of Ralph Bathurst,* Warton, p. 214.
9. *CCEd,* 'John Gardiner'; *Kidder,* pp. 72–3.

11. A Turning Point

1. Accounts, 1692–7; *Strode* v. *Dean of Wells* (1684): TNA, *C 6/74/61* & *C 8/721/51*; *Dean & Chapter,* II, pp. 453–4; Serel, 'On the Strodes', pp. 6–20.
2. Copy of Ned's pardon, 1686: SHC, *DD/X/LDD/1;* Quarter Session order book: SHC, *Q/SO/8/122a–186a*; Wills of Edward Strode and his daughter Elizabeth, 24 September 1697 & 24 March 1713: *PROB 11/475/10* & *PROB 11/547/309*; Green, *March of William of Orange,* pp. 33–8 & 45; Davis, *Shepton Mallet Story,* pp. 50–60.
3. *Evelyn,* 14 December 1692.
4. Luttrell, II, pp. 543, 564 & 567.
5. Bathing in and drinking the mineral waters appeared to cure a wide range of ailments: see Dr Robert Pierce's *Bath Memoirs. A Step to the Bath,* by Ward, pp. 16 & 163–4; Wroughton, *Stuart Bath,* pp. 200–8.
6. Accounts, 31 May & 23 December 1693; *Canonical Houses,* pp. 68–70; *Dean & Chapter,* II, p. 465; Venn, *Alumni Cantabrigienses,* I, p. 416.

7. *A Sermon Preached … Fifth of November, 1692,* by Kidder, p. 18; Luttrell, II, p. 610.
8. *A Sermon Preached … March 12, 1692[3],* by Kidder, p. 8.
9. *Kidder,* p. 82.
10. Miscellaneous notes (1693): SHC, *DD/SAS/795/SE/28*; Luttrell, II, p. 550.
11. Of Kidder's later children, Paul, Richard and Katherine were buried in May 1680, and John was born and buried in 1684. Ann was born in 1686 and her sister, Susanna, in 1680: *Registers of St Martin Outwich,* ed. Bannerman, pp. 4–6 & 104–5; *Allegations for Marriage Licences issued by the Bishop,* ed. Armytage, p. 334; *London Marriage Licences,* ed. Foster, p. 463.
12. *Registers of Marriages of St. Mary le Bone,* ed. Bannerman, p. 161; Ditcheat PR: SHC, *D/P/dit.2/1/1–3;* Newman, *Records of the Jeanes-Janes Family,* pp. 24 & 134–5; Will of Robert Jeanes, 20 September 1694: *PROB 11/423/236*; *Cathedral Monuments,* p. 185.

12. Secret Marriage & Courtship

1. Luttrell, III, p. 363.
2. *Kidder,* pp. 83–98 & 193–6.
3. The father, but not the son, is listed as an apothecary in *Eighteenth Century Medics,* ed. Wallis, p. 148.
4. Consistory Court depositions, '*Cupper* v. *Lovett*': SHC, *D/D/Cd/106,* ff. 10–53.
5. An 'Elizabeth' was baptised at Bruton on 25 March 1694, with an empty space probably left for later inclusion of the father's name. Illegitimate children were usually marked as 'base' after the mother's name. A Mary Lovett was married at Bruton two years later. *Registers of Bruton,* ed. Hayward, II, pp. 2 & 36.
6. *Somerset Incumbents,* ed. Weaver, p. 162; *CCEd,* 'Aylesbury'; Alsbury, *Undignified Exits,* pp. 21–5.
7. *Charge of Richard,* by Kidder, pp. 32–3.
8. Diocesan Court act book, 1692–7: SHC, *D/D/Ca/366.* Having moved from Sadler Street, Frances was living with her mother and sister in the High Street in 1699: SHC, *DD/FS/Box 72.*
9. Quarter Sessions order book, 'Christmas 1697': SHC, *Q/SO/8/364a, 365* & *564.* In 1696, A'Court had been with a group of men who had stood outside a young widow's house in Axbridge where one of them, Mr Hall, claimed 'yt he had fuckd ye said widow, Syms, and swore By God he had fuckd her many a time, and yt he would fuck her again yt night'. Syms won her case, as she had done against Hall at the Taunton assize a few months earlier, winning costs and damages of 40 shillings for defamation: Consistory Court depositions, '*Sims* v. *Hall*': SHC, *D/D/Cd/118,* ff. 34–5. It may be that A'Court went on to marry Frances Lovett, as a 'Richardus Courtis' is recorded as marrying Anna Lovell in 1705: *Wedmore Parish Registers,* ed, Sydenham, p. 55.
10. *Evelyn,* 29 December 1694–20 January 1695.
11. Luttrell, III, p. 423.
12. *Wills,* I, p. 76; *Cathedral Monuments,* pp. 112–3; *Canonical Houses,* p. 179.

13. Will of Edmund Dawe, 20 March 1695: *PROB 11/426/42.*
14. He was buried at Orchard Wyndham on 29 June 1695: St Decuman PR.
15. *Kidder,* pp. 134–44; Will of Richard Kidder, 25 February 1695: *PROB 11/474/498.*
16. *Canonical Houses,* pp. 24 & 33; *Kidder,* pp. 99–127, 203–10 & 213.
17. *Kidder,* p. 120.
18. St Cuthbert's PR, October 1695.

13. William Penn

1. Penn had preached in Bath in 1687, but it was not until after the Act of Toleration (1689) that a few Quaker meeting houses were established in Somerset: Wroughton, *Stuart Bath,* pp. 184–6. *Papers of William Penn,* ed. Dunn, III pp. 420–2; Dunning (ed.), *Christianity in Somerset,* pp. 50–55; Morland, 'Mid-Somerset Friends', pp. 249–76; Murphy, *William Penn,* pp. 228–9; Defoe, *A Tour,* I, pp. 266–70.
2. *Persecution Expos'd,* by Whiting, pp. 240–3.
3. Ashton, *Social Life,* pp. 351–3.
4. *Collection of the Works of William Penn,* I, pp. 142–3; WCA, CAB 1687–1709, ff. 58 & 67.
5. *Papers of William Penn,* ed. Dunn, III, p. 421.
6. *Persecution Expos'd,* by Whiting, p. 243.
7. A license to meet at the house of Nicholas Thomas in Wells was granted in January 1696: SHC, *D/D/ol/51. Persecution Expos'd,* by Whiting, pp. 243–4; *Somersetshire Quarterly Meetings,* ed. Morland, pp. 242–3. Hannah married another Quaker, John Banks, later in the year.
8. *Kidder,* pp. 143–4.
9. Consistory Court depositions, '*Taylor* v. *Hippesley*': SHC, *D/D/Cd/108,* ff. 2–7, & *D/D/Pd/6;* Morris, 'Defamation and Sexual Reputation', pp. 323–4.
10. *Kidder,* pp. 129–32 & 193–6.
11. Accounts, 4 October 1697; Recepta, 1699–1701.
12. Defoe, *A Tour,* I, p. 40.
13. Accounts, 24 November 1696 & 9 January 1697.

Part Two, 1697–1718

14. Baby Betty

1. Medical recipes: SHC, *DD/WO/56/10/3; Midwives Book,* by Sharp, pp. 33, 104–5 & 109.
2. Cressy, *Birth, Marriage and Death,* p. 47.
3. Accounts, 1697.
4. *Illustrated Journeys of Celia Fiennes,* ed. Morris, p. 195. Defoe, *A Tour,* I, pp. 272–6; Collinson, II, pp. 255–6.

5. Accounts, 1697; West Bradley manor: SHC, *DD/SAS/C/114/33* & *DD/TRANS/s/29.*
6. Yelling, *Common Field and Enclosure,* pp. 3–10; Williams, *Draining of the Somerset Levels,* pp. 95–110; Thirsk (ed.), *Agrarian History,* p. 361; SHC, *D/P/balt/23/28;* Diary, 14 November 1709.
7. Luttrell, IV, pp. 480 & 495; *Commons Journals,* XII, pp. 610 & 658; *Lords Journals,* XVI, pp. 414 & 430.
8. Accounts, 23 September 1697; Agreement, 26 October 1699: SHC, *DD/SAS/C/114/33; Morris* v. *Foxwell* (1699): TNA, *C 8/361/48.*
9. Accounts, 1697.
10. *London Gazette,* 3346, 2 December 1697.
11. *Midwives Book,* by Sharp, pp. 167, 353 & 367.

15. Bad Omens

1. Cressy, *Birth, Marriage and Death,* pp. 197–229; Abbott, *Life Cycles,* pp. 155–7; Astbury, 'Being Well'.
2. Accounts, December 1697; Expensa, 1699.
3. Expensa, 'In Books', 1699.
4. *The First Book,* by Palladio, p. 1.
5. Will of William Morris, 15 October 1690: DHC, *D238/F2;* Recepta, 9 January 1699.
6. *Evelyn,* 26 March, 25 June & 23 July 1699; Luttrell, IV, p. 544.
7. *Evelyn,* 3 September 1699; *Mr. Knight's Strange and Amazing Prophesy,* p. 8.
8. Holmes, *Making of a Great Power,* pp. 231 & 435–6.
9. Expensa, August 1699.
10. The pall-bearers were Richard Healy, William Westley, Philip Hodges, William Hughes, John Davis (the mayor) and Colonel Berkeley. Other friends included Claver's cousin, the attorney Andrew Shirley, a bachelor from Bristol who often sent ox tongues for Claver's table: Accounts 1697–1698; *Inhabitants of Bristol,* ed. Ralph, p. 4.
11. *Chapter Book 1666–1683,* p. 25; Crawford, *Vicars,* p. 71.
12. The monument to Elizabeth survives at Ditcheat. Expensa, 23 May 1704, 20 June & 17 July 1711; Floor slab to Harvey in Bath Abbey; Diary, 23 April 1719 & 4 November 1725; Bishop, 'Bath's Second Guildhall', p. 59.
13. *Canonical Houses,* pp. 24 & 78–9; *Kidder,* pp. 99–127; Expensa, October 1699.

16. A New Home

1. Expensa, 'In Building at Wells', 1698–1702.
2. Expensa, March 1701 & October 1702.
3. Recepta, March 1701; Expensa, 1702 & December 1703.
4. Claver thought that the new lease included 'the Ground I took in for enlarging my Garden': Expensa, 1 October 1702. The additional costs of improving the

stables, coach-house and garden amounted to £75: Expensa, December 1703. House lease, 1 October 1702: SHC, *DD/SAS/C/114/18/1; Canonical Houses,* pp. 74–5 & 178–83; *Dean & Chapter,* II, pp. 480–1;

5. Expensa, 1701–2.
6. Expensa, 6 May 1701.
7. Collinson, II, pp. 406–10; White (ed.), *Keynsham and Saltford,* pp. 1–5; Lowe, 'Demise of Keynsham's Great House', pp. 3–11.
8. Saracen's Head indentures, 1690–1706: Morgan Library and Museum, USA; Chamberlain Street taxes, 1703, 1706 & 1708: SHC, *DD/FS/72/2/15, 29–30 & 43;* Holmes, *History of the Parish,* pp. 151–2; *Wookey Manor,* ed. Hasler, pp. 105 & 122–3; Hasler & Luker, *Parish of Wookey,* p. 48.
9. *Kidder,* pp. 145–9. Later, Harry Bridges (cousin of the Duke of Chandos) was a dinner guest along with Claver at Kelston, though it appears that Harry and his son were only once at Claver's home: Diary, 28 April 1709.
10. SHC, Consistory Court depositions, '*Quirke* v. *Dunn*': SHC, *D/D/Cd/118,* ff. 87–8.
11. Will of Thomas Bridges, 9 May 1705, plus codicils: *PROB 11/494/173.* A few months before his death at the age of 81 in October 1728, Harry Bridges left everything he could to his illegitimate son, James, an attorney. He left his second wife, Elizabeth Freeman, daughter of a Bristol merchant, 'for her rude and unmannerly behaviour, her indecent & impudent language, her vile & notorious lewdnesse & viciousnes', one shilling. He explained that she 'hath lately been delivered of two daughters', though 'for several years past I have not been capable of carnal copulation with womankind': will of Bridges, 7 July 1728: *PROB 11/630/317.*
12. *Kidder,* pp. 149–52; *Bishop of Bath* v. *Bridges*, 12 Mod. 401, 88 *English Reports* 1408 (1700).
13. *Flying Post,* 799, 21 June 1700; *History of England,* by Oldmixon, p. 210; Luttrell, IV, pp. 658–9.
14. *Kidder,* pp. 152–9.
15. *Kidder,* pp. 159–79; Collinson, I, pp. 212–3.
16. Mayor's letter, January 1702: *Voices of Eighteenth-Century Bath,* ed. Fawcett, p. 165; Mayor's order, October 1700: SHC, *DD/SAS/C/151/2/5.*
17. *Evelyn,* September 1701.

17. Wedding Bells

1. Thoms, *Book of the Court,* p. 411; *London Gazette,* 3804, 27 April 1702.
2. Luttrell, V, pp. 201, 204 & 210; *History of the Reign,* by Boyer, I, pp. 75–9; *Voices of Eighteenth-Century Bath*, ed. Fawcett, pp. 17 & 175; Bucholz, 'Nothing but Ceremony', pp. 295–7.
3. Seyer, *Memoirs,* II, pp. 551–2; Latimer, *Annals of Bristol,* pp. 43–6.
4. *Kidder,* pp. 149 & 156.

5. West Bradley contract, 11 November 1702: SHC, *DD/SAS/C/114/33/3; Morris* v. *Hood* (1701): TNA, *C 8/595/69; Gregory* v. *Morris* (1703): TNA, *C 10/264/28;* Expensa, March 1703.
6. Miscellaneous notes, 14 September 1702: SHC, *DD/SAS/795/SE/28; Cathedral Monuments,* pp. 183 & 281; Heard, *Shepton Mallet,* pp. 26–33.
7. *Lexicon Technicum*, by Harris, I, Preface. Most of the subscribers in the Wells region were Claver's friends, including William Hughes, Richard Healy and Christopher Lucas.
8. Cook, *Decline of the Old Medical Regime,* pp. 233–53; Ellis, 'Background of the London Dispensary', pp. 197–212. A decade later, Claver gave a guinea 'toward procuring an Act of Parliament for suppressing Empiricks [Quacks]': Expensa, 13 March 1714.
9. *Craft and Frauds,* by Pitt, 'Preface' and pp. 72, 127 & 149.
10. William had married Edith Larder in 1689 with marriage portion of £3,000: BRO, *0028F/33.* Accounts, 19 February 1686; Squibb, 'Bragge Family', pp. 58–66; Prowse marriage settlement, 1701: DHC, *D-MHM/8836A;* Collinson, III, pp. 582–3.
11. Thomas Cook was married to Richard Healy's eldest daughter, Mary.
12. Expensa, Autumn 1703.

18. The Great Storm

1. Collinson, III, pp. 562–3; Indentures, 23 & 24 September 1703: SHC, *DD/SAS/C/114/35.* The Prowses had properties in Wells; survey of Wells Manor, 1684: SHC, *DD/CB/36.*
2. Expensa, 6 November 1703.
3. *Evelyn,* 26 & 27 November 1703.
4. *Chronicles of John Cannon,* ed. Money, I, p. 46.
5. Luttrell, V, pp. 364–5; Seyer, *Memoirs,* II, pp. 552–7; Defoe, *A Tour,* I, p. 270; *An Exact Relation of the Terrible Tempest,* p. 3.
6. *The Shortest-Way,* p. 18.
7. *London Gazette,* 3972, 6 December 1703; *Marriage Allegation Bonds,* ed. Jewers, p. 89. Claver (and the Cuppers) administered to the Conyers: Recepta, 6 November 1698.
8. *The Storm,* pp. 60–1; *Life of Ken,* II, pp. 129–30.
9. *An Exact Relation of the Late Terrible Tempest,* pp. 15–6.
10. *The Storm,* p. 270.
11. *Evelyn,* May 1704; Will of Ralph Bathurst, 25 August 1703: *PROB 11/476/427;* Parker, *Architectural Antiquities,* p. 83; *Life of Ken,* I, pp. 201–2.
12. Will of Archibald Harper, 5 May 1711: *PROB 11/539/29.* Claver prescribed for him a few days before his death on 11 May 1713: Expensa, 2 & 4 May 1713.
13. Will of Richard Kidder, 25 February 1695: *PROB 11/474/498.*
14. *Life of Ken,* II, pp. 119, 123 & 131–5; Marshall, *George Hooper,* pp. 97–103.

15. Cassan, *Lives of the Bishops,* II, p. 172; *History of My Own Time,* by Burnet, II, p. 282; *Dean & Chapter,* II, pp. 483–4.
16. Expensa, 1704–5.
17. *Wells Manor,* pp. 194–7; Expensa, 1704; Recepta, 1709.
18. Ebdon deeds, 1706–1837: SHC, *DD/BR/mt/2, Parts 1 & 2;* 'Ashe Wyndham', *Hist. Parl., 1690–1715*; Wyndham, *A Family History,* pp. 33–5; Recepta, 1709.
19. Recepta, 1703–5; Expensa, 1703–7, 24 December 1708.
20. Expensa, 5 February 1706.
21. Consistory Court depositions, '*Quirke* v. *Day*': SHC, *D/D/Cd/109; Wells Manor,* pp. 79, 98–99 & 136.
22. WCA, CAB 1687–1709, f. 155.

19. The Tolling Bell

1. Expensa, 'In Books', 1705–6. Most books came from John Miller of Sherborne, and 13 'Setts of Instrumental Music' were bought from Henry Hammond at Bath.
2. *A Treatise upon the Small-Pox,* by Blackmore, pp. 11–12 & 43; *A Treatise of the Small-Pox,* by Harvey, p. 159.
3. *A Treatise upon the Small-Pox,* by Blackmore, pp. 42 & 52–80.
4. Expensa, 'Expended', 1706; *Dean & Chapter,* II, p. 489. Gardner, *Wells Capitals,* pp. 11–12; Dearmer, *Cathedral Church,* pp. 128–34; Colchester, *Stained Glass.*
5. Howgrave-Graham, *Wells Clock.*
6. Wells Cathedral, *Misericords;* Gardner, *Wells Capitals.*
7. *Cathedral Monuments,* pp. 110–1; Expensa, 13 June 1711; *Dean & Chapter,* II, p. 497.
8. Will of Edward Berkeley, 20 January 1701: *PROB 11/495/307.* For Edward's estate, see Ashford and Webb, 'Edward Berkeley's Diary', and Webb, 'Edward Berkeley's Diary, 1684'.
9. *Cathedral Monuments,* p. 36; WCA, CAB 1687–1709, ff. 186 & 223.
10. Diary, 1 November 1725.
11. Abigail's uncle, Charles Guilford, who had died earlier in the year, left £1,000 to each of his two nieces, Abigail and Rebecca, and his properties in Lambeth to his elder sister and her husband. *Cathedral Monuments,* p. 217; *Dean & Chapter,* II, p. 489; Marshall, *George Hooper,* p. 184.
12. *Instructions,* by Fénelon, pp. 1 & 3.
13. Expensa, 'In Clothes for my Daughter & Schooling', 1708.
14. Expensa, 'Miscellaneous Expenses', 1707–1708.
15. *Mysteries,* by Venette, pp. 1, 98, 107, 141 & 291.

20. 'Drink If You Please'

1. Claver was an executor: will of Edmund Dawe, 3 September 1708: *PROB 11/543/251.*
2. Seyer, *Memoirs,* II, p. 558; Latimer, *Annals of Bristol,* pp. 78–9.

3. Diary, 17 May 1709; Expensa, 12 August 1708 & 1709–10. Molly or her sister Elizabeth may have been responsible for the recipes recorded in the Bragge 'Cookery Book' (over 100 pages, *c.*1690–1720) that was auctioned in London in 2019.
4. Diary, 29 December 1709.
5. Expensa, 3 May 1710; Diary, 11 February 1721; Lympsham deeds: SHC, *DD/DN/2/14/1–4.*
6. Diary, 30 & 31 December 1709, 7 January 1710; Expensa, 7 January 1710 & 1713–14.
7. Regular members included John Prowse and John Tuthill of Axbridge, Mr Hill of Banwell, Mr White of Shapwick, and Henry Mills the schoolmaster. Others included Mr Hunt of Chewton Mendip and Mr Uphill of Bristol, and the clergymen John Pope, Eldridge Aris, Edward Wotton, Henry Gapper and John Whitehand.
8. Accounts, 20 March 1695; Johnstone, 'Instruments', pp. 33–6.
9. Diary, 27 December 1709; Crawford, *Vicars,* pp. 15, 28–9, 53, 64 & 76.
10. Diary, 6 July 1709.
11. WCL, ChAB 1704–25, ff. 20, 24 & 99; Diary, 25 January 1710.
12. *Parish Register of Horsington,* ed. Daniel, p. 29; Diary, 28 April–20 July 1709; *Dean & Chapter,* II, p. 491.
13. Diary, July–October 1709; Newton, *Misery to Mirth,* pp. 193–230.
14. Claver often entertained the Harringtons on their trips to Wells, including John's daughter, Helena and her husband Lawson Huddleston, rector of Kelston.
15. Gent, *Trial of the Bideford Witches;* Barry, *Witchcraft and Demonology;* Pickering, *Hellish Knot.*
16. Diary, 6 September 1709; Granvill, *A Blow at Modern Saduccism,* pp. 95–125; Hunter, 'New Light', pp. 311–53. There had been reports of a woman possessed by the devil at Ditcheat in the sixteenth century: *A True and Most Dreadfull Discourse,* anon.
17. *Dean & Chapter,* II, pp. 475–80; Cathedral Registers, 17 March 1700, p. 8; Diary, 12 April 1725.

21. High Crimes & Misdemeanours

1. WCL, ChAB 1683–1704, f. 314 *et passim*; Cathedral Registers, 4 March 1709, p. 9; Expensa, 17 November 1709. Jane Nooth had several other children, though Mary died in 1713. James Nooth was witness to a dispute at the Crown in 1716 and would later become deputy-clerk and gamekeeper for the dean and chapter: SHC, *D/D/Cd/114/a*; WCL, ChAB 1704–25, f. 169 *et passim.*
2. Nooth's copy of the Statutes, 1703: SHC, *DD/SAS/C795/SE/11*; Parker, *Architectural Antiquities,* pp. 27–38; Reynolds, *Wells Cathedral,* pp. clxx–clxxix; Crawford, *Vicars,* pp. 14–29.

3. Diary, 4 & 11 June 1709, 11, 27 & 28 January and 16 February 1710; Expensa, 28 January 1710; Crawford, *Vicars,* pp. 124–6.
4. Diary, June 1709–February 1710; Henry's marriage, 3 February 1704: Cathedral Registers, p. 77; Barnes, 'Church and Education in Wells', pp. 765–6; Colchester (ed.), *Wells Cathedral School,* pp. 33–4; *Kidder,* pp. 197–201; *Dean & Chapter,* II, pp. 494–5; *Canonical Houses,* pp. 68–70 & 163. The letter of commendation, dated 11 June 1711, was published when Mills became embroiled in a controversy with the bishop of Bangor: *Post Boy,* 8 February 1717, p. 5.
5. Diary, 2 January & 1 February 1710; Expensa, 6 January, 1710.
6. Diary, 9 February 1710; *Canonical Houses,* pp. 33–4; 'Autobiography of the Rev. Elias Rebotier', ed. Fry, pp. 110–11; Marshall, *George Hooper,* 120–1.
7. Diary, 23 December 1709. Claver also had a disagreement with Prater over a right of way near Wells: Expensa, 17 & 21 July 1710.
8. Will of John Prowse, 31 March 1710: *PROB 11/515/92;* Marshall, *George Hooper,* p. 186; Expensa, 5 May 1710.
9. Collinson, III, p. 563; Expensa, August 1710 & October 1713.
10. *Perils of False Brethren,* pp. 7–8.
11. *Speech of Henry Sacheverell,* p. 3.
12. Diary, March 1710; Holmes, *Trial,* pp. 234–6; Holmes, 'Sacheverell Riots', p. 56.
13. Marshall, *George Hooper,* pp. 148–9.
14. Expensa, 26 April & July 1710, 4 July 1711; Watchet PR: SHC, *D/P/St.d;* Locke, *Seymour Family,* pp. 148–92.
15. The Wells MP, Edward Colston had been elected a member of the Woolcombers' Company and a burgess of the city in 1707. WCA, Serel's book, 22 April 1707: SHC, *DD/SAS/795/SE28*; Latimer, *Annals of Bristol,* pp. 85–6; 'Bristol' & 'Wells', *Hist. Parl., 1690–1715.*
16. Wyndham, *Family History,* pp. 36–45.

22. Among the Gentry

1. Expensa, 14 February 1712.
2. Holmes, *British Politics,* pp. 69–72, 79–80, 105–6, 140–2 & 178–81.
3. Diary, 2 November 1709; Expensa, 5 July 1711.
4. Diary, 3 July 1720, 3 June 1721, 2 May & 21 July 1722, 3 May 1726. Claver also knew Baptists at Croscombe, three miles from Wells. Armstrong, *Story of Croscombe.*
5. Accounts, 4 October 1686; *Life of Ken,* I, pp. 239–48; Nishikawa, 'English Attitudes', pp. 29–34, 43 & 86–105. Ken died in March 1711.
6. Mayo, *Huguenots in Bristol,* pp. 20–31.
7. Accounts, April 1689–February 1691; Recepta, 4 February 1707; *Protestant Exiles,* ed. Agnew, p. 44; *Cathedral Monuments,* pp. 122–3. Under the government's Tontine scheme, Gendrault invested £100 for his three-year-old son, Charles, in 1693; Diary, May–July 1709.

8. Expensa, November 1709–June 1714.
9. Diary, November–December 1709; Expensa, November 1709–June 1714; Locke, *Seymour Family,* pp. 203–51; 'Edward Seymour', *Hist. Parl., 1690–1715.*
10. Diary, August 1709–November 1710; Expensa, July–December 1714; *A Transcription of George Horner's Lease Book,* ed. Morris, pp. 5–7; Collinson, II, pp. 461–4; 'Thomas Horner', *Hist Parl., 1715–1754*; BHO, *History of Somerset,* 7, pp. 42–50.
11. Expensa, May 1710–May 1713; *Cathedral Monuments,* pp. 25–26; Will of William Westley, 11 March 1718 & 30 July 1719: *PROB 11/570/323.* In 1709, William left £125 to endow a charity for the widows and children of poor clergymen: SHC, *A/AMV/1.*
12. Expensa, 25 July 1711, 24 January 1713 & 9 December 1712.
13. Expensa, 7 February 1712, 3 September 1710 & 6 January 1713.
14. Expensa, 11 June 1712, 22 June 1713 & 21 August 1714.
15. Diary, 22 September 1709; Expensa, 13 September 1709 & 1 April 1711.
16. Expensa, 18 May 1709 & 14 January 1710–July 1711.
17. Expensa, 28 August 1712; 1 May, 4 & 13 December 1713; 2 April 1714. Claver also owned Westholme, at Pilton: Phelps, *History,* II, p. 241.
18. West Bradley PR & Overseer's Accounts: SHC, *D/P/brad.w.2/1/1* & *13/2/1;* Expensa, 21 March 1713 & 13 May 1714. The elder Henry Bull died in June 1711, leaving the farm to his widow, son and daughters.
19. Orders of penance for Grace Hurly, 6 October 1712; Martha Denmead, 7 August 1719; Hannah Strode, 15 May 1723; William Hawkins, 8 November 1724: SHC, *D/D/Ppr/3.*

23. Queen Anne's Peace

1. Expensa, 1 September 1712, 30 July & 20 October 1713.
2. Expensa, 2 May, 4 August, 24 October & 8 December 1712; 'Bath', www.freshford.com.
3. Will of William Bragge, 9 October 1712: *PROB 11/533/29;* Expensa, 23 March 1713.
4. Bowers, *Organs and Organists; Dean & Chapter,* II, p. 495; Expensa, 1713 & 29 April 1714.
5. Expensa, April–July 1713; *Pharma.,* pp. 198–9 & 226–7.
6. *London Gazette,* 5136, 7 July 1713; WCA, CAB 1709–21, f. 51; Johnstone, 'Claver Morris', p. 98; *A Sermon Preach'd,* by Hooper, p. 5; Expensa, 6–7 July 1713.
7. Hyland, 'Richard Steele', pp. 59–80.
8. Expensa, 14 August 1714 & 22 February 1715; Hatton, *George I,* pp. 170–80.
9. Seyer, *Memoirs,* II, pp. 561–71; Latimer, *Annals of Bristol,* pp. 106–8; Rogers, 'Riot and Popular Jacobitism', pp. 70–80.
10. Expensa, 2 November 1714, 23 March 1715 & 5 November 1716; *A Cat may look on a Queen,* by Dunton, p. 12.

11. Hippisley, *Some Notes on the Hippisley Family,* pp. 27–9.
12. Richard Mogg, marriage settlement: SHC, *DD/MGG/1/1/11*; Will of John Mogg, 20 May 1727: *PROB 11/ 800/257;* Johnson, *Brief History of the Manor House,* pp. 16–22. John, Dorothy and Richard Mogg were always patients, and they outlived Claver: memorial plaque, St John the Baptist church, Farrington.
13. After Ann's death in childbirth in 1707, Edward married her sister Elizabeth, in 1720. Rogers, *Montacute House,* pp. 8 & 20; 'Edward Phelips', *Hist. Parl., 1660–1690.*
14. Expensa, 11 October 1714; Wills of William Helyar and son, 1 February 1695, 18 September 1710 & 19 August 1723: *PROB 11/442/367* & SHC, *DD/WHL/25* & *26.* Dunning, *Somerset Families,* pp. 52–7.
15. Holmes, *Electorate and the National Will,* p. 11. The list of freeholders at the November meetings in Wells included many of Claver's friends, men like William Westley, Thomas Horner and Gerard Martin, as well as acquaintances such as Harry Bridges: SHC, *DD/WY/15/2/6.*
16. Expensa, 9 February & 12 August 1715; 'William Helyar', *Hist. Parl., 1660–1690*; 'Somerset', 'Wells' & 'Minehead', *Hist. Parl., 1715–1754.* On 1 February 1715, William Wyndham was also elected MP for Minehead, though the election was declared void in September.
17. *Flying Post,* 3658, 16 June 1715; Wilson, *Sense of the People,* pp. 101–13; Rogers, 'Riot and Popular Jacobitism', pp. 76–7.
18. Petrie, 'Jacobite Activities', pp. 85–106; *Political State,* by Boyer, p. 341; Wyndham, *A Family History,* pp. 46–62.

24. Family & Friends

1. 'Wells', *Hist. Parl., 1715–1754.*
2. Mary Evans' estates, 1717, & Power of Attorney, 1747: SHC, *Q/RRP/1/31* & *Q/SR/315/104–106; Registers of the Abbey Church,* II, ed. Jewers, p. 435; *Wells Manor,* p. 180; Bendall, *Dulcote History.*
3. Recepta, 19 December 1716; Expensa, 20 & 28 December 1716.
4. Expensa, 19 & 21 May, 19 August 1715; 5, 17 & 19 December 1716.
5. Expensa, 20 June 1715, 19 December 1716, 27 June & 14 November 1717; WCL, ChAB 1683–1704, ff. 301 & 306; *Cathedral Monuments,* pp. 10 & 281.
6. Expensa, 5 March & 16 April 1716.
7. Johnstone, 'Claver Morris', pp. 108–10.
8. Recepta, 16 July 1715–31 October 1718; Expensa, 8 July 1715–5 October 1717.
9. *Dean & Chapter,* II, p. 499; Marshall, *George Hooper,* pp. 153–7.
10. Margaret Muttlebury was married to John Evans of Wells in 1681: SHC, *DD/SAS/C795/PR/364.* Williams (ed.), *Post Reformation Catholicism,* p. 46; Hasler, *Parish of Wookey,* pp. 68 & 122–3; Land Tax & Presentment for High Street, 1709 & 1712: SHC, *DD/SAS/PR.162* & *DD/GS/4/145;* Haydon, *Anti-Catholicism,* pp. 76–116. There were many more Catholics in Wells in

the early 1680s: SHC, *Q/SO/7/220a & 259.* Higgins (ed.), *Margaret Higgins Database.*

11. Recepta, Spring 1705.
12. *Catholic Spectator,* II, pp. 254–8; Estcourt (ed.), *English Catholic Nonjurors,* pp. 24 & 229; Expensa, October 1715; *Cathedral Monuments,* p. 95; Williams (ed.), *Papist Estates in Wiltshire;* Williams, *Catholic Recusancy*; Lancaster, 'Nonconformity and Anglican Dissent', pp. 260–6 & 372; *Wells Corporation,* ed. Scrase, pp. 178–9; Loxton, *Ston Easton*, p. 120.
13. Diary, June 1723–December 1724; *Devon and Exeter Oath Rolls;* Haydon, *Anti-Catholicism,* pp. 122–4. Coplestone Bampfylde was made burgess of Wells in April 1718: WCA, CAB 1709–1721, f. 108.
14. WCA, CAB 1709–1721, ff. 86–106; Expensa, 25 November–2 December 1717.
15. Robert Taylor collected over £4 in donations from Claver, William Bragge and other new burgesses: Imray, *Wells Old Almshouse,* p. 79.
16. Will of Maurice Berkeley, 19 May 1712: *PROB 11/558/50;* Expensa, 1716–1717.
17. Will of George Farewell, 31 March 1717: *PROB 11/559/324*; Dispute over the will and purchase of Hadspen estate, 1717 & 1720: TNA, *C/11/17/11,* SHC, *DD/YB/ box 52 & DD/FC/21; Parish Register of Horsington,* ed. Daniel, pp. 71–3; Expensa, 5 October 1717.

Part Three, 1718–1727

25. The Letter

1. *Chronicles of John Cannon,* ed. Money, I, p. 147. Claver's fee was two shillings and sixpence: Recepta, 23 January 1718. Oak is listed as 'Oke' in *Eighteenth Century Medics*, ed. Wallis, p. 440.
2. *Whole Duty,* Allestree, 'Author to Printer'; Spurr, *Restoration Church,* pp. 281–96.
3. *Dean & Chapter,* II, pp. 500–1. WCL, ChAB 1683–1704, ff. 329 & 340; *CCEd,* 'William Hill'.
4. Diary, 20 July 1718; WCL, ChAB 1704–1725, ff. 124, 128. Perry was finally dismissed for 'great neglect of duty and contemptuous conduct', in 1723: *Dean & Chapter,* II, p. 509. Will of Matthew Brailsford, 30 July 1730: *PROB 11/663/371; Cathedral Monuments,* p. 107.
5. Diary, 12 March 1710; West Quantoxhead PR, baptisms, 11 May 1675; Will of Lucas, 4 August 1752: SHC, *DD/BR/ho/35; Cathedral Monuments,* p. 106.
6. Diary, 26–29 August 1718; Salmon, *Salmon Chronicles,* documents 143–52.
7. Claver had visited the Leighs on the Isle of Wight in May 1711: Expensa, 6 & 12 June 1711.
8. Diary, 21–23 November 1718; Johnstone, 'Claver Morris', p. 101.
9. Recepta, 1718; Diary, 24 November 1718.

10. Diary, 25–29 November 1718; Recepta, 28 November 1718; 'John Trevelyan', *Hist. Parl., 1690–1715;* Dunning, *Somerset Families,* pp. 137–40.
11. Diary, 29–30 November 1718; Recepta, 1 December 1718; 'Francis Warre', *Hist Parl., 1715–1754*; *Recipes and Remedies,* ed. White, pp. 25–6.
12. Diary, 1 December 1718.
13. Recepta, 15 December 1712 & 18 December 1714; Marriage of Burland to Cridland, 29 June 1682: St Mary's East Barnet PR; Burland debts, 1702: SHC, *DD/SAS/C112/9/3*; Collinson, I, pp. 249 & 256–7; BHO, *History of Somerset,* 6, pp. 113–8 & 145–6.
14. *Dean & Chapter,* II, pp. 487–8. Cooper had a wife and children to support. In 1718, he gave £1 towards the new charity school: Barnes, 'Church and Education in Wells', pp. 557 & 597.
15. *Dean & Chapter,* II, p. 502; Will of Samuel Hill, 3 March 1716: *PROB 11/533/45; CCEd,* 'Samuel Hill'.
16. Diary, 11–25 December, 1718; Expensa, 25 December 1718.

26. The Severance

1. Diary, 11 January 1719. Mary Evans stayed with the Hoskins family in April 1724.
2. Diary, 16 & 17 January 1719; Expensa, 24 January 1719.
3. Expensa, 12 & 13 February 1719; Diary, 12 February 1719.
4. Diary, 17 February 1719; Johnstone, 'Claver Morris', p. 117.
5. Diary, 18 March 1718. Claver probably recommended John Harvey, the stonemason from Bath, for the design of the monument to Frances in 1723: Easter, 'Church Monuments', pp. 154 & 294.
6. Diary, 19 March 1719; 'An Account of the Extraordinary Meteor', by Halley, p. 988.
7. Diary, 7 May 1719; Expensa, 7 May 1719; Crellin, 'Gascoigne's Powder', pp. 1–15.
8. Diary, 6 March & 29 June 1719; Collinson, III, pp. 478–9.
9. Account of Burland's debts, 21 May 1719: SHC, *DD/SAS/C112/9/4.*
10. Diary, 21 May, 15 & 18 June 1720; BHO, *History of Somerset,* 6, pp. 76–85; *Burland* v. *Waldegrave* (1721): TNA, *C 11/2168/3.*
11. Diary, July–August 1719; Expensa, 31 December 1719; Thorncombe PR, 22 July 1719; Will of Elizabeth Bragge, 28 June 1719: *PROB 11/570/462;* BHO, *History of Somerset,* 4, pp. 68–75. Children at Wayford were 'put to school' within months of Elizabeth's death: SHC, *D/P/WA, 2/9/2.*
12. Alicia was the sister of Dorothy, Frank Newman's wife. Alicia's marriage settlement, 1728: SHC, *DD/SX/38/2;* Diary, 2 July 1710; Collinson, II, pp. 371–3.
13. Diary, 20 & 26 September 1719; Will of William Westley, 11 March 1718 & 30 July 1719: *PROB 11/570/323.*
14. Ann, a spinster, lived in Kensington until her death in 1728 (aged 38). She was buried in the cathedral, and left £300 for the creation of an extravagant

marble monument to her parents, in which she is depicted as the reclining figure. Susanna and her four children were Ann's main beneficiaries. See the wills of Ann and Susanna, 30 April 1728 & 6 August 1739: *PROB 11/622/186 & PROB 11/698/218; Allegations for Marriage Licences issued by the Bishop,* ed. Armytage, p. 334; *Londinium Redivivum,* by Malcolm, p. 24.

15. Diary and Expensa, September 1719; Wills of Marshall & William Brydges, 25 August 1711 & 30 May 1734: *PROB 11/635/74* & *PROB 11/680/227.*
16. Convocation Book, 7 December 1719: SHC, *DD/SAS/C795/SE 32* & *DD/SAS/795/SE29.*
17. Marriage settlement, 15 October 1715: North Devon Record Office, *48/25/22/4;* Chichester, *History of the Family,* p. 48.

27. Loss & Reconciliation

1. Diary, 20–23 October 1719.
2. Will of Gabriel Odingsells, 20 January 1713: *PROB 11/540/266;* Odingsells trust, 1716: SHC, *DD/SAS/H/70/11/1;* Lympsham deeds, 1700–1716: SHC, *DD/DN/2/14/1–4;* Chancery disputes, 1717–1722: TNA, *C 11/221/15, C 11/2368/19* & *C 11/1429/45.* Gabriel (1690–1734) was author of three unsuccessful comedies, the first being a satire, *The Bath Unmask'd* (1725).
3. Tate, *Somerset Enclosure,* pp. 28 & 39.
4. Diary, 2 June & 4 November 1719; *Butleigh Ancestry*, 'Creech'; Case of Butleigh Inhabitants, 1627: SHC, *DD/DN/168*; Consistory Court depositions, *Uphill* v. *Sparrow*, 1719–20: SHC, *D/D/Cd/114,* ff. 119–22; BHO, *History of Somerset,* 9, pp. 59–75. Claver paid Mattocks 11 guineas to fight Creech's case: Expensa, 31 August 1723.
5. Quarter Session rolls, 1708 & 1719: SHC, *Q/SR/Rolls 249* & *290.* There was another case at Pilton, in 1717: SHC, *Q/SR/Roll 284.*
6. Diary, 23, 24 & 28 December 1719; Will of William Malet, 11 June 1722: *PROB 11/600/264;* Mattocks inventory, 1736, SHC, *D/D/Cti/106.*
7. Wills of William Coward, father and son, 5 March 1705 & 28 April 1715: *PROB 11/483/133* & *PROB 11/546/358; Cathedral Monuments,* pp. 132–4 & 236; WCA, Serel's book, 'Cowards'; Reid and Scrase, 'A Great House', pp. 35–37.
8. 'William Piers', 'William Coward I', 'William Coward II' & 'Wells', *Hist. Parl., 1715–1754.*
9. Claver composed the epitaph: Diary, October–December 1719; Collinson, II, p. 73.
10. Robert and Joseph were grocers, Charles a builder, and Benjamin an innkeeper. The Taylors had properties throughout the city: see the will of Robert Taylor, 6 August 1726: *PROB 11/634/262;* Taylor wills and deeds, 1660–1720s: SHC, *DD/FS/27;* High Street land tax, 1720: SHC, *DD/SAS/PR/162; Cathedral Monuments,* pp. 227–9; *Wells Corporation,* ed. Scrase, pp. 186 & 198.
11. Claver often hired horses from Tudway: Diary, 13 December 1719; Colchester (ed.), *Wells Cathedral School,* pp. 58–9.

12. Diary and Expensa, November–December 1719; WCA, Serel's book, 'Mayors'; Jones, 'New Light', pp. 275–6.
13. Diary, November 1719–January 1720; Expensa, 16 January 1720; 'Anne Daw' in Cathedral Registers, 20 January 1720, p. 152. Charles Dawe believed he had left 'a handsome maintenance' for all his children. Aside from his son and heir, John, he left £500 each for Charles, Edmund, Nancy and Elizabeth when they came of age: his will, 18 April 1717: *PROB 11/576/374.*
14. Diary, 15 June & 14 December 1722.
15. Indenture of Chichester and Leigh, 20 October 1717: SHC, *DD/SAS/C432/29*; *Lords Journals,* XXI, 1 February–6 April 1720;
16. Diary, 8 March 1720.

28. The Common Lands

1. Diary, January–February 1720; *Lords Journals,* XXI, 17 February–7 April 1720.
2. Petition and Act, 1720: SHC, *DD/DN/176* & *Q/RDe/79.*
3. Convocation Book, 14 & 19 March 1720: SHC, *DD/SAS/795/SE/28* & *29; Dean & Chapter,* II, pp. 506–8.
4. Diary, 26 & 30 March 1720.
5. Annuity agreement between Claver and his mother, 15 June 1721: SHC, *DD/WM/1/112.*
6. Diary, 15 October 1720; *Wells Manor,* pp. 90 & 97–8; *Dean & Chapter,* II, p. 503.
7. Diary, esp. 24 June, 10 & 22 September 1720; Paul, 'South Sea Bubble'.
8. Diary, 14 & 21 May 1720.
9. Diary & Expensa, 23 July 1720.
10. Diary, 7 September 1720.
11. Enclosure map, 1720–1721: SHC, *Q/RDe/79.*
12. WCL, ChAB 1704–1725, f. 152; Diary, 8 & 20 September 1720. It was not until 1723 that Claver renewed the lease on his house: Diary, 25–26 June 1723.
13. Some of the drawings (on paper with Italian watermarks) were based on the *Codex Bellunensis.* The album (sold by Sothebys in 1992) is inscribed in Latin, '19th October 1719, Claver Morris / a gift from the Chancellor of the diocese of Wells, John Pope'. Pope was married to Robert Creighton's second daughter, Margaret (died 1717), by whom he had five children, though none reached adulthood. The gift was probably in recognition of Claver's efforts to save their last surviving child, 'Willey Pope, who died about 5 a clock, being in Convulsions & senseless when I came to him': Diary, 9 September 1719.
14. Diary, 1 September 1720; *Fielding* v. *Fielding* (1720): TNA, *C 11/259/37; Fielding* v. *Gould* (1721): TNA, *C 11/2283/45.*
15. Diary, 24 November 1720; WCL, ChAB, 1704–25, f. 45 *et passim*; Cathedral Registers, p. 152; *Cathedral Monuments,* p. 292; *Dean & Chapter,* II, p. 506.
16. Diary, 7 & 21 January 1720, 19 October 1721.
17. Diary, November–December 1720; Will of Bower, 30 December 1725: *PROB 11/622/203.*

18. Claver's accounts for costs of enclosure and his agreement with Bower, 1720: SHC, *DD/SAS/C/114/ 33/3* & *DD/SAS/C/114/33/3*; Enclosure poor-rate, 1778: SHC, *DD/DN/168.*
19. Diary & Expensa, January–March 1721; West Bradley contracts: *SHC, DD/SAS/C/114/33/3.*
20. Diary, 9 May 1723.
21. Diary, 16 March, 27 July, 2 August & 14 September 1720. Piers, born in May 1686, was still only thirty-three at the time of his second marriage in March 1720. His first wife, Elizabeth, by whom he had several children, was the eldest daughter of Elizabeth Greene of Westminster and Hervey Ekins, lord of the manor of Weston Favell near Northampton. After her marriage to Piers, the Ekins family visited Wells where they were entertained by Claver: Diary, April–May 1709; Cole, *History and Antiquities of Weston Favell.* After his marriage to Mary in 1720, Piers had more children and built a new manor house at West Bradley in 1726: Hasler, 'The Peirs Family', pp. 7–10.

29. A Contested Election

1. Diary, 22 February & 3, 14 & 19 August 1721; Expensa, 9 March 1720 & 25 March 1721; Eklund, 'The Incompleat Chymist'.
2. Diary, March–May 1721. Joseph Norton died in 1722, having made his will on 26 June 1720: *PROB 11/584/347.*
3. Diary, 27 March & 23 July 1719; Expensa, 23 July 1719 & 15 December 1722.
4. Diary, 21 February, 21 & 29 April 1721; Expensa, 29 April 1721.
5. Diary, 30 January, 16 September & 27 December 1721; Expensa, 27 January 1722; Bellchambers, *Somerset Clockmakers,* pp. 32–5.
6. Expensa, 27 July & 24 December 1721; Diary, 4 December 1721.
7. The violin cost 3 guineas and the bow 5 shillings, from William Hill in London: Expensa, 20 January 1721; Johnstone, 'Claver Morris', pp. 114–16.
8. Diary & Expensa, May 1721.
9. Expensa, 4 April & 13 August 1720; Diary, 8–18 March, 30 June & 4 July 1721, 20 February 1722.
10. Diary, 31 May–5 June 1721. Having taken over his father's business, Cupper was very much 'my Apothecary' for Claver, though 15 other apothecaries are named in the diary, including Salmon, Taylor and Worrall in Wells: Diary, digital.
11. Expensa, 5 September 1721.
12. *Cathedral Monuments,* p. 83; Diary, 11 September 1721.
13. Diary, 14 September, 17 & 22 December 1721.
14. Diary, 2–9 December 1721; Expensa, 3 October 1721.
15. Diary, 29 January & 7 March 1722; Enclosure Act, 1722: SHC, *DD/DN/176; Lords Journals,* XXI, 27 November 1721–7 March 1722.
16. Diary, 2 August 1720 & 13 October 1721.

17. Reid, 'A Great House', pp. 35–9; 'Francis Gwyn', *Hist. Parl., 1715–1754*; Admission of freemen, January–February 1722: WCA, CAB 1709–21, ff. 166–82; Luff report, 5 March 1722: SHC, *DD/SAS/795/SE29.*
18. Diary, 15–16 March 1722; Wyndham letters, 26 February 1722: SHC, *DD/SH/77/1* & *DD/WY/15/2/6*; Admission of Wyndham & Gwyn, 16 March 1722: WCA, CAB 1721–1745, ff. 1–4.
19. There were 44 signatories, including George Hamilton, William Berkeley, Harry Bridges, Thomas Strangways and John Burland: SHC, *DD/WY/15/2/6.* Claver's name also appears on similar lists.
20. Diary, 23 & 26 March, 8 & 11 April 1722, 13 May 1723; 'Wells', *Hist. Parl., 1715–1754*; Hanham, 'Early Whig Opposition', pp. 335–7. On 24 March 1722, Gwyn was also re-elected (uncontested) to his old seat at Christchurch, which he gave up to be MP for Wells.

30. The Glastonbury Enclosure

1. Enclosure Act, 1722: SHC, *DD/DN/176* & *DD/SLt/7.*
2. A year later, parliament passed the notorious Waltham Black Act (1723), introducing over fifty new capital offences for poaching. For 'the rule of law', see Thompson's *Whigs and Hunters,* pp. 258–69, and Peluso, 'Whigs and hunters'.
3. Notes on Glastonbury CAB, *post* October 1715: SHC, *DD/SAS/795/SE/28;* Glastonbury land tax, 1728: SHC, *DD/DN/176.*
4. Diary, April–June 1722. Fear was awarded two shares in the common moor. *Moxham* v. *Hamilton* (1722): TNA, *C 11/2285/71;* Moxham's will, 1729: SHC, *DD/S/BT/4/6/6.* Claver prescribed for Moxam's wife in August 1722, and his son was buried by the Quakers in 1733*: Parish Registers of Street,* ed. Jewers, pp. 77–8.
5. Rates for Enclosure, 1722: SHC, *DD/DN/177.*
6. Diary, July–September 1722. The precision of Claver's measurements can be seen in his drawings, to which a scrap of a prescription is attached: SHC, *DD/SAS/C/114/33/3.*
7. Enclosure map and documents, 1722: SHC, *Q/RDe/63;* Hamilton's estate, 1759: SHC, *DD/DN/176.*
8. Diary, 28 July & 8 December 1722; Expensa, 28 July 1722.
9. Diary, 14 January, 10 March & 22 May 1722; Expensa, 21 July 1722.
10. Gourlay, *History of Sherborne School,* pp. 45–52; *Sherborne Registers,* ed. Pick, pp. li & 12.
11. Dairy & Expensa, June 1722.
12. Diary, 30 May 1722.
13. Diary, 13–25 August 1722; Will of Fox, 11 July 1735: *PROB 11/674/381.* It was probably at Cook's that Claver bought a copy of Sir John Floyer's *A Comment on Forty Two Histories described by Hippocrates in the First and Third Books of his Epidemics* (1726), which he signed and dated '1726': information received from Dr Denis Gibbs, Oxford.
14. Expensa, 28 May & 15 December 1722.

31. 'A Very Hot Dry Summer'

1. Diary, 3 January–24 May 1723; *Hamilton* v. *Coward*, 1723: TNA, *C 11/2170.*
2. Diary, December 1722; *Cathedral Monuments,* pp. 165–6; Legacies of Mary Healy, 1744: SHC, *DD/CR/24;* Copy of will of Richard Healy, 14 October 1734: SHC, *DD/GIL/13.*
3. Diary, 10–11 February 1723.
4. Diary, 20 February & 6 June 1723; Loxton, *Ston Easton,* p. 120.
5. Diary, March–May 1723; Wills of Henry and Edward Strode, 17 February 1721 & 28 February 1723: *PROB 11 589/442* & *PROB 11/590/266;* Pilton deeds, *post* 1705: SHC, *DD/SVL/2/10/3.*
6. Diary, 1 & 3 May 1723, 28 March 1724; Will of Anne Starr, 10 & 25 April 1723: *PROB 11/653/272.*
7. Diary, 18 January 1718 & 27 April 1721; Matthews, *A Brief History.*
8. Diary, 4 June 1723; Expensa, 1 April & 10 August 1723.
9. Diary, 14 June 1723 & 10 March 1724, and Diary notes.
10. 'Diary of Thomas Smith', 26 November 1722, in *Charters and Records,* ed. Neale, p. 207.
11. Diary, 13 August & 14 September 1723, 16 January & 9 March 1724.
12. Diary, 22 August 1723; Pye, *Some Observations,* p. 21. Lucas gave Claver a copy: Diary, 27 June 1724. Although Claver refers to other surgeons in his diary, Lucas is by far the most important both as a friend and colleague. He is referred to over 625 times: Diary, digital.
13. Inscription on a floor slab in St Cuthbert's; Diary, 8 June 1724; Will of John Irish, 12 December 1701: *PROB 11/463/284; Cathedral Monuments,* p. 126. In 1707, Claver bought Gay a present, 'a silver vent-pipe': Expensa, 9 April 1707.
14. Diary, 29 January, 22 June & 11 October 1723.
15. Expensa & Diary, 17 December 1723.
16. Claver did not always record the names of the patients for whom he prescribed, but according to his diary, for the period 1718–26 he made over 2,500 prescriptions: Diary, digital.
17. Diary, 15 May–26 July 1723, 30 January & 18 May 1724; *A Sermon Preach'd,* by Archer; Will of Archer, 24 March 1736: *PROB 11/699/133.*

32. Seen by Candlelight

1. Diary, 19 November 1723.
2. Diary, 5 March 1724; Gourlay, *A History,* p. 51.
3. The original benefactors included William Bragge, Jane and Christopher Keen, Christopher Lucas, William Piers and William Westley. Claver donated £2 each year. The greatest benefactors were Bishop Hooper (£10 per year), and his daughter Abigail Prowse (£3). Wells Blue School papers: SHC, *DD/WBS/1 & 21;* Minutes, 5 August 1713: WCA, CAB 1709–21, f. 55; Wells tax records, 1698 & 1699: SHC, *DD/FS/Box 72; Cathedral Monuments,* p. 281;

Barnes, 'Church and Education in Wells', pp. 46–50, 228–356 & 523–720. A very similar school had been set up at Bath in 1711: BRO, *103/1/2/1.*

4. Quarter Session roll, 1718: SHC, *Q/SR/Roll 285*; Diary, 14 March 1720, 14 April–12 November 1724; *Dean & Chapter,* II, p. 514; Colchester (ed.), *Wells Cathedral School,* p. 38.
5. On the way to Lydlinch, one of Claver's horses got so badly stuck in mud, oxen were required to pull the calèche from the ditch. Diary, 9 May 1723, 20–26 March & 6 October 1724.
6. Johnstone, 'Claver Morris', pp. 110–112.
7. Diary, 20–22 May 1724.
8. Diary, 9–14 July 1724.
9. Contract with Paddock, 19 December 1724: SHC, *DD/SAS/C/114/33/3.*
10. Diary, esp. 7 October 1724 & 12 May 1725.
11. Diary, 25 June, 12 November–22 December 1724.
12. Diary, 30 October 1724–2 February 1725.
13. *Compleat Chymist,* by Glaser, pp. 143–4; Diary, 2 December 1724 & 24 March 1725.
14. Diary, 5 April 1725.

33. Dining Alone

1. Diary, 27 March 1725; Cathedral Registers, p. 12; *Cathedral Monuments,* p. 249.
2. Diary, 26 October 1724 & 1 February 1726; St Cuthbert's PR: SHC, *D/P/W. St.C.*
3. Diary, 20 September 1725 & 19 April 1726; *Cathedral Monuments,* pp. 5–7 & 282–3.
4. Diary, 8 September 1725–23 June 1726; *Vicars Choral* v. *Morris* (1726): TNA, *C 11/317/26;* WCL, ChAB 1704–25, f. 199; Crawford, *Vicars,* pp. 124–6.
5. Diary, 28 June & 11 July 1726; Johnstone, 'Claver Morris', p. 119. Grace Pierce lived until 1736: Cathedral Registers, p. 153. The Crown and the Mitre were Claver's favourite haunts during the last decade of his life; mentioned over 300 times in his diary, 1718–26: Diary, digital.
6. Diary, 3–5 November 1725; Fawcett, *Bath Entertain'd,* pp. 4 & 20. Greenway delivered the three-foot urns and two large flowerpots (which he placed in the 'oval' of Claver's garden) in the Spring: Diary, 7 January, 10–11 March, 25 & 27 May 1726.
7. Diary, 12–14 March 1726.
8. No guests were invited to the funeral, but Claver received gloves, a ring and other accoutrements of a pall-bearer: Diary, 29 March 1726.
9. Diary, 28 March 1725; *Wills.* IV, pp. 112 & 132; McGarvie, *Book of Frome,* pp. 72–83. Claver had treated members of the Whitchurch and Leversedge families at least since 1700: Recepta, 'Advice', 1700.
10. 'Thomas Palmer', *Hist. Parl., 1715–1754; Cathedral Monuments,* pp. 65–7; *Wills.,* II, pp. 87–9.

11. *Watson* v. *Morris* (1722 & 1725): TNA, *C 11/1429/45* & *C 11/1449/31.*
12. *Hall* v. *Morris* (1725): TNA, *C 11/2262/18.*
13. Jane Pitt, William's wife, was the sister of Honora, married to Davidge Gould. Diary, 17 January 1724 & 21 March 1726; Wills of William (16 & 19 May 1724) & Jane (10 August 1731) Pitt: *PROB 11/604/15* & *PROB 11/695/396;* Inquisition of lunacy (1726): TNA, *C 211/19/P41.*
14. Claver went to New Street to prescribe for the nine-year-old Anne 27 times in April 1726. St Cuthbert's PR baptisms: SHC, *D/P/W.St.C; Cathedral Monuments,* pp. 55–8; *Pharmacopoeia,* by Culpeper, p. 131; 'Baron', *Marriages at Bristol,* ed. Price.
15. Diary, 5 October 1725 & 7 March 1726; Wallis, 'Exotic Drugs'.
16. John Ravenhill's bill, 1720: BRO, *0028F/17.* Diary, 26–27 January 1726.
17. Bragge papers: DHC, *D-MHM* & *RGB/LL;* Squibb, 'Bragge Family', pp. 62–3.
18. Will of William Bragge, 2 July 1726: *PROB 11/612/242;* Thorncombe PR, 20 October 1726: DHC, *PE/THO.* John Bragge restored the family's finances.
19. Diary, 8 August 1726.
20. Will of Gerard Martin, 29 August 1721: *PROB 11/614/282.* A floor-slab at West Bradley church records Gerard's death on 2 December 1726 (aged 56), and that of Mary his widow on 15 March 1734 (aged 51).
21. Pre-marriage settlement, 1725: SHC, *DD/X/FRC/5.*
22. When Lucas died in 1756 (aged 81), he left no children, and his wife had died in 1740: *Cathedral Monuments,* p. 106. His practice and most of the estate was left to his nephew, the physician Benjamin Pulsford, though he also left £30 to be invested for the poor of West Quantoxhead: copy of will, 24 August 1752: *SHC, DD/BR/ho/35* & *DD/FS/58/1/11;* Benjamin and William Pulsford's daybook, 1756–66: SHC, *DD/FS/48/6/1;* Allen, 'Medical Practice'; Loudon, 'Nature of Provincial Medical Practice', pp. 4–6.
23. Mary lived at Dulcote until her death in 1746. Her estate was inherited by Brailsford Hughes of Monmouthshire who claimed to be her 'next protestant heir' as her Catholic cousin, John Evans, was debarred. Quarter Session roll, 1747: SHC, *Q/SR/315/104–106;* Goddard, *An Extract from the Sessions-Rolls,* pp. 63–5; Williams (ed.), *Post Reformation Catholicism,* p. 46.
24. Diary, 15 May 1726; St Cuthbert's PR, baptisms: SHC, *D/P/W.St.C.*
25. Later in the year, when he lost his wife Grace, he buried her in the cathedral. WCA, CAB 1721–45, ff. 40–4; St Cuthbert's pew register, 1670–1755: SHC, *D/B/wls/35/1; Cathedral Monuments,* p. 35.
26. Diary, 25 November 1725; *Dean & Chapter,* II, pp. 506–15. Hooper died in September 1727 (aged 87); Creighton in February 1734 (aged 96); and Archer in October 1739 (aged 66).
27. 'Clark's List'; '7 April 1727', *Remarks and Collections,* IX, ed. Salter, p. 295.
28. Claver's will, 18 May 1725: *PROB 11/617/369.* From a letter, dated 30th March 1727, written by John Tottenham, a prebend of Wells and one of Claver's patients, we know that Claver's final wish was granted: *Remarks and*

Collections, IX, ed. Salter, p. 295. Some of the music played may have been by the Moravian composer Gottfried Finger and the Italian Giovanni Battista Bassani. After a concert at his house on 20th November 1725 Claver noted in his diary that the music included 'Finger's two Sonatas which I would should be Play'd at my Funeral, & two of Bassani's Sonatas'.

Epilogue

1. Claver's executors were granted permission to erect the monument next to his grave in May 1730. *Dean & Chapter,* II, pp. 517 & 520; *Cathedral Monuments,* pp. 96 & 184–5. A translation of the epitaph is provided in *Diary of a West Country Physician,* ed. Hobhouse, pp. 46–7.
2. Cathedral Registers, pp. 11–13 & 153–5; *Cathedral Monuments,* pp. 101–2 & 230–1.
3. John Burland (b. 1724) letter, 1746: SHC, *DD/SF/2998(3); Cathedral Monuments,* pp. 99–100; *Canonical Houses,* pp. 178–83.

SOURCES

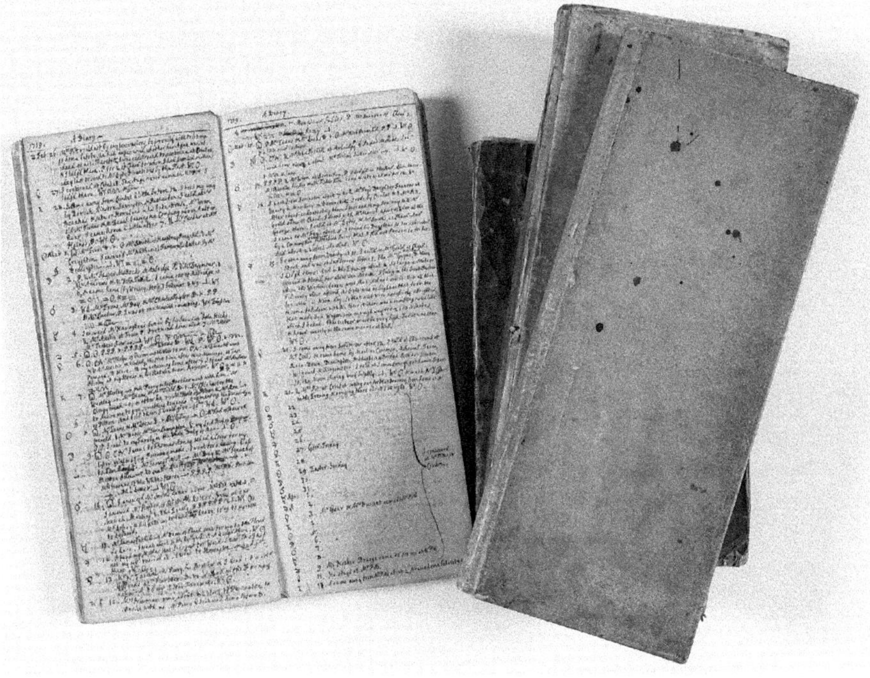

FIGURE 23 The Claver Morris Manuscript Books

The story of Claver Morris's life is based on the private diaries and accounts he kept, from his marriage to Grace Greene in 1685 until a few months before his death in 1727. Not all of his writings have survived, but there are diaries for the periods 1709–1710 and 1718–1726, and daily accounts of income and expenditure throughout the period 1685–1723. These writings, penned in his home-made black ink, are contained in four unpaged books, each bound in vellum.

- **Book 1** (*c.*144 pages, 40 × 16cm). In 1674, when Grace Greene became an orphan, her legal guardian, Thoresby Hardres, began to keep a book of accounts recording his management of her inheritance. As soon as Grace married in 1685, Hardres handed this book to Claver who used it to record his own accounts until Lady Day, 24th March 1698 (the day traditionally regarded as marking the end of the year). Claver's main headings were 'Money Received for my Advice & Prescriptions in Physick' and 'Money Laid Out'. Almost a quarter of Book 1 was kept by Hardres, and his entries are cited here as 'Hardres Accounts'. Thereafter, all the entries are by Claver and are cited here as 'Accounts'. Folded into the Book is a loose sheet, dated 8th July 1692, certifying the award of Claver's MD.
- **Book 2** (*c.*200 pages, 32 × 20cm). Following his entries in Book 1, on 25th March 1698 Claver began a new book of accounts which he maintained for eleven years, until 24th March 1709. Opening from the side of the book marked 'EXPENSA' is a ledger of expenditure (*c.*140 pages, each page with two lined columns) kept under various headings such as 'In Housekeeping', 'In Clothes and Household Stuff', 'About Horses and their Keeping', and 'Miscellaneous Expenses'. Inside the 'EXPENSA' there is also a special section of twenty-seven pages detailing the costs of work and materials 'In Building my House at Wells' from 1698 to 1702, and another six-page section for further 'Building Work' from April 1702 to December 1703. Opening from the other side of Book 2, marked 'RECEPTA', is Claver's account of his income (*c.*60 pages, each with two columns) under headings such as 'Debts & their Interest' and 'For Advice in Physick'. Inside the cover Claver noted the four letters that would open the combination lock on the hall closet door. All references to Book 2 are cited here as 'Expensa' or 'Recepta'.
- **Book 3** (*c.*464 pages, 40 × 16cm). This book contains accounts for the period 25th March 1709 to 31st December 1723, and a diary for the year 25th March 1709 to 24th March 1710. Opening from the side of the book marked 'EXPENSA', records of expenditure (*c.*316 pages) are kept under headings such as 'In Household Keeping', 'In Household Stuff & Books', 'In Taxes & Disbursements', 'About my Horses', 'Money Given besides of the Dedicated Part', and 'Miscellaneous Expenses'. Opening from the side marked 'RECEPTA', the book begins with 'A Diary' (*c.*15,000 words over 24 pages) consisting of a daily record of key activities briefly noted alongside the astrological sign for the day of the week, often with a few simple ideographs indicating when Claver was at home or called out to visit patients. The book continues (*c.*124 pages) with accounts of income received from landed estates,

'Advice in Physick', 'Debts, & their Interest' and 'Miscellaneous Receipts'. All expenditure, income, and diary entries are cited here as 'Expensa', Recepta' or 'Diary'.

- **Book 4** (*c.*280 pages, 40 × 16cm). This book contains the diary that Claver kept almost every day from 25th June 1718 until 12th August 1726. It contains over 280 pages of writing (though two pages are missing, for the periods 7–22 June 1721 and 1–16 January 1722), amounting to about 164,000 words. In addition to the abbreviations and ideographs of the 1709–1710 diary, several new ones are included, representing activities such as attending church, writing prescriptions, and working in the laboratory or study. A weather report is also regularly included as a series of ideographs at the end of each day. Altogether, with the 1709–1710 diary, the word count for both diaries amounts to over 179,000 words. All of the dairy entries are cited here as 'Diary'.

Throughout his books, Claver's handwriting is usually neat, quite small and clear; often sloping slightly to the right and rarely crossed out or corrected. Occasionally, his writing becomes quite ragged, perhaps after he had been drinking. His words and phrases are not studied, but those that came to mind when he sat down every day or so to make a private record of the key facts and figures for each day. A few additional entries, such as his summaries of his annual income from 'Advice & Prescriptions', are undated, written in the margins or flyleaves on the books. In keeping with this relaxed manner of composition, the spelling of common words, especially the names of people and places, is often inconsistent, as Claver simply adopts what appear to be phonetic spellings. Alchemical and medical symbols are also often used to represent common elements or compounds, such as copper or aqua fortis (nitric acid).

It is clear from the internal evidence of the surviving books that some parts of Claver's diary have been lost. From notes to himself in his accounts, such as 'see my Diary' and 'as might be seen in my Diary', we know that a diary was kept at least for some, and probably for the whole, of the period 25th March 1710 to 24th June 1718. The last diary entry that survives (for 12th August 1726) coincides with the last page of Book 4, and there is no indication that Claver was not intending to continue. So it is probable that a diary for the last months of his life is also lost.

In 1934, Edmund Hobhouse published a selection of Claver's diary (about 18 per cent of the total word-count) and a few extracts from his accounts, *The Diary of a West Country Physician A.D. 1684–1726*. Earlier, in 1932, he had published an article 'The Library of a Physician *circa* 1700' consisting of a verbatim record of most of the books that Claver recorded as having purchased between 1685 and 1723. Later, from 1936 to 1942, Hobhouse also published a series of short notes, 'Dr. Claver Morris' Accounts', taken from Books 2 and 3. To date, these are the only parts of Claver's writings that have been printed.

In recent years, H. Diack Johnstone has published a study of Claver's musical activities, 'Claver Morris, an Early Eighteenth-Century English Physician and Amateur Musician *Extraordinaire*' (2008), in which there is an appendix of the music purchased by Claver. Johnstone also published an article, 'Instruments, Strings, Wire and Other Musical Miscellanea in the Account Books of Claver Morris (1659–1727)', which includes a chronological list of items purchased. Johnstone's essays are based upon Books 1, 3 and 4, but at the time of his research, Book 2 was missing.

Aside from the great body of writings in over 1,000 pages of diaries and accounts, some further papers in Claver's hand have survived, and many more include just his name or signature. Most of these papers are cited on the Notes and Sources here. A typescript of all diary entries has been created to support research for this book, and this is referred to in the Notes as 'Diary, digital'. Copies of Books 1, 3 and 4 can be found at the Somerset Heritage Centre, Taunton.

Manuscript Sources

Bath Record Office

Bath: Minute book of the charity school, 1711–1773: *103/1/2/1.* **Bragge:** William's marriage agreement (1688), letters & legal costs (1716–1720): *0028F/17* & *33;* John's will (copy): *0028F/41.*

Dorset History Centre

Bragge Family

Prowse & Bragge marriage settlement, 1701: *D-MHM/8836A*; Survey of Bragge estates, 1722: *D-MHM/8335;* Mortgage of Thorncombe manor, 1724: *D-MHM/8968;* Lease of Thorncombe manor, 1725: *D-MHM/8971;* Inventory of William Bragge, 1726: *RGB/LL/116;* Legacy of William Bragge, 1731: *RGB/LL/468.*

Parish Records

Bishop's Caundle: Parish registers & overseer's accounts: *PE/BCD* & *PE/BCD/OV1/1.* **Lydlinch:** Parish registers & churchwarden's accounts: *PE/LYD* & *PE/LYD/CW1/1* & *CW2/1.* **Manston:** Parish registers & papers: *PE/MAN* & *MAN RE4/1.* **Thorncombe:** Parish registers: *PE/THO.*

Wills

Claver: John (1739): *MIC/R/207/DA/22;* Susan (1729): *MIC/R/198/DA/38;* William (1686): *MIC/R/258/DA/30.* **Gillingham:** Elizabeth (1699): *MIC/R/183/DA/30.* **Morris:** William (1690): *D238/F2.*

The National Archives

Court of Chancery

Strode v *Dean of Wells* (1684): *C 6/74/61* & *C 8/721/51; Morris* v *Shirley* (1687): *C 7/223/36*; *Morris* v *Goddard* (1690): *C 8/418/99; Morris* v *Foxwell* (1699): *C 8/361/48; Morris* v *Hood* (1701): *C 8/595/69; Gregory* v *Morris* (1703): *C 10/264/28; Farewell* v *Farewell* (1717): *C 11/17/11*; *Goldfinch* v *Odingsells* (1717): *C 11/221/15; Fisher* v *Odingsells* (1720): *C 11/2368/19; Fielding* v *Fielding* (1720): *C 11/259/37; Burland* v *Waldegrave* (1721): *C 11/2168/3; Fielding* v *Gould* (1721): *C 11/2283/45; Watson* v *Morris* (1722 & 1725): *C 11/1429/45* & *C 11/1449/31*; *Moxham* v *Hamilton* (1722): *C 11/2285/71; Hamilton* v *Coward* (1723 & 1725): *C 11/2170/20* & *C 11/850/82; Principals of Vicars Choral* v *Morris* (1726): *C 11/317/26; Hall* v *Morris* (1725–34): *C 11/2262/18*; *Samuel Pitt, Inquisition of lunacy* (1726): *C 211/19/P41.*

Wills

Aish, William (1725): *PROB 11/606/147.* **Archer,** Edmund (1739): *PROB 11/699/133.* **Bampfylde,** Coplestone Warwick (1727): *PROB 11/621/6.* **Bathurst,** Ralph (1704): *PROB 11/476/427.* **Bave,** Charles (1733): *PROB 11/667/241.* **Berkeley,** Edward (1707) *PROB 11/495/307;* Maurice (1717) *PROB 11/558/50;* William (1737): *PROB 11/645/410.* **Bower,** Edmund (1728): *PROB 11/622/203.* **Bragge,** Elizabeth (1719): *PROB 11/570/462;* Matthew (1691): *PROB 11/405/113;* William (1713): *PROB 11/533/29;* William (1726): *PROB 11/612/242.* **Brailsford,** Mathew (1732): *PROB 11/663/371.* **Brewer,** Thomas (1723): *PROB 11/599/433.* **Bridges,** Harry (1729): *PROB 11/630/317;* Thomas (1707): *PROB 11/494/173.* **Brydges,** Marshall (1711): *PROB 11/635/74;* William (1736): *PROB 11/680/227.* **Bull,** Henry (1687): *PROB 11/410/135;* Henry (1694): *PROB 11/428/402;* Henry (1732): *PROB 11/706/335;* Joanna (1721): *PROB 11/581/439;* John (1704): *PROB 11/483/242;* Richard (1709): *PROB 11/516/65.* **Burge,** Thomas (1718): *PROB 11/570/316.* **Cannington,** Thomas (1705): *PROB 11/481/411.* **Claver,** James (1709): *PROB 11/509/309.* **Comes,** Richard (1733): *PROB 11/714/334.* **Cooke,** Hodges (1706): *PROB 11/491/161.* **Cooth,** John (1712): *PROB 11/538/101.* **Coward,** William (1705): *PROB 11/483/133;* William (1715): *PROB 11/546/358.* **Davis,** John (1694): *PROB 11/461/40.* **Dawe,** Charles (1720): *PROB 11/576/374;* Edmund (1695): *PROB 11/426/42;* Edmund (1708): *PROB 11/543/251.* **Day,** John (1701): *PROB 11/479/236.* **Dennett,** John (1695): *PROB 11/20/726.* **Evans,** William (1632): *PROB 11/162/104;* William (1683): *PROB 11/374/408;* William (1705): *PROB 11/540/280.* **Farewell,** George (1717): *PROB 11/559/324.* **Fox,** Baruch (1735): *PROB 11/674/381.* **Greene,** Mary (1674): *PROB 11/345/95.* **Gutch,** Robert (1681): *PROB 11/393/158.* **Harper,** Archibald (1714): *PROB11/539/29.* **Hardres,** Thoresby (1691): *PROB 11/405/124;* Thorseby (1685): *PROB*

11/386/54. **Healy,** Richard (1706): *PROB 11/535/318.* **Helyar,** William (1697): *PROB 11/442/367;* William (1723): *PROB 11/594/389.* **Hill,** Samuel (1715): *PROB 11/553/45.* **Hodges,** Richard (1729): *PROB 11/632/465.* **Hooper,** George (1727): *PROB 11/618/316.* **Horner,** Samuel (1703): *PROB 11/571/320.* **Hughes,** William (1715): *PROB 11/551/280.* **Hunt,** William (1719): *PROB 11/663/166.* **Iliffe,** Edith (1718): *PROB 11/582/180.* **Irish,** John (1701): *PROB 11/463/284;* Matthew (1705): *PROB 11/488/316.* **Jeanes,** Philipa (1704): *PROB 11/477/352;* Robert (1694): *PROB 11/423/236.* **Keen,** Francis (1664): *PROB 11/304/410.* **Kidder,** Richard (1703): *PROB 11/474/498;* Anne (1728): *PROB/11/622/186;* Susanna [Everard] (1739): *PROB 11/698/218.* **Layng,** Henry (1726): *PROB 11/613/190.* **Long,** William (1737): *PROB 11/699/77.* **Malet,** William (1724): *PROB 11/600/264.* **Martin,** Gerard (1721): *PROB 11/614/282.* **Mattocks,** Elizabeth (1682): *PROB 11/376/333.* **Mogg,** John (1675): *PROB 11/354/536;* John (1728): *PROB 11/800/257.* **Morris,** Claver (1725): *PROB 11/617/369.* **Newman,** Richard (1696): *PROB 11 433/11;* Henry (1726): *PROB 11610/99.* **Nichols,** Thomas (1724): *PROB 11/624/41.* **Norton,** Joseph (1720): *PROB 11/584/347.* **Odingsells,** Gabriel (1714): *PROB 11/540/266.* **Paine,** John (1741): *PROB 11/715/155.* **Pitt,** Jane (1739): *PROB 11/695/396*; William (1724): *PROB 11/604/15;* Samuel (1729): *PROB 11/631/242;* Samuel (1738): *PROB 11/691/85.* **Prickman,** John (1693): *PROB 11/420/115.* **Prowse,** John (1710): *PROB 11/515/92.* **Rebotier,** Elias (1766): *PROB 11/915/250.* **Seymour,** Edward (1707): *PROB 11/495/231.* **Shirley,** Andrew (1719): *PROB 11/573/411;* Andrew (1740): *PROB 11/753/235.* **Starr,** Anne (1732): *PROB 11/653/272.* **Strode,** Edward (1704): *PROB 11/475/10;* Edward (1723): *PROB 11/590/266;* Elizabeth (1713): *PROB 11/547/309;* Henry (1721): *PROB 11/589/442.* **Taylor,** Robert (1729): *PROB 11/634/262.* **Tuthill,** John (1636): *PROB 11/176/294.* **Webb,** Katherine (1713): *PROB 11/537/173;* Thomas (1711): *PROB 11/551/302.* **Wells,** Samuel (1709); *PROB 11/510/34.* **Westley,** Thomas (1661): *PROB 11/309/275;* William (1719): *PROB 11/570/323.* **White,** William (1725): *PROB 11/608/72.* **Willoughby,** William (1730): *PROB 11/643/39.*

North Devon Record Office

Chichester: marriage settlement, 1715: *48/25/22/4.* **Drewe:** will of Thomas (copy), 1705: *826M/E3a.* **Wills:** 'Copies of Transcripts and Extracts […] collected by Miss Olive Moger', 22 vols: *Moger Catalogue;* 'Devon Will Abstracts', typescript by Cliff Webb, May 1979: *16/2/GEN.*

Somerset Heritage Centre

Families

Bragge: Elizabeth's will, 1719: *D/P/WA/2/9/2.* **Burland:** Spaxton farm deeds, 1680s: *DD/HI/A/118* & *DD/SAS/C112/5.* Documents relating to John's estate &

debts: *DD/SAS/C112/9/3 & 4;* Deeds & letter of administration, 1697–1770: *DD/SAS/C114/18/1.* **Chichester:** Family papers, 18th century: *DD/SF/2997-8, 3855.* **Davis:** Manuscript book of cases by Peter Davis, 1720s: *DD/S/HP/1.* **Dawe:** Deeds for estate at Ditcheat, 1701–1771: *DD/HYD/2.* **Evans:** Miscellaneous deeds, Godney manor & Westbury: *DD/BR/mmd/11 & 12.* Godney manor at Mere, 1705-72: *DD/SAS/C/795/SE/2.* Mary Evans, Papist estates, 1717: *Q/RRP/1/31;* Quarter Session roll, 1747: *Q/SR/315/104-106.* **Farewell:** Chancery dispute over George's will, 1717: *DD/YB/ box 52.* Estate, 1720: *DD/FC/21.* **Fisher:** *Wills* & estate at Somerton: *DD/DN/153.* Will extracts & Somerton charities, 1675–1924: *DD/SMC/12.* **Gifford:** Alicia, marriage settlement, 1728: *DD/SX/38/2.* **Greene:** Lease of house at Crane Court, 25 February 1675: *DD/WM/1/52.* **Hardres:** Thoresby, 'TH's Accounts' 1674–85: *A/AHZ.* **Healy:** Administration of Mary's estate, 1744; Baltonsborough indenture, 1712: *DD/CR/24.* Documents & will of Rev. Richard, 1705–1734: *DD/GIL/13.* **Helyar:** William's wills, 1710 & 1723: *DD/WHL/25 & 26.* **Jeanes:** Robert's will, 20 September 1694: *DD/WM/1/127h.* **Keen:** Marriage settlement, 1725: *DD/X/FRC/5.* **Leigh:** Family papers: *DD/SAS/C432/29.* **Lucas:** Leases & copy of Christopher's will, signed in 1752: *DD/BR/ho/35* & *DD/FS/58/1/11.* **Mattocks:** Inventory of George, 1736: *D/D/Cti/106.* **Mogg:** Richard, marriage settlement, 1719: *DD/MGG/1/1/11.* **Morris:** Claver, CM Accounts, 1674–1698; Diary, 1709–10 & 1718–26; Expensa, 1709–1723; Recepta, 1709–1723: *A/AHZ.* Beast leases for commons, no date: *D/P/Lav/23/1.* House lease, 1702: *DD/SAS/C/114/18/1.* Leases & commons papers, 1698–1720: *DD/SAS/C/114/33/3.* **Morris:** Hannah, annuity for North Cadbury, 1721: *DD/WM/1/112.* **Morris:** Ruth, lease of land at Felton, 2 November 1678: *DD/WM/1/105 & 114.* **Morris:** William, mortgage of house at Abbas Combe, 1672: *DD/WM/1/109.* Articles of agreement for Manston, 29 August 1661: *DD/WM/1/111.* **Moxham,** William, copy of will, 1729: *DD/S/BT/4/6/6.* **Muttlebury:** marriage bond, 1681: *DD/SAS/C/795/PR/364.* **Nash:** documents, 1718–1812: *DD/WM/39.* **Odingsells:** Deeds, 1711: *DD/NN/91*; Trust, 1716: *DD/SAS/H/70/11/1.* **Parfitt:** Wells deeds, 1665–1728: *DD/WM/55*. **Piers [Peirs]:** Deed of Trust, 1686: *DD/PINC/9/5.* **Salmon:** Estate papers, 17–18th century: *DD/TD/31.* **Strode:** copy of Edward's pardon, 1686: *DD/X/LDD/1.* **Taylor:** Wills & deeds, 1660–1720s: *DD/FS/27.* **Tuthill:** Marriage settlement, 1699: *D/B/bw.* **Walrond:** Will of Henry, 26 December 1720: *DD/LC/53/3.* **Westley:** William's charity bequest, 1709: *A/AMV/1.* **Wyndham:** Correspondence on election, 1722: *DD/SH/77/1.*

Wells

Cathedral Records: Cathedral statutes & charters of vicars choral: *DD/SAS/C/795/SE/11.* Deeds & leases of vicars choral, 1686–1866: *DD/WM/52.* Transcripts of registers of baptisms, marriages & burials, 1660–1982: *DD/WCL/69.* Britton's 'History of Wells Cathedral & Bath Abbey' (1825) with notes: *DD/SAS/C/795/SE/83.* Records of the Peculiar of the Dean of Wells, 1693–1749: *D/D/Pd/1,13 & 21.* **City Records:** Benjamin & William Pulsford's daybook, 1756–1766: *DD/FS/48/6/1*. Cordwainers' Company, 1606–1720: *DD/SAS/C/795/SE/50/1* & *2*. Convocation books (copies): *DD/SAS/C/795/SE/32/1*. Deeds, 1701–19: *DD/SAS/C/151/2/1*. Deeds for Healey, Paine & Bathurst, 1679–1726: *DD/SAS/C/114/19*. Elections: *DD/SAS/C/795/SE/118*. Mayor's orders, 1700: *DD/SAS/C/151/2/5*. Miscellaneous notes & extracts, 1189–1855: *DD/SAS/795/SE/28*. Miscellaneous notes & extracts, 1315–1875: *DD/SAS/795/SE/29*. Plan of Wells, by William Symes [Simes], 1735: *DD/SAS/PR/504*. Presentment of verderers of the High Street, 1712: *DD/GS/4/145*. Properties in the Liberty & New Street, 1700s: *DD/TD/41/3*. Properties in East Wells, 1688–1836: *DD/WM/16*. Records of various taxes, 1699–1808: *DD/FS/Boxes 71* & *72*. Records of lands, taxes & poor rates, 1699–1720s: *DD/SAS/PR/160, 162–164*. Survey of Wells Manor, 1684: *DD/CB/36*. Wells Blue School, 1641–1996: *DD/WBS/1* & *21*. Illustrations of Wells: *A/DAS/1/420*. **St Cuthbert's Parish Records:** *D/P/W.St.C.* Marriages, 1609-1754, transcript: *DD/X/CPL/29*. Parish records, 1668–1727: *T/PH/lanc/17*. Pew register, 1670–1755: *D/B/wls/35/1*. Poor rates, 1698–1726: *D/P/w.st.c/13/2/1*. Subscription books for surgeons & schoolmasters, 1672–1695 & 1685–1730: *D/D/Bs/42 & 43*. Vestry book: *D/B/Wls/35/11*.

Somerset & Other Places

Somerset: Consistory Court deposition books, 1686–1726: *D/D/Cd/101-115, 126, 128*. Diocesan Court records, 1671: *D/D/ca/350*. Diocesan Court act book, 1692–1697: *D/D/Ca/366*. Medical recipe MS books: *DD/X/FW/C/1751* & *DD/WO/56/10/3*. Quarter Session rolls & examinations, 1693–1727: *Q/SR/Rolls 193–295*. Quarter Session order books, 1676–1687, 1688–1708 & 1708–29: *Q/SO/7, 8* & *9*. Certificates for Dissenters' meetings, 1694–1705: *D/D/ol/51*. Miscellaneous election papers, 1714–1727: *DD/WY/15//2/6*. **Axbridge:** Churchwarden's accounts: *D/P/Ax.4/1/1*. **Baltonsborough:** Parish records: *D/P/balt*. Documents on manor & parish: *DD/DN/168*. Enclosure Act for Baltonsborough, 1719–1720: *DD/SAS/C/795/SE/10*. Map & roll of enclosure, 1720–1721: *Q/RDe/79*. Commissioners' accounts, 1706–1720: *DD/SAS/c/61*. **Banwell:** Parish records: *D/P/ban*. **Bruton:** Parish records: *D/P/brut*. **Chewton Mendip:** Bastardy documents: *D/P/Chewt.m.13/5/5*. **Dinder:** Land & tenements, 1639–1687: *DD/WM/75–78, 82*. **Ditcheat:** Parish records: *D/P/dit.2/1/1–3*. **Glastonbury & Butleigh:** Deeds (Davis, Hamilton, Odingsells, Coward), 1662–1730: *DD/DN/90* & *91*. Documents on rates, estates, leases & enclosure, 1662–1789: *DD/DN/175–177* & *180*. Enclosure documents, 1721: *DD/SLT/7*. Map & Roll of Enclosure, 1722: *Q/RDe/63*. **Godney:** Manor & Wills of Ivyleafe family, 1698–1797: *DD/OB/43*. **Keynsham:** Parish Registers: *DD/SOG/1225*. **Lympsham:** Deeds, 1699–1758: *DD/DN/2/14/1–4*. **Pilton:** Parish records: *D/P/pilt.2/1/1-2, 4/1/4, 23/18*. Land, 1698: *DD/WM/1/123*. Records of the Peculiars (Pilton & North Wootton): *D/D/Ppr/3* & *8*. Land Claver Morris leased, 30 July 1714: *DD/WM/1/94*. Deeds, post 1705: *DD/SVL/2/10/3*.

Shepton Mallet: Parish records: *D/P/She.2/1/2.* **Watchet:** Parish records: *D/P/St.d.* **Wedmore:** John Westover's diary (1685–1700) & documents: *DD/X/HKN/1-2.* **West Bradley:** Registers of baptisms, burials & marriages: *D/P/brad.w.2/1/1.* Overseer's accounts: *D/P/brad.w.13/2/1.* Manor, 1705–1732: *DD/SAS/C/114/35.* Manor & tenants, 1674 & 1691: *DD/SAS/C/114/33.* Leases & commons papers, 1698–1720: *DD/SAS/C/114/33/3.* **Worle:** Parish records: *D/P/wor.* Ebdon Farm documents, 1706–1837: *DD/BR/mt/2, Parts 1 & 2.*

Wells Cathedral Library

Chapter Act Books for 1683–1704, 1705–1725 & 1725–1744. Manuscript Music Books from the Vicars Choral Library: *VC/Music MS. 1–9.*

Wells City Archives

Corporation Act Books: 1687–1709; 1709–1721; 1721–1745. Thomas Serel's book on Wells: mayors, recorders & historical notes.

Printed Primary Sources

'An Account of the Extraordinary Meteor seen all over England', by Edmund Halley, *Philosophical Transactions of the Royal Society,* 30 (1719), pp. 978–90.

Abstracts of Somerset Wills, etc., copied from the manuscript collections of the late Rev. Frederick Brown, ed. Frederick Arthur Crisp, 6 vols (1887–1890).

Acts and Ordinances of the Interregnum, 1642–1660, ed. C.H. Firth (1911).

Allegations for Marriage Licences issued by the Bishop of London, 1611 to 1828, ed. G.J. Armytage (1887).

Allegations for Marriage Licences issued from the Faculty Office of the Archbishop of Canterbury at London, 1543–1869, ed. G.J. Armytage (1886).

'Articles of Visitation and Enquiry', in *The Prose Works of Thomas Ken,* ed. J.T. Round (1838).

'The Autobiography of the Rev. Elias Rebotier, Rector of Axbridge, Somerset', ed. E.A. Fry, *Proceedings of the Somerset Archaeological and Natural History Society,* XX (1894), pp. 91–112.

Bath Memoirs; or, observations in three and forty years practice, by R. Pierce (Bath, 1697).

Bishop's Transcripts at Wells, copied from the originals by Arthur J. Jewers, ed. E. Dwelly, vols 1 & 2 (Herne Bay, 1913–14), vol. 5 (Fleet, Hants, 1917).

A Blow at Modern Sadducism in some Philosophical Considerations about Witchcraft, by Thomas Glanvill (1688).

A Brief Historical Relation of State Affairs from September 1678 to April 1714, by Narcissus Luttrell, 6 vols (Oxford, 1857).

British History Online: www.british-history.ac.uk

Butleigh Ancestry, Genealogy and Family History: butleigh.org

Calendar of the Manuscripts of the Dean and Chapter of Wells, Historical Manuscripts Commission, 2 vols (1907–1914).

Calendar of Wills and Administrations in the Court of the Archdeacon of Taunton, 1537–1799, ed. E.A. Fry (1912).

A Cat may look on a Queen; or, a Satyr on her Present Majesty, by John Dunton (1708).

The Charge of Richard, Lord Bishop of Bath and Wells [...] 1692, by R. Kidder (1693).

Charters and Records of Neales of Berkeley, Yate and Corsham, ed. J. A. Neale (Warrington, 1907).

The Chronicles of John Cannon, Excise Officer and Writing Master, ed. John Money, 2 vols (Oxford, 2010).

'Clark's List of Admissions to Balliol College, VII, 1720–1738': http://archives.balliol.ox.ac.uk/Past%20members/trace.asp

A Collection of the Works of William Penn, by William Penn, 2 vols (1726).

A Collection of the Yearly Bills of Mortality from 1657 to 1758 inclusive (1759).

The Compleat Chymist, or, a New Treatise of Chymistry, by Christophe Glaser (1667 edn).

The Craft and Frauds of Physick Expos'd, by R. Pitt (1702).

Daffy's Original and Famous Elixir Salutis, by Anthony Daffy (1681).

The Desires and Resolutions of the Club-Men of the Counties of Dorset, and Wilts. [...] 25 May 1645 (1645).

Devon and Exeter Oath Rolls, 1723, Friends of Devon Archives: www.foda.org.uk/oaths/intro/introduction1.htm

Devonshire Wills: a collection of annotated testamentary abstracts, by Charles Worthy (1896).

The Diary of a West Country Physician A.D. 1684–1726, ed. Edmund Hobhouse (1934).

The Diary of John Evelyn, ed. E.S. de Beer, 6 vols (Oxford, 1955).

Directions for Prayer, for the Diocess of Bath and Wells, by Thomas Kenn (1685).

Directory of Somerset, XVII Century [Hearth Tax Exemptions], ed. E. Dwelly (Weston-super-Mare, 1994 edn).

Dorset Incumbents, 1542–1731, by G.D. Squibb (Dorchester, 1953).

Dorset Hearth Tax Assessments 1662–1664, ed. C.A.F. Meekings (Dorchester, 1951).

'Dr. Claver Morris' Accounts', ed. Edmund Hobhouse, in *SDNQ,* 22 (1936–1938), pp. 78–81, 100–2, 147–51, 172–5, 199–203 & 230–2; 23 (1939–1942), pp. 40–1, 100–3, 134–40, 164–6, 182–5 & 345–7.

An Exact Relation of the Late Terrible Tempest, anon. (1704).

An Extract from the Sessions-Rolls of the County of Somerset, by William Goddard (1765).

The First Book of Architecture, by Andrea Palladio, ed. G. Richards (1693).

'Hearth Tax: Middlesex 1666, Chelsea', in *London Hearth Tax: City of London and Middlesex, 1666* (2011), BHO.

Hearth Tax for Somerset 1664–5, ed. R. Holworthy (Weston-super-Mare, 1994 edn).

The History and Antiquities of the County of Somerset, by John Collinson, 3 vols (Bath, 1791; Gloucester, 1983 edn).

The History of England, by John Oldmixon (1730).
History of My Own Time, by Gilbert Burnet, 2 vols (1724 & 1734).
The History of the Reign of Queen Anne, digested into Annals, by Abel Boyer (1703–1713).
The History of Taunton, by Joshua Toulmin (1791).
The Humble Petition of the Widdows and Fatherless Children the West of England, by Clubmen (1689).
The Illustrated Journeys of Celia Fiennes, 1682–1712, ed. C. Morris (1984).
The Inhabitants of Bristol in 1696, ed. Elizabeth Ralph & Mary E. Williams (Bristol, 1968).
Instructions for the Education of a Daughter, by François Fénelon (1708).
Inventory of the Historical Monuments in the County of Dorset, by Royal Commission, III (1970).
Journals of the House of Commons (1803).
Journals of the House of Lords (1767–1830).
The Ladies Cabinet Enlarged and Opened, by Patrick Ruthven (1654).
'The Library of a Physician *circa* 1700', by Edmund Hobhouse, *The Library,* XIII (1932), pp. 89–96.
Lexicon Technicum, by John Harris, I (1704).
The Life and Literary Remains of Ralph Bathurst, M.D., Dean of Wells, by Thomas Warton (1761).
The Life of Richard Kidder, D.D. Bishop of Bath and Wells. Written by Himself, ed. Amy Edith Robinson (Frome, 1924).
Londinium Redivivum, by J.P. Malcolm (1812).
The London Gazette, 1665–1727: www.thegazette.co.uk
London Inhabitants within the Walls, 1695, ed. D.V. Glass (1966).
London Marriage Licences 1521–1869, ed. J. Foster (1887).
The London Spy, by Ned Ward, ed. Paul Hyland (Michigan, 1993).
Marriage Allegation Bonds of the Bishops of Bath and Wells, ed. Arthur J. Jewers (Exeter, 1909).
Marriages at Bristol Cathedral, 1615–1754, ed. Roger Price (Bristol, 2015).
The Midwives Book: or the Whole Art of Midwifery Discovered, by Jane Sharp (1671, new edn 1999).
The Minute Books of the Dorset Standing Committee, 23rd Sept. 1646 to 8th May 1650, ed. C.H. Mayo (Exeter, 1902).
'Monumental Inscriptions of St Cuthbert's, Wells, Somerset', typescript by Mervyn Medlycott & Pat Jenkins for Somerset & Dorset Family History Society (1996).
Mr. Knight's Strange and Amazeing Prophesy, for Three Years to Come, by William Knight (1699).
The Mysteries of Conjugal Love Reveal'd, by Nicolas Venette (1707).
Obedience Due to the Present King, Notwithstanding our Oaths to the Former, by Francis Fullwood (1689).
The Papers of William Penn, volume 3: 1685–1700, ed. R. Dunn & M. Dunn (Pennsylvania, 1986).

The Parish Register of Horsington, in the County of Somerset, 1558–1836, ed. W.E. Daniel (Frome, 1907).
The Parish Registers of Street, in the County of Somerset, ed. Arthur J. Jewers (Exeter, 1898).
The Perils of False Brethren, both in Church, and State, by Henry Sacheverell (1709).
Persecution Expos'd, in Some Memoirs Relating to the Sufferings of John Whiting, and many others of the people called Quakers, by John Whiting (1715).
Pharmacopoeia Londinensis, or the New London Dispensatory, by William Salmon (1682 edn).
Pharmacopoeia Londinensis [...] Further Adorned, by Nicholas Culpeper (1653 & 1720 edns).
The Political State of Great Britain, X, by Abel Boyer (1715).
The Proceedings of the Old Bailey, London's Central Criminal Court, 1674–1913: oldbaileyonline.org
Protestant Exiles from France in the Reign of Louis XIV, I, ed. D.C.A. Agnew (1871).
Quarter Session Records for the County of Somerset, ed. W. H. Bates Harbin, 4 vols (1907–1919).
Recipes and Remedies. An 18th century collection by Margaret Bampfylde of Hestercombe, ed. Philip White (Hestercombe, 2006).
The Registers of the Abbey Church of SS. Peter and Paul, Bath, ed. Arthur J. Jewers, 2 vols (1900–1901).
The Registers of Bruton, Co. Somerset, 2 vols, ed. D.L. Hayward (1911).
The Registers of Caundle Bishop, Dorset, from 1570 to 1814, ed. C.H. Mayo (Hertford, 1895).
The Registers of Lydlinch, Co. Dorset, 1559 to 1812, ed. C.H. Mayo & F.G. Henley (1899).
The Registers of Marriages of St. Mary le Bone, Middlesex, 1668–1812, ed. W.B. Bannerman (1917).
The Registers of St Martin Outwich, London, ed. W.B. Bannerman (1905).
Remarks and Collections of Thomas Hearne, IX, ed. H.E. Salter (Oxford, 1914).
Report on the Manuscripts of Wells Cathedral, ed. J.A. Bennett, Historical Manuscripts Commission (1885).
A Sermon at the Funeral of the Right Honourable the Lady Jane [...] Wife to the Honourable Charles Cheyne Esq. at Chelsey, by Adam Littleton (1669).
A Sermon Preach'd before Both Houses of Parliament [...] July 7, 1713, by George Hooper (1713).
A Sermon Preached before the King & Queen at Whitehall, the Fifth of November, 1692, by Richard Kidder (1693).
A Sermon Preached before the King and Queen at White-Hall, March 12, 1692[3], by Richard Kidder (1693).
A Sermon Preach'd in King Henry VII's Chapel at Westminster, by Edmund Archer (1710).
The Sherborne Register, 1550–1950, ed. P. Pick (Winchester, 1950 edn).
A Short Account of the Life of the Right Reverend Father in God, Thomas Ken, by W. Hawkins (1713).

The Shortest-Way with the Dissenters, by Daniel Defoe (1702).
Some Observations on the Several Methods of Lithotomy, by Samuel Pye (1724).
Somerset Incumbents, ed. F. W. Weaver (Bristol, 1889).
The Somerset Protestation Returns and Lay Subsidy Rolls, 1641–1642, ed. A.J. Howard (Almondsbury, 1975).
The Somerset Quarterly Meeting of the Society of Friends 1668–1699, ed. Stephen C. Morland (Taunton, 1978).
The Speech of Henry Sacheverell, D.D. made in Westminster Hall on Tuesday, March 7, 1709/10, by Henry Sacheverell (1710).
A Step to the Bath with a Character of the Place, by Ned Ward (1700).
The Storm, by Daniel Defoe (1704).
A Survey of Dorsetshire, ed. John Coker (1732; Sherborne, 1980 edn).
A Tour Through the Whole Island of Great Britain, by Daniel Defoe, 2 vols (1724–1727; 1962 edn).
A Transcription of George Horner's Lease Book, typescript by S. & M. Morris (Kenilworth, 1992).
A Treatise of the Small-Pox and Measles, by Gideon Harvey (1696).
A Treatise upon the Small-Pox, in Two Parts, by Richard Blackmore (1722).
A True and Most Dreadfull Discourse of a Woman Possessed with the Devill [...] at Ditchet, anon. (1584).
A True Relation of A Monstrous Female Child, anon. (1680).
A True Relation of Two Prodigious Births, anon. (1680): SHC, *A/AEP/12.*
The Tryal of Dr. Henry Sacheverell, House of Peers (1710).
The Vanity of the Dissenters' Plea for their Separation from the Church of England, by Robert Creighton (1682).
Voices of Eighteenth-Century Bath, ed. Trevor Fawcett (Bath, 1995).
Wedmore Parish Registers, 3 vols, ed. H.A.H. Sydenham (1899–1890).
Wells Cathedral: its monumental inscriptions and heraldry, ed. A. J. Jewers (1892).
Wells Cathedral Chapter Act Book 1666–1683, ed. D.S. Bailey (1973).
Wells Corporation Properties, ed. A.J. Scrase & J. Hasler (Taunton, 2002).
West Somerset Parish Register Transcriptions: wsom.org.uk
The Whole Duty of Man, by Richard Allestree (1658).
Wookey Manor and Parish, 1544–1841, ed. Joan Hasler (Gloucester, 1995).

Secondary Sources

Abbott, Mary, *Life Cycles in England 1560–1720* (1996).
Allen, Margaret, 'Medical Practice in Eighteenth-Century Wells', *Somerset Historical Studies* (1969), pp. 25–35.
Allen, Phyllis, 'Medical Education in 17th Century England', *Journal of the History of Medicine and the Allied Sciences*, 1 (1946), pp. 115–143.
Allen, Phyllis, 'Scientific Studies in the English Universities of the Seventeenth Century, *Journal of the History of Ideas*, 10 (1949), pp. 219–53.
Alsbury, Colin, *Undignified Exits: a Colourful Selection of Tales of Seventeenth Century Clergy* (Frome, 2003).

Andrews, William, *Famous Frosts and Frost Fairs in Great Britain* (1887).

Anon, *The Catholic Spectator*, II (1824).

Armstrong, Keith, *The Story of Croscombe* (Wells, 1997).

Armytage, W.H.G., 'The Royal Society and the Apothecaries 1660–1722', *Notes and Records of the Royal Society of London*, 11 (1954), pp. 22–37.

Ashford, P. & Webb, A.J., 'Edward Berkeley's Diary, 1684', *SDNQ*, 37 (2019), pp. 426–36.

Ashton, John, *Social Life in the Reign of Queen Anne* (1897 edn).

Astbury, Leah, 'Being Well, Looking Ill: Childbirth and the Return to Health in Seventeenth-Century England', *Social History of Medicine*, 30 (2017), pp. 500–19.

Atthill, Robin, *Mendip: a New Study* (Newton Abbot, 1976).

Bailey, D.S., *The Canonical Houses of Wells* (Gloucester, 1982).

Bailey, D.S., *Wells Manor of Canon Grange* (Gloucester, 1985).

Baines, Anna, *The Monmouth Rebellion in Wells* (Wells, n.d.).

Barnes, A.D., 'The Church and Education in Wells, Somerset, from the Eve of the Reformation Until 1891', M.Phil. thesis, University of Manchester, 1990.

Barry, Jonathan, *Witchcraft and Demonology in South-West England, 1640–1789* (Basingstoke, 2012).

Barry, Jonathan, 'John Houghton and Medical Practice in London c.1700', *Bulletin of the History of Medicine*, 92 (2018), pp. 575–603.

Barry, Jonathan, 'Educating Physicians in Seventeenth-Century England', *Science in Context*, 32 (2019), pp. 137–54.

Bayley, A.R., *The Great Civil War in Dorset, 1642–1669* (Taunton, 1910).

Bellchambers, J. K., *Somerset Clockmakers* (Ramsgate, 1968).

Bendall, N. & I., *Dulcote History*: www.dulcote.com

Berrios, German E., 'Madness from the Womb', *History of Psychiatry*, 17 (2006), pp. 223–35.

Bishop, M., 'Bath's Second Guildhall, c. 1630 to 1776', *Survey of Bath and District*, 5 (1996), pp. 48–71.

Bloom, J.H. & James, R.R., *Medical Practitioners in the Diocese of London [...] 1529-1725* (Cambridge, 1935).

Bondeson, J., 'The Isle Brewers Conjoined Twins of 1680', *Journal of the Royal Society of Medicine*, 86 (1993), pp. 106–9.

Bowers, R., Colchester, L.S. & Crossland, A., *Organs and Organists of Wells Cathedral* (Wells, 1998 edn).

Bryan, George, *Chelsea in Olden and Present Times* (Chelsea, 1869).

Bucholz, R.O., '"Nothing but Ceremony": Queen Anne and the Limitations of Royal Ritual', *Journal of British Studies*, 30 (1991), pp. 288–323.

Burnby, J.G.L., *A Study of the English Apothecary from 1660 to 1760, Medical History, Supplement* 3 (1983).

Bush, Robin, *Somerset Stories* (Wimborne, 1990).

Capp, Bernard, *When Gossips Meet: Women, Family and Neighbourhood in Early Modern England* (Oxford, 2003).

Cassan, Stephen Hyde, *Lives of the Bishops of Bath and Wells*, 2 vols (1829–1830).

Chandler, David G., *Sedgemoor 1685: an Account and an Anthology* (1985).

Chichester, A.P.B., *History of the Family of Chichester, from AD 1066 to 1870* (1871).

Clergy of the Church of England Database: n.d. www.theclergydatabase.org.uk

Colchester, L. S., *Stained Glass in Wells Cathedral* (Wells, 1973).

Colchester, L.S. (ed.), *Wells Cathedral: a History* (Wells, 1982).

Colchester, L.S. (ed.), *Wells Cathedral School* (Wells, 1985).

Cole, John, *The History and Antiquities of Weston Favell in the County of Northampton* (1827).

Cook, Harold, *The Decline of the Old Medical Regime in Stuart London* (1986).

Cook, Harold, 'Physicians and the New Philosophy', in *The Medical Revolution of the Seventeenth Century*, ed. R. French & A. Wear (Cambridge, 1989), pp. 246–71.
Cook, Harold, 'Good Advice and Little Medicine: the Professional Authority of Early Modern English Physicians', *Journal of British Studies*, 33 (1994), pp. 1–33.
Crawford, Anne, *The Vicars of Wells: a History of the College of Vicars Choral* (Wells, 2016).
Crellin, J.K., 'Gascoigne's Powder: a British prescription and home medicine, 1600s to early 1900s', *Pharmaceutical Historian*, 49 (2019), pp. 1–15.
Cressy, David, *Birth, Marriage & Death: Ritual, Religion and the Life-Cycle in Tudor and Stuart England* (Oxford, 1997).
Croot, Patricia E.C. (ed.), *A History of the County of Middlesex, XII: Chelsea* (2004).
Croot, Patricia, *The World of the Small Farmer: tenure, profit and politics in the early modern Somerset Levels* (Hatfield, 2017).
Curth, Louise, 'The Medical Content of English Almanacs 1640–1700', *Journal of the History of Medical and Allied Sciences*, 60 (2005), pp. 255–82.
Davies, Randall, *Chelsea Old Church* (1904).
Davis, Fred, *The Shepton Mallet Story* (Oakhill, 1977 edn).
Dearmer, Percy, *The Cathedral Church of Wells* (1889).
Debus, Allen, 'Chemistry and the Universities in the Seventeenth Century', *Estudos Avancados*, 4 (1990), pp. 173–96.
Delay, Margaret, *The Germ of an Idea: Contagion, Religion and Society in Britain, 1660–1730* (New York, 1716).
Dominiguez-Rodrguez, M.V., '"Profiting Those that Cannot Understand the Latine": Exploring the Motives for Medical Translation in 17th-Century England', *Neuphilologische Mitteilungen*, 115 (2014), pp. 131–52.
Dunning, Robert (ed.), *Christianity in Somerset* (Taunton, 1975).
Dunning, Robert, 'The Bishop's Palace' in *Wells Cathedral: a History*, ed. Colchester, pp. 227–47.
Dunning, Robert, *Somerset Families* (Tiverton, 2002).
Easter, C.J., 'Church Monuments of Devon and Cornwall, c. 1660 c. 1730', Ph.D. thesis, University of Plymouth, 2006.
Eklund, Jon, 'The Incompleat Chymist: being an essay on the eighteenth-century chemist in his laboratory, with a dictionary of obsolete chemical terms of the period', *Smithonian Studies in History and Technology* (1975), pp. 1–49.
Ellis, F.H., 'The Background of the London Dispensary', *Journal of the History of Medicine and Allied Sciences*, 20 (1965), pp. 197–212.
Estcourt, E.E. (ed.), *The English Catholic Nonjurors of 1715, being a summary of their estates* (1885).
Evans, John, *A Chronological Outline of the History of Bristol* (Bristol, 1824).
Faulkner, T., *An Historical and Topographical Description of Chelsea and its Environs*, 2 vols (1810–1829).
Fawcett, Trevor, *Bath Entertain'd* (Bath, 1998).
Foster, Joseph (ed.), *Alumni Oxoniensis* (Oxford, 1888–1891).
Frank, Robert G., 'Medicine', in *History of the University of Oxford*, IV, ed. Nicholas Tyacke (Oxford, 1997), pp. 505–58.
Fuller-Eliot-Drake, Elizabeth, *The Family and Heirs of Sir Francis Drake*, 2 vols (1911).
Gadd, Trixie, 'The impact of the landscape on the clergy of seventeenth-century Dorset', in *Church and People in Interregnum Britain*, ed. F. McCall (2021), pp. 87–110.
Gardner, Arthur, *Wells Capitals* (Wells, 1998 edn).
Gent, Frank J., *The Trial of the Bideford Witches* (Crediton, 1998 edn).
Gourlay, A.B., *A History of Sherborne School* (Sherborne, 1971).

Green, Emanuel, *The March of William of Orange through Somerset* (1892).
Grigson, Francis, *Genealogical Memoranda relating to the Family of Bisse* (1886).
Hall, William G., 'Pills, Potions and Plasters: A Country Surgeon at Work in Wedmore Somerset from 1686–1706.' (revised August 1998) tutton.org/content/Pills-potions-vs-1
Hall, William G., 'The Casebook of John Westover of Wedmore, Surgeon, 1686-1700.' (revised July 1999) tutton.org/content/Westover_journal
Hanham, Andrew, 'Early Whig Opposition to the Walpole Administration; The Evidence of Francis Gwyn's Division List on the Wells Election Case, 1723', *Parliamentary History*, 15 (1996), pp. 333–60.
Haskins, Charles, *The Ancient Trade Guilds and Companies of Salisbury* (Salisbury, 1912).
Hasler, Joan & Luker, Brian, *The Parish of Wookey* (Gloucestershire, 1997).
Hasler, Joan, 'The Peirs Family of Wells', *SDNQ*, 23 (2001), pp. 3–10.
Hatton, Ragnhild, *George I, Elector and King* (1978).
Haydon, Colin, *Anti-Catholicism in Eighteenth-Century England, 1714–80* (Manchester, 1993).
Hayton, D., Cruikshanks, E., Handley, S. (ed.), *The History of Parliament: the House of Commons 1690–1715* (2002).
Heard, Herbert, *Shepton Mallet. Notes on the Charities of the Town* (Shepton Mallet, 1903).
Henning, B.D. (ed.), *The History of Parliament: the House of Commons 1660–1690* (1983).
Hervey, S.H.A., *The Wedmore Chronicle*, 2 vols (Wells, 1881–1898).
Higgins, Rory (ed.), *The Margaret Higgins Database of Catholics in England and their Friends, 1607–1840* (2017): catholicfhs.online
Hippisley, A.E., *Some Notes on the Hippisley Family* (Taunton, 1952).
Hobhouse, Edmund, 'The Library of a Physician *circa* 1700', *The Library*, 13 (1932), pp. 89–96.
Holmes, Geoffrey, *British Politics in the Age of Anne* (1967).
Holmes, Geoffrey, *The Trial of Doctor Sacheverell* (1973).
Holmes, Geoffrey, *The Electorate and the National Will in the First Age of Party* (Lancaster, 1975).
Holmes, Geoffrey, 'The Sacheverell Riots: The Crowd and the Church in Early Eighteenth-Century London', *Past & Present*, 72 (1976), pp. 55–85.
Holmes, Geoffrey, *The Making of a Great Power: late Stuart and early Georgian Britain, 1660–1722* (1993).
Holmes, Thomas Scott, *The History of the Parish and Manor of Wookey* (Bristol, 1885).
Homan, Peter G., 'Daffy: a legend in his own preparation', *Pharmaceutical Journal*, 23 Dec. 2006.
Howgrave-Graham, R.P., *The Wells Clock* (Wells, 1973 edn).
Hunter, Michael, 'New Light on the "Drummer of Tedworth": conflicting narratives of witchcraft in Restoration England', *Historical Research*, 78 (2005), pp. 311–53.
Hutchins, J., *The History and Antiquities of the County of Dorset* (1774; 3rd edn, 4 vols, 1861–1874).
Hyland, Paul, 'Richard Steele: scandal and sedition', in *Writing and Censorship in Britain*, ed. P. Hyland & N. Sammells (1992), pp. 59–80.
Imray, Jean, *Wells Old Almshouse* (Wells, 2022).
Johnson, M. & Fallon, B., *A Brief History of the Manor House, Farrington Gurney, Somerset* (Cornwall, 1998).
Johnson, Robert, 'Wells and the Monmouth Rebellion', *History Round Wells*, no. 5 (2002), pp. 3–10.
Johnstone, H. Diack, 'Claver Morris, an Early Eighteenth-Century English Physician and Amateur Musician *Extraordinaire*', *Journal of the Royal Musical Association*, 133 (2008), pp. 93–127.

Johnstone, H. Diack, 'Instruments, Strings, Wire and Other Musical Miscellanea in the Account Books of Claver Morris (1659–1727)', *Galpin Society Journal*, 60 (2007), pp. 29–35.

Jones, C., 'New Light on the Wells By-election of 1719', *SDNQ*, 31 (1983), pp. 275–6.

Lancaster, Henry, 'Nonconformity and Anglican Dissent in Restoration Wiltshire, 1600-1689', Ph.D. thesis, University of Bristol, 1995.

Lasocki, David & Helen Neate, 'The Life and Works of Robert Woodcock, 1690–1728', *American Recorder*, 29 (1988), pp. 92–104.

Latimer, John, *The Annals of Bristol in the Eighteenth Century* (1893).

Le Fanu, W.R., 'The Lost Half-Century in English Medicine, 1700–1750', *Bulletin of the History of Medicine*, 46 (1972), pp. 319–48.

Leong, Elaine, *Recipes and Everyday Knowledge: Medicine, Science, and the Household in Early Modern England* (Chicago, 2018).

Locke, A. Audrey, *The Seymour Family: History and Romance* (1911).

Loudon, Irvine, 'The Nature of Provincial Medical Practice in Eighteenth-century England', *Medical History*, 29 (1985), pp. 1–32.

Lowe, Barbara, 'The Demise of Keynsham's Great House', *North Wansdyke Past and Present*, no. 7 (1995), pp. 3–11.

Loxton, G.A.J., *Ston Easton Perambulation*. (Ston Easton, 2000).

Lysons, Daniel, *The Environs of London, II: County of Middlesex* (1795).

Macaulay, T.B., *The History of England from the Accession of James II*, II (1848).

Malone, C.M., *Façade as Spectacle: Ritual and Ideology at Wells Cathedral* (Leiden, 2004).

Marshall William, M., *George Hooper, 1640–1727, Bishop of Bath and Wells* (Milborne Port, 1976).

Matthews, M., *A Brief History of the Hippisley Family*: boddyparts.co.uk

Mayo, Ronald, *The Huguenots in Bristol* (Bristol, 1985).

Meek, Marion, *The Wells Liberty and Bishop's Palace* (Wells, 1982).

Morland, Stephen C., 'Mid-Somerset Friends in the Eighteenth Century', *Journal of the Friends' Historical Society*, 52 (1971), pp. 249–76.

Morris, Polly, 'Defamation and Sexual Reputation in Somerset, 1733-1850', Ph.D. thesis, University of Warwick, 1985.

Mortimer, Ian, 'Diocesan Licensing and Medical Practitioners in South-West England 1660–1780', *Medical History*, 48 (2004), pp. 49–68.

Mortimer, Ian, *The Time Traveller's Guide to Restoration Britain* (2017).

Muddiman, J.G. (ed.), *The Bloody Assizes* (Edinburgh, 1929).

Murphy, Andrew, *William Penn. A Life* (Oxford, 2019).

Neale, Frances, 'A Seventeenth-Century Doctor: John Westover of Wedmore', *The Practitioner*, 203 (1969), pp. 699–704.

Newman, Angela, *Records of the Jeanes-Janes Family of England and 'Parts Beyond The Seas'* (2008).

Newton, H., 'Children's Physic: Medical Perceptions and Treatment of Sick Children in Early Modern England, c. 1580–1720', *Social History of Medicine*, 23 (2012), pp. 456–74.

Newton, H., *Misery to Mirth: Recovery from Illness in Early Modern England* (Oxford, 2018).

Nishikawa, Sugiko, 'English Attitudes toward Continental Protestants with Particular Reference to Church Briefs c.1680-1740', Ph.D. thesis, University of London, 1998.

Nott, Anthony, *Under God's Visitation: a Study of the City of Wells from the Civil War to the Restoration* (Wells, 2010).

Osborn, Sally, 'The Role of Domestic Knowledge in an Era of Professionalisation: Eighteenth-Century Manuscript Medical Recipe Collections', Ph.D. thesis, University of Roehampton (2016).

Parker, J.H., *The Architectural Antiquities of the City of Wells* (Oxford, 1866)
Paul, Helen, 'The "South Sea Bubble", 1720', *European History Online* (2015).
Peluso, Nancy Lee, 'Whigs and hunters: the origins of the Black Act, by E.P. Thompson', *Journal of Peasant Studies*, 44 (2017), pp. 309–21.
Petrie, Charles, 'The Jacobite Activities in South and West England in the Summer of 1715', *Transactions of the Royal Historical Society*, 18 (1935), pp. 85–106.
Phelps, William, *The History and Antiquities of Somersetshire*, 4 vols (1835–1839).
Pickering, Andrew, *The Hellish Knot: Witches and Demons in Seventeenth Century Somerset* (Devizes, 2013).
Plumptre, E.H., *The Life of Thomas Ken, DD. Bishop of Bath and Wells*, 2 vols (1888-9).
Porter, Roy, *Quacks: Fakers and Charlatans in English Medicine* (2000).
Powell, A.H., *The Ancient Borough of Bridgwater in the County of Somerset* (Bridgwater, 1907).
Reid, R.D. & Scrase, A.J., 'A Great House and Two Lanes in Wells', *Somerset Archaeological and Natural History*, 125 (1981), pp. 31–43.
Reynolds, H.E., *Wells Cathedral: its foundation, constitutional history and statutes* (Wells, 1881).
Rogers, Malcolm, *Montacute House, Somerset* (1991).
Rogers, Nicholas, 'Riot and Popular Jacobitism in Early Hanoverian England', in *Ideology and Conspiracy: Aspects of Jacobitism, 1689-1759*, ed. E. Cruickshanks (Edinburgh, 1982), pp. 70–88.
Salmon, H.J.D., *Salmon Chronicles* (privately printed, n.d.).
Scrase, Tony, 'Wells Inns', *SDNQ*, 31 (1984), pp. 378–95.
Scrase, Tony, 'The Inhabitants of Wells 1600-1649,' *History Round Wells*, no. 7 (Wells, 2003), pp. 3–22.
Scrase, Tony, *Somerset Towns: Changing Fortunes 800–1800* (Stroud, 2005).
Sedgwick, R. (ed.), *The History of Parliament: the House of Commons 1715–1754* (1970).
Sellers, R.V., 'The Chantry College in the Mountroy of Wells', *Wells Natural History and Archaeology Society Report* (Wells, 1959–1960), pp. 5–17.
Serel, Thomas, 'On the Strodes of Somerset', *Proceedings of the Somerset Archaeological Society*, 13 (1865), pp. 6–20.
Seyer, S., *Memoirs Historical and Topographical of Bristol*, 2 vols (Bristol, 1821).
Sloan, A.W., *English Medicine in the Seventeenth Century* (Durham, 1996).
Smith, Hannah, 'Mary Astell, *A Serious Proposal to the Ladies* (1694) and the Anglican Reformation of Manners in Late-Seventeenth-Century England', in *Mary Astell: Reason, Gender, Faith*, ed. W. Kolbener & M. Michelson (Aldershot, 2007), pp. 31–48.
Spring, Matthew, 'The Reverend Robert Creighton's Seven Pieces for Twelve-course Lute in British Library Additional Manuscript 37074', *The Lute: Journal of the Lute Society*, 55 (2015), pp. 32–48.
Spurr, John, *The Restoration Church of England, 1640–1689* (New Haven, 1991).
Squibb, G.D., 'The Bragge Family of Sadborow and their Muniments', *Proceedings of Dorset Natural History and Archaeological Society*, 64 (1943), pp. 58–68.
Squibb, G.D., *Dorset Incumbents, 1542–1731* (Dorchester, 1953).
Stevenson, John, *Two Centuries of Life in Down, 1600–1800* (Belfast, 1920).
Stobart, Anne, *Household Medicine in Seventeenth-Century England* (2016).
Tate, W.E., *Somerset Enclosure Acts and Awards* (Frome, 1948).
Tate, W.E., *The English Village Community and the Enclosure Movements* (1967).
Thirsk, Joan (ed.), *The Agrarian History of England and Wales*, V (Cambridge, 1984).
Thompson, E.P., *Whigs and Hunters: the origin of the Black Act* (New York, 1975).
Thoms, W.J., *The Book of the Court* (1844 edn).
Timmons, Stephen A., 'Executions following Monmouth's rebellion: a missing link', *Historical Research*, 76 (2003), pp. 286–91.

Venn, J.A. (ed.), *Alumni Cantabrigienses*, Part 1, 4 vols (Cambridge, 1922–1954).
Waller, Maureen, 'Disease and death in late Stuart London', Gresham College, 2004: gresham.ac.uk/lecture/transcript/print/disease-and-death-in-late-stuart-london/
Wallis, P.J. et al. (ed.), *Eighteenth Century Medics* (Newcastle-upon-Tyne, 1988 edn).
Wallis, Patrick, 'Exotic Drugs and English Medicine: England's Drug Trade, c.1550-c.1800', London School of Economics, Working Papers, no. 143 (2010).
Wear, Andrew, *Knowledge and Practice in English Medicine, 1550–1680* (Cambridge, 2000).
Webb, A.J., 'Edward Berkeley's Diary and Notebook, 1690', *SDNQ*, 37 (2015), pp. 412–24.
Wells Cathedral Publications, *Misericords of Wells Cathedral* (Wells, 1998 edn).
White, E. (ed.), *Keynsham and Saltford Life and Work in Times Past, 1539–1945* (Keynsham, 1990).
Wicks, A.T., 'The Creighton Family of Somerset', *SDNQ*, 23 (1942), pp. 335–6.
Wigfield, W. Macdonald, *The Monmouth Rebellion: A Social History* (Bradford-on-Avon, 1980).
Wigfield, W. Macdonald, *The Monmouth Rebels 1685* (Gloucester, 1985).
Williams, J.A., *Catholic Recusancy in Wiltshire, 1660–1791* (1968).
Williams, J.A. (ed.), *Post Reformation Catholicism in Bath*, I (1975).
Williams, J.A. (ed.), *Papist Estates in Wiltshire in the Eighteenth Century*: www.wiltshirerecord society.org.uk/research/texts/papist-estates-wiltshire-eighteenth-century/
Williams, M., *The Draining of the Somerset Levels* (Cambridge, 1970).
Wilson, Kathleen, *The Sense of The People: Politics, Culture and Imperialism in England, 1715–1785* (Cambridge, 1994).
Winn, Colin G., *The Pouletts of Hinton St. George* (1976).
Wroughton, John, *Stuart Bath: Life in the Forgotten City, 1603–1714* (Bath, 2004).
Wyndham, H.A., *A Family History, 1688–1837: the Wyndhams of Somerset, Sussex and Wiltshire* (Oxford, 1950).
Yelling, J.A., *Common Field and Enclosure in England 1450–1850* (1977).
Zook, Melinda, 'The Bloody Assizes: Whig Martyrdom and Memory after the Glorious Revolution', *Albion*, 27 (1995), pp. 373–96.

INDEX

Pages in *italics* refer figures and pages followed by n refer notes.

For Product Safety Concerns and Information please contact our EU representative GPSR@taylorandfrancis.com
Taylor & Francis Verlag GmbH, Kaufingerstraße 24, 80331 München, Germany

www.ingramcontent.com/pod-product-compliance
Ingram Content Group UK Ltd.
Pitfield, Milton Keynes, MK11 3LW, UK
UKHW021308260926
475702UK00048B/914

9781032367644